Principles of Veterinary Parasitology

Principles of Veterinary Parasitology

Dennis Jacobs

Mark Fox

Lynda Gibbons

Carlos Hermosilla

WILEY Blackwell

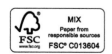

Contents

About the Authors

Dennis Jacobs qualified from the University of Glasgow Veterinary School in 1964 and studied for his PhD in Glasgow and Copenhagen. He is Emeritus Professor of Veterinary Parasitology at The Royal Veterinary College (University of London) and a Fellow of the Royal College of Veterinary Surgeons, the Royal College of Pathologists and the Higher Education Academy. He has been Visiting Professor at the University of the West Indies, Trinidad; St George's University Medical School, Grenada; Ross University School of Veterinary Medicine, St Kitts; the South China Agricultural University, Guangzhou, Peoples Republic of China; and at the University of Melbourne, Australia. He was Vice-president of the World Association for the Advancement of Veterinary Parasitology from 2003 to 2007 and Secretary of the European Veterinary Parasitology College from its foundation in 2003 to 2009. He has published one book and co-edited another, written several book chapters and more than 150 peer-reviewed scientific papers and reviews.

Mark Fox graduated from The Royal Veterinary College (University of London) in 1977 and, after a period in small animal practice, studied for a PhD at the same college where he is currently Professor of Veterinary Parasitology. He is a Member of the Royal College of Veterinary Surgeons, Diplomat and Board Member of the European Veterinary Parasitology College, Fellow of the Higher Education Academy and a past Honorary Secretary of the Association for Veterinary Teaching and Research Work and British Veterinary Association Council member. He established Masters degree courses in Wild Animal Biology and Wild Animal Health with the Institute of Zoology (London Zoo) and was jointly-awarded the BVA William Hunting medal in 2005 for research on coccidial infection in wild birds of prey. His current research interests focus on the epidemiology of parasite infections in both domestic and wild animals.

Lynda Gibbons graduated with a BSc Honours degree from the University of Leicester in 1969 and studied for a PhD at the London School of Hygiene and Tropical Medicine, University of London. She is a Chartered Biologist and Fellow of the Royal Society of Biology and was a council member of the Systematics Association from 1993 to 1995. She was head of the Animal Helminthology Biosystematics Unit of the CAB International Institute of Parasitology from 1992 to 1997 and an attached senior lecturer at The Royal Veterinary College until 2010. She was awarded the Elsdon-Dew medal in 1993 by the Parasitological Society of Southern Africa and the Betts prize by The Royal Veterinary College in 2006. She has run training programmes and courses for overseas students and developed a joint RVC/FAO on-line programme on faecal diagnosis of helminth infection. She has published two books, a book chapter and 78 scientific papers.

Carlos Hermosilla entered the Faculty of Veterinary Medicine at the University Austral of Chile in 1984 and achieved the degree of DVM in 1989. He obtained his doctoral degree (Dr med. vet.) in 1998 at the Justus Liebig University, Giessen, Germany where he is currently Professor of Veterinary Parasitology. From January 2008 to March 2011 he held the position of Senior Lecturer for Veterinary Parasitology at The Royal Veterinary College, London, United Kingdom and since 2009 has held a position as Visiting Professor of the University Austral of Chile. In 2009 he finished his habilitation thesis (Dr habil.) in Parasitology. In the last 14 years he has mainly been involved in the field of coccidian parasites (*Eimeria bovis*, *E. ninakohlyakimovae*, *E. arloingi*, *Neospora caninum*, *Toxoplasma gondii*, *Besnoitia besnoiti*). He has so far published more than 80 papers in international scientific journals.

Foreword

Parasites are not only scientifically fascinating but when they infect humans or animals they present sophisticated and highly evolved targets that are difficult to control even in the technically advanced world in which we live. Moreover parasitic diseases of domestic animals (in contrast to those of humans) are a real and present danger to the health and welfare of animals throughout the globe, in rich and in poor countries, in temperate as well as in tropical climates. The nature of parasitic diseases of livestock, whilst occasionally acute and lethal, is frequently chronic and endemic leading to the continual detriment of welfare and productivity. This is critical given the rapidly expanding global population and the equally rapidly expanding demand for meat and dairy products. Of current importance, the effects of parasitism on morbidity, mortality and productivity exacerbate the greenhouse gas emissions from ruminants, and the successful control of parasitism mitigates such emissions. Apart from affecting the production of food, some parasites of animals infect humans and are of considerable public health importance. So a new, up to date textbook on this subject is to be welcomed.

This book fills an important niche. It is unashamedly written for students, in its broadest sense, of the subject. These are, of course, mainly those studying to become veterinary clinicians, veterinary nurses or following other veterinary-related courses. But it is also ideal for other types of "learner" such as the qualified professional pursuing continuing education. The authors are highly experienced and knowledgeable university teachers, and it shows. The approach is clinically relevant and highly practical. The text anticipates the misunderstandings and errors that learners can easily make. For example, it makes clear that humans get infected with hydatid disease only from the ingestion of eggs (excreted by dogs) and not from accidental ingestion of hydatid cysts in meat! There is an admirable use of apt analogies to clarify concepts and frequent use of text boxes to expand, explain or expound particular issues or historical examples – for example the history of sheep scab in the UK. As experienced teachers ourselves, we recognise the care with which terms sometimes taken for granted are explained, e.g. formulation in the context of drugs. And there is even a pronunciation guide on the associated website.

The lay out, we suspect, may owe some debt to Angus Dunn's wonderful and out of print book *Veterinary Helminthology* (Professor Jacobs was a PhD student with Dunn when he was writing his classic). After an initial chapter describing basic concepts, the rest is divided into two broad sections. The first part deals with the subject matter taxonomically, although always with clinical relevance in mind; the second then approaches the subject from the perspective of the animal host species or group, and the organ(s) affected and associated syndromes, which is how parasitic diseases are presented to the clinician. In the appropriate places there are sections specifically dealing with ectoparasiticides, anthelmintics and antiprotozoal drugs. The discussions of treatments and control are suitably detailed for the target audience and their rationales are thoroughly explained; it is a lot easier to remember when one does what, if one understands the underlying reasons!

This book is a valuable addition to the literature on veterinary parasitology. Although three of the authors are based in the UK, all the authors have extensive international experience and the book reflects this with comprehensive cover of all the major parasitic diseases of domestic animals worldwide. It will be of use to students of the subject throughout the world.

Professor the Lord Trees and
Professor Diana J.L. Williams

Preface

Between us, the authors of this textbook have accumulated a century's worth of teaching experience. This has culminated in a set of undergraduate course-notes crafted to match the learning requirements of our British and American students. Always sensitive to feedback, we have, over the years, progressively honed content and eliminated ambiguity, thereby providing a solid foundation for the present more ambitious enterprise, intended as a 'student-friendly' introduction to Veterinary Parasitology.

Our teaching has been enhanced by ideas avidly gathered from many national and international sources, including visits to other institutions and attendances at meetings such as those organized by the World Association for the Advancement of Veterinary Parasitology (Eckert, 2013). We are privileged to have had the opportunity to gain inspiration from so many gifted colleagues and we thank them for sharing their knowledge and expertise.

A number of friends have contributed more directly to the evolution of our course-notes. In particular, we wish to thank Dr Manice Stallbaumer, Professor Mike Taylor, Professor Phillip Duffus and Dr Rachel Lawrence for their various inputs. Professor Taylor's authoritative book *Veterinary Parasitology, Third Edition* (Taylor, Coop and Wall, 2007) has been an invaluable reference work during the preparation of our text.

An ever-expanding knowledge-base has lead progressive universities to reappraise veterinary education. A comprehensive knowledge of every component discipline is no longer a feasible aspiration for the student nor is it a realistic expectation for examination boards. Modern approaches encourage students to become problem-solvers by instilling an understanding of basic principles rather than 'drowning' their intellect in a mass of detail. Factual information is of course important to support 'professional day 1 competencies' but it should be carefully selected and restricted to that actually required to meet defined educational and professional objectives.

Another trend in veterinary education is the adoption of 'integrated' curricula which aim to unify component strands of expertise needed for clinical practice. The downside of this otherwise commendable approach is that it tends to fragment the presentation of discipline-based subjects, dispersing information throughout 'systems' modules based on alimentary, respiratory and other body functions, or between 'species' modules focussed on equine, ruminant and small animal medicine. This makes underlying concepts and inter-relationships in Veterinary Parasitology and other disciplines more difficult to appreciate, to the detriment of understanding and clinical application.

The aims of this textbook are therefore to provide a guide to learning that:

i) is straightforward, easy to comprehend and informative without being encyclopaedic;

ii) is useful for students whether engaged in traditional or integrated modular educational systems;

iii) provides knowledge relevant for the immediate needs of the veterinary student uncluttered by unnecessarily detailed or advanced information;

iv) supports learning and enhances understanding by clearly illustrating conceptual relationships between parasitic organisms, their biology and the diseases they cause.

The scope of the original course-notes has been broadened to encompass a wider geographical coverage. In this regard, teaching experience gained by the authors in Europe, South America, the Caribbean, South-East Asia and Australasia has proved a valuable asset.

Finally, attention is drawn to a quotation from a poem by the Scottish bard, Robert Burns, that some believe to be a satire on 18th-century medicine (Nicolson, 2010): 'Some books are lies frae end to end'. Or, in modern parlance: 'Textbooks ... can vary in their quality and will almost always include some form of bias, reflecting the authors' experience, opinion and interpretation of the evidence' (Dean, 2013). We have endeavoured to keep our text on a sound footing but, in accord with the 21st-century emphasis on evidence-based medicine, the reader is encouraged to use this book as a springboard for independent enquiry, to delve deeper and to challenge our assertions.

Dennis Jacobs, Mark Fox,
Lynda Gibbons, Carlos Hermosilla
The Royal Veterinary College (University of London)
January 2015

Acknowledgements

The authors are grateful to the many colleagues who assisted in various ways during the preparation of this book. In particular, Dr Damer Blake, Dr Siân Mitchell, Dr Sonja Jeckel, Professor Laura Kramer, Dr Martin Nielsen, Professor Tammi Krecek, Professor Michael K. Rust, Dr Felipe Torres-Acosta, Dr Constantin Constantinoiu, Mr Brian Cox, Ms Lisa Harber and Mr 'Don' Donald all gave generously of their time in support of this project.

We also express our gratitude to Bayer Animal Health and Elanco Animal Health for kind donations to offset costs incurred during the preparation of this book.

Our sincere thanks are due to all those who provided photographs or images, including:

Peter Bates, Surrey, UK (Figure 8.19). Graham Bilbrough, IDEXX Laboratories Europe BV (Figure 9.26). Ross Bond, The Royal Veterinary College, University of London (Figures 9.10, 9.31 and 9.34). Jackie Bowman and A. Gray, Lincolnshire, UK (Figure 9.20). David Brown, Northamptonshire, UK (Figure 8.10). David Buxton, Midlothian, Scotland (Figures 4.36 and 4.38). Luis Canseco, Elanco Animal Health, UK (Figures 8.32, 8.33, 8.34 and 8.35). Colin Capner, Novartis Animal Health, UK (Figure 7.41). Brian Catchpole, The Royal Veterinary College, University of London (Figure 1.8). Dong-Hwan Choe and Michael K. Rust, University of California Riverside, USA (Figures 2.19, 2.20, 2.21 and 9.44). Peta Clode, University of Western Australia (Figure 4.16). Doug Colwell, Agriculture and Agri-Food Canada (Figures 2.46, 2.47, 2.48, 8,21 and 8.22). Constantin Constantinoiu, James Cook University, Australia (Figures 3.2 and 3.6). Luisa Cornegliani, Milan, Italy (Figures 9.29 and 9.30). Arwid Daugschies, University of Leipzig, Germany (Figures 7.11 and 7.30). Luisa De Risio, Animal Health Trust, UK (Figure 9.37). Theo de Waal, University College Dublin, Ireland (Figures 5.2, 5.42 and 8.4). Ian Denholm, University of Hertfordshire, UK (Figure 7.42). Peter Deplazes, University of Zurich, Switzerland (Figure 5.21). David Ferguson, Nuffield Department of Clinical Laboratory Science, Oxford, UK (Figures 1.7 and 4.5). Juan Antonio Figueroa-Castillo, FMVZ-UNAM, Mexico (Figure 8.12). Ronan Fitzgerald, Bayer Animal Health, UK (Figures 2.15, 2.16 and 3.1). Michael Frank, http://www.mickfrank.com/ and Nick Short, The Royal Veterinary College, University of London (Figures 2.49 and 9.40). Chris Gardiner, James Cook University, Australia (Figure 8.18). Arcangelo Gentile, University of Bologna, Italy (Figures 4.33 and 8.23). Edward Greaves, The National Sweet Itch Centre, Wrexham, Wales (Figure 9.11). Thomas Geurden and Edwin Claerebout, University of Ghent, Belgium (Figure 9.21). Martin Hall, The Natural History Museum, London (Figure 2.43). Peter Irwin, Murdoch University, Australia (Figures 4.44 and 4.45). Sonja Jeckel, AHVLA at The Royal Veterinary College, University of London (Figures 2.24, 4.32, 6.44, 8.27 and 8.31). Anja Joachim, University of Veterinary Medicine, Vienna, Austria (Figure 8.29). Arlene Jones, Powys, Wales (Figures 7.37 and 7.38). Wayne Jorgensen, Department of Agriculture, Fisheries and Forestry, Queensland, Australia (Figure 8.16). Lofti Khalil, St Albans, UK (Figures 5.32 and 6.9). Thomas R. Klei, Louisiana State University, USA (Figures 6.34, 6.36, 6.38, 7.24 and 9.3). Derek Knottenbelt, University of Liverpool, UK (Figures 2.29, 9.8, 9.12, 9.13 and 9.15). Alexander Koutinas, Aristotle University of Thessaloniki, Greece (Figure 9.35). Laura Kramer, University of Parma, Italy (Figures 4.13, 5.13, 7.28, 7.29, 9.27, 9.28, 9.33 and 9.38). Eddy Krecek, eddy@mcmaster.co.za (Figure 1.4). Tammi Krecek, Ross University School of Veterinary Medicine, St Kitts, West Indies (Figures 3.9, 5.11, 6.10, 7.21, 9.19 and 9.42). Chris Lewis, Sheep Veterinary Services, Cheshire, UK (Figure 3.27). James Logan and Christina Due, London School of Hygiene and Tropical Medicine, UK (Figures 2.32 and 9.45). London Scientific Films, Braughing, Herts, UK (Figures 2.44, 2.50, 5.22, 5.39, 6.11, 6.37, 6.39, 6.41, 6.42, 6.43, 7.17 and 9.2). Adrian Longstaffe, Bristol, UK (Figure 5.14). Vincenzo Lorusso, University of Edinburgh Medical School, Scotland (Figure 8.17). Bertrand Losson, University of Liège, Belgium (Figure 9.14). Calum Macpherson, St George's University, Grenada, West Indies (Figure 6.56).

Vince McDonald and Farah Barakat, Kings College, University of London, UK (Figure 8.5). John McGarry, University of Liverpool, UK (Figures 4.30, 9.22 and 9.24). James McGoldrick, University of Glasgow, Scotland (Figures 6.23 and 8.1). Gianfranco Militerno, University of Bologna, Italy (Figures 4.34 and 8.24). Siân Mitchell, AHVLA, Carmarthen, Wales (Figures 2.24, 4.14, 5.40, 5.41, 5.43, 6.24 and 6.27). Ivan Morrison, Roslin Institute, Edinburgh, Scotland (Figure 3.8). Martin Nielsen, University of Kentucky, USA (Figures 5.24, 5.25, 6.32, 6.35, 7.4, 9.5 and 9.7). Domenico Otranto, University of Bari, Italy (Figures 7.22 and 7.25). Chandra Panchadcharam and Mohamed Faizal Hassan, Veterinary Research Institute, Ipoh, Malaysia (Figure 7.39). David Parsons, Poultry Health Centre, Trowbridge, UK (Figures 8.37, 8.39, 8.40, 8.41 and 8.43). Bill Pomroy, Massey University, New Zealand (Figure 8.7). Steffan Rehbein, Merial Gmbh (Figures 5.17, 6.25, 8.28 and 8.30). Sandra Scholes, AHVLA, Carmarthen, Wales (Figure 4.14). Brian Smyth, The Royal Veterinary College, London, UK (Figures 6.51, 6.53, 6.57 and 9.23). Karen Snowden, Texas A&M University, USA (Figures 6.10 and 9.19). Dan Snyder, Elanco Animal Health, USA (Figure 2.38). Natalia Soto-Barrientos, St José, Costa Rica (Figure 1.12). Manice Stallbaumer, Cornwall,

UK (Figure 8.25). Peter Stevenson, Hampshire, UK (Figures 5.1 and 5.16). Russell Stothard, Liverpool School of Tropical Medicine, UK (Figure 5.49). Christina Strube, University of Veterinary Medicine, Hannover, Germany (Figure 7.10). Anja Taubert and Christian Bauer, Justus Leibig University, Giessen, Germany (Figures 6.50 and 8.38). Andrew Thompson, Murdoch University, Australia (Figure 4.16 and 5.18). Manuela Tittarelli, Instituto 'G. Caporale', Teramo, Italy (Figures 9.16, 9.17 and 9.18). Felipe Torres-Acosta, Autonomous University of Yucatan, Mexico (Figure 8.6). Chris Tucker and Tom Yazwinski, University of Arkansas, USA (Figures 7.32 and 8.36). Luigi Venco, Cremona, Italy (Figures 6.1 and 7.26). Jozef Vercruysse, University of Ghent, Belgium (Figures 5.44, 5.47, 5.48 and 8.15). Larry Wadsworth, Texas A&M University, USA (Figure 3.9). Mike Walker, Norfolk, UK (Figures 5.28 and 6.16). Richard Wall and Matthew Walters, University of Bristol, UK (Figure 8.20).

Despite their best endeavours, the authors were unable to identify copyright holders for source materials used to prepare the following: Figures 2.6, 2.11, 2.12, 2.42, 3.16, 3.17, 3.21, 3.22, 3.23, 6.33, 6.58 and 7.14. Anyone owning rights to these is asked to contact John Wiley and Sons, Ltd.

List of abbreviations

AAD	Amino-acetonitrile derivative	**MHC**	Major histocompatability complex
ACh	Acetylcholine	**ML**	Macrocyclic lactone
AIDS	Acquired immunodeficiency syndrome	**Na**	Sodium
BZD	Benzimidazole	**nAChR**	Nicotinic acetylcholine receptor binding site
Ca	Calcium	**NK**	Natural killer cell
CFT	Complement fixation test	**NLM**	Neural larva migrans
CNS	Central nervous system	**NO**	Nitric oxide
CO$_2$	Carbon dioxide	**o.p.g.**	Oocysts per gram of faeces
DNA	Deoxyribonucleic acid	**OLM**	Ocular larva migrans
e.p.g.	Eggs per gram of faeces	**OP**	Organophosphate
EL$_3$	Early parasitic third stage larva	**PABA**	Para-amino benzoic acid
ELISA	Enzyme-linked immunosorbent assay	**PCR**	Polymerase chain reaction
EPM	Protozoal myeloencephalitis	**PGE**	Parasitic gastroenteritis
ERP	Egg reappearance period	**PP**	Period of persistency
FAD	Flea allergic dermatitis	**PPP**	Prepatent period
Fe	Iron	**RBC**	Red blood cell
HIV	Human immunodeficiency virus	**RNA**	Ribonucleic acid
HWD	Canine heartworm disease	**SEM**	Scanning electron micrograph
IDI	Insect Development Inhibitor	**SP**	Synthetic pyrethroid
IFAT	Indirect fluorescence antibody test	**sp., spp.**	species (singular and plural)
IgM, IgG, IgE, IgA, etc. Different classes of immunoglobulin		**Th1, Th2**	Two categories of helper T-lymphocytes
IGR	Insect Growth Regulator	**UV**	Ultraviolet
IL-2, IFN-γ, etc. Names given to different cytokines		**VLM**	Visceral larva migrans
KOH	Potassium hydroxide	**ZnSO$_4$**	Zinc sulphate
L$_1$, L$_2$ etc First stage larva, second stage etc.		**3D**	Three-dimensional
Mf	Microfilariae		

About the companion website

This book is accompanied by a companion website:

www.wiley.com/go/jacobs/principles-veterinary-parasitology

The website includes:

- Glossary

- Parasites listed by host and body system

- Pronunciation guide

- Parasite recognition: fleas, flies, worms and worm eggs

- Revision questions and answers

- Further reading list: books, articles and websites

- Powerpoint files of all diagrams for downloading

CHAPTER 1

Veterinary Parasitology: basic concepts

1.1 Introduction

The primary aim of this book is to provide a 'student-friendly' introduction to Veterinary Parasitology for those aspiring to become veterinarians, veterinary nurses or veterinary scientists. It also offers an accessible resource for those already qualified and wishing to refresh or expand their general knowledge of the topic. Others engaged in the many and varied facets of animal health and veterinary public health will also find information relevant to their interests.

This first chapter explores the nature of parasitism while Chapters 2–7 examine clinically relevant relationships and interactions between the parasite, its host and the environment. Finally, Chapters 8 and 9 recognise that, in the real world, veterinarians and animal health workers are not usually presented with a parasite as such, but with a problem concerning some bodily dysfunction affecting a flock, herd or individual.

To fulfil the aims of this book, the emphasis throughout has a clinical bias. Academic information is restricted to that necessary to gain a broad understanding of the pathogenesis, epidemiology, diagnosis and control of the commonest parasitic diseases. Key words are defined in the text or, if printed in a blue typeface, explained in a nearby 'Help box'. A glossary is provided on the website that accompanies this book.

Wherever possible, concepts are described in straightforward language, and unnecessary jargon or detail is avoided. Further aids to learning are provided in 'Help boxes', while

Principles of Veterinary Parasitology, First Edition. By Dennis Jacobs, Mark Fox, Lynda Gibbons and Carlos Hermosilla.
© 2016 John Wiley & Sons, Ltd. Published 2016 by John Wiley & Sons, Ltd.
Companion website: www.wiley.com/go/jacobs/principles-veterinary-parasitology

'Extra Information Boxes' offer additional insights for more advanced readers. Cross-references within the book are given in the format (see Section 9.2.3), (see Table 9.10) etc. These are to assist readers who may wish to follow up on particular points, but they can otherwise be ignored.

The emphasis with regard to parasite identification and the diagnosis of associated disease is on 'how it's done' rather than 'how to do it'. Latin names and taxonomic relationships are introduced only where these provide a useful foundation for comprehension, learning or further reading. The number of parasites that might be encountered in veterinary practice is so great that to mention them all would transform this 'guide to

learning' into an encyclopaedia, which would defeat the purpose of the book. Selected examples are therefore given to provide an understanding of underlying principles and to illustrate the range and diversity that exists within the wonderful world of Veterinary Parasitology.

1.1.1 What is Veterinary Parasitology?

Animal disease can have noninfectious or infectious origins. Noninfectious diseases result from genetic defect, physiological abnormality, structural dysfunction or external factors such as injury, radiation or poisoning. In contrast, infectious diseases are associated with invasive self-replicating agents that have evolved to occupy an animal body as their ecological niche in just the same way as a koala bear has become adapted for life in a particular species of *Eucalyptus* tree.

By convention, the study of infectious agents is divided into Microbiology, which embraces noncellular and prokaryotic organisms, like viruses and bacteria, and Parasitology, which is concerned with eukaryotic life-forms. Fungi are an anomaly in this scheme as, although they are eukaryotes, they are traditionally taught as part of Microbiology in most veterinary schools and so have been omitted from this book.

Veterinary Parasitology is a composite of three distinct disciplines, each with its own set of host–parasite interactions, clinical considerations and vocabulary. The three topics that make up the bulk of Veterinary Parasitology are:

a – Veterinary entomology: the study of parasitic arthropods, including insects, ticks and mites (see Chapters 2 and 3);

b – Veterinary protozoology: a subject that embraces the wide range of single-celled eukaryotic organisms that comprise the parasitic protozoa (see Chapter 4);

c – Veterinary helminthology: which covers three main groups of parasitic worms – trematodes (flukes), cestodes (tapeworms) and nematodes (roundworms), as well as some minor groups such as the thorny-headed worms (see Chapters 5–7).

1.2 Parasitism and parasites

1.2.1 Parasitism

Parasitism is part of a spectrum of intimate zoological relationships between unrelated organisms which includes:

a – Commensalism: two species living together for the benefit of one or both, but without detriment to either

Help box 1.1

Definition of some key technical terms

Aetiology/ aetiological agent: the cause or origin of a disease.

Biotic potential: an expression of the rate at which a parasitic species can multiply. It depends on the number of offspring produced ('fecundity') and the number of generations each year ('generation time').

Endemic: a term used to describe a population or area within which a pathogen is established, replicating and being transmitted between hosts.

Epidemiology: the science that describes and explains patterns of disease in the host population (i.e. the distribution and determinants of disease).

Eukaryote: an organism with a cytoskeleton and complex subcellular structures enclosed within membranes (including a nucleus containing chromosomes). Examples: protozoa and metazoa.

Incidence: the number of new cases of infection per unit time.

Pathogen/pathogenicity/pathogenesis: an organism that causes disease / the severity of the damage caused / the mechanism of the disease process.

Prevalence: proportion of host population infected at a point in time.

Prokaryote: an organism without a nucleus or other membrane-bound subcellular structures; DNA in circular plasmid. Example: bacteria.

Species: the basic unit of biodiversity. Although everyone knows what a species is, there is no exact definition as boundaries are often blurred. Two commonly cited definitions are: 'a group of organisms capable of interbreeding and producing fertile off-spring' and 'a separately evolving lineage that forms a single gene-pool'.

Taxonomic: relating to the laws and science of describing, identifying, naming and classifying organisms.

party, and without any metabolic dependence (e.g. cattle egrets and cattle).

b – Symbiosis: two species living together, each dependent on the other for their mutual well-being and survival (e.g. cellulose-digesting organisms in the caecum of a horse).

c – Parasitism: two species living together, where one of the pair (the parasite) is living at the expense of the other (the host).

d – Parasitoidism: two species living together as in parasitism except that the host invariably dies (or is at least rendered incapable of functioning) once the parasitoid has extracted the sustenance it needs for that stage of its development. Familiar examples include parasitoidal wasps used in horticulture that lay their eggs on or in other insects to provide a food-source for their larvae.

Parasitism implies nutritional dependence on the host for at least part of the life-cycle. It also involves a high degree of specialised adaptation as the animal body is not a passive ecological niche (like a rotten tree-trunk harbouring beetles, for example) but is responsive and hostile to foreign invasion. A parasite must be able to overcome host defences and evade immunological attack. Mechanisms must also be in place to ensure transfer of infection, both geographically from host to host ('horizontal transmission') and temporally from generation to generation ('vertical transmission'). This often entails an intricate integration of the life-cycle of the parasite with that of its host.

Parasites can themselves be victims or beneficiaries of invading organisms. Fleas, for example, are exploited by larval stages of both tapeworms and nematodes, while the canine heartworm, *Dirofilaria*, is metabolically dependent on a symbiotic bacterium, *Wohlbachia*.

1.2.2 Classification

The unwise student could approach every parasitic infection as a separate entity, but this would be an enormous task and a very inefficient approach to learning. It would soon become apparent that similarities exist between some diseases and this would prompt the question: 'what are the common factors?' So, classification is an inherent attribute of human curiosity. It has been noted already that Veterinary Parasitology embraces at least three types of arthropod, several types of protozoa and at least three types of parasitic worm, and so the value of classifying aetiological agents of disease is already becoming apparent.

Taxonomy is a powerful and essential component of biological understanding, although, from a clinician's viewpoint, it is a tool rather than an end in itself. Knowledge of the relationship between parasites often allows similarities in life-cycle, epidemiology, pathogenesis and drug susceptibility to be predicted. Thus, if used intelligently, classification provides a valuable framework for learning and reduces considerably the amount that has to be committed to memory. The classification in this book is kept at the simplest level compatible with this objective.

Help box 1.2

Classification

The animal kingdom is divided into some 35 phyla (singular 'phylum'), which in turn are subdivided successively into Class, Order, Family, Genus and Species, with a species being the basic replicating entity. Subclass, Suborder and Superfamily groupings are also useful in some contexts. Relationships are deduced from morphological, biological and, more recently, molecular evidence and so taxonomic charts (and, confusingly, parasite names on occasion) have to be revised as knowledge accumulates. This can lead to discrepancies between different information sources.

Nomenclature

The identity of every organism is defined by using a combination of its genus and species names. Thus, the protozoan parasite that causes redwater fever in northern European cattle is *Babesia divergens*, while the related species *Babesia bovis* and *Babesia bigemina* cause similar diseases in warmer regions. By international agreement, the ending -osis is placed on a parasite name to indicate the disease caused by that parasite, e.g. babesiosis. By tradition, the ending -iasis is sometimes preferred in human medicine and may occasionally be found in veterinary publications.

It is sometimes useful in Veterinary Parasitology to refer to the common characteristics of a larger grouping of parasites such as a family, which always has a technical name ending in -idae (e.g. the Ixodidae, which is anglicised as 'ixodid ticks'), or even a superfamily with the suffix -oidea (e.g. the Trichostrongyloidea, which becomes 'trichostrongyloid worms').

Writing parasite names

When writing parasite names, the genus name always starts with a capital letter while the species name is lower case throughout. The convention in parasitology as in all biological disciplines is to italicise these. The first time a parasite is mentioned in a text, the full name is used, but thereafter the genus name is abbreviated, e.g. *Babesia divergens* becomes *B. divergens*. The word 'species' can be abbreviated to sp. (singular) or spp. (plural), so '*Babesia* sp.' means an unnamed *Babesia* species, while '*Babesia* spp.' refers to more than one species in that genus.

Why use Latin names?

Latin names are universal, whatever language is being used for communication. Local names can be parochial (for example, babesiosis is known as 'Red-water fever' in the UK but as 'Texas fever' in the USA) or ambiguous ('sand-fly' for example refers to phlebotomine sand-flies in most countries, but is the colloquial term for biting midges in some others).

Pronouncing Latin names

There is no right or wrong way to pronounce a Latin scientific name. Some are tongue-twisters and with these it helps to know how the word can be broken down into syllables. Some of the most troublesome Latin names are listed in the Pronunciation Guide on the website that accompanies this book.

1.2.3 Host–parasite relationships

Parasites and their hosts have evolved together over many millions of years. Every host is vulnerable to infection by several, if not many, parasitic species. Thus, there are many more parasitic species on this planet than host species! It is not surprising, therefore, that a great diversity of host–parasite relationships exists. These are often amazingly intricate and are part of the fascination of parasitology, as will become apparent when the life-cycles of individual parasites are described in later chapters.

Parasites

Parasites can be broadly categorised according to their location on or in the body of their host:

a – Ectoparasites: live or feed on the surface of the host, or embed themselves into superficial or adjacent underlying tissues. Ectoparasites engage in host–parasite

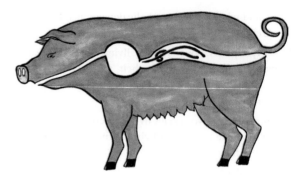

Figure 1.1 Gastrointestinal parasites such as the worms depicted here in black are technically 'outside' of any body tissue.

associations ranging from flies that land fleetingly to feed on secretions from the eyes, nose or other orifices to mites that spend nearly their whole lives in skin tunnels.

b – Endoparasites: live within the body of the host. Parasites may be found in every body tissue except, perhaps, bone and keratin. Those free in the lumen of the gastrointestinal tract are, technically speaking, lying outside of any host tissue (see Figure 1.1), but they are nevertheless included in this category.

A fundamental distinction that influences both the pathogenesis of infection and options for control is the relationship of the parasite to the tissue it inhabits:

a – Extracellular parasites: these live on or within host tissues but do not penetrate into host cells. Examples include almost all metazoan and also many protozoan parasites.

b – Intracellular parasites: these live inside a host cell modifying its genomic expression to cater for their needs, e.g. many protozoan parasites and at least one nematode genus (*Trichinella*).

Parasites can also be differentiated on the basis of their reproductive behaviour in the final host (see Figure 1.2). This distinction is useful as it points towards fundamental biological differences that influence pathogenesis, epidemiology, control and treatment:

a – Microparasites: these multiply within their host. Consequently, each organism that enters the body is capable of initiating a massive infection if not checked by host defences or by chemotherapy. This category includes the parasitic protozoa (as well as microorganisms such as bacteria).

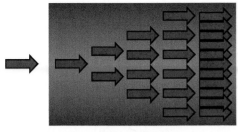

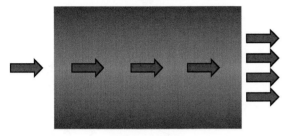

Microparasites

Macroparasites

Figure 1.2 Microparasites (above) multiply their numbers within the host; whereas the number of mature macroparasites (below) never exceeds the number that invaded the host (with a few exceptions).

b – Macroparasites: these do not generally increase in number while they are on or within the final host. They may produce eggs or larvae but these are dispersed into the environment. Thus, the number of mature parasites on or in the final host never exceeds the number of infective units that originally invaded the body. This category includes arthropods and helminths, although there are a few species that break the general rule by multiplying on or in the host (for example: lice, mites and a few nematodes, e.g. some *Strongyloides* species).

c – Microcarnivores: these visit the host transiently to feed but leave again before undergoing any development or producing offspring. Many parasitic arthropods, such as mosquitoes, can be included in this designation.

With such a diverse spectrum of host–parasite associations, there are inevitably some organisms that do not fit conveniently into these broad groupings.

Hosts

Some parasites require just one host to complete their developmental cycle and produce progeny. Others utilise two or more animals. Hosts can be exploited in different ways and the following terminology is used to differentiate between these:

a – Final (or definitive) host: a term used to identify the host in which sexual reproduction of the parasite takes place.

b – Intermediate host: this is a host in which only immature stages grow and develop. Asexual replication may occur (but not sexual reproduction).

c – Transport and paratenic hosts: no parasitic development of any kind takes place in these and they are not a necessary part of the life-cycle. The parasite takes advantage of another animal by using it as a vehicle to increase its chances of reaching its next essential host. The word 'paratenic' implies an intimate relationship in which the parasite becomes embedded within the tissues of its host. The corresponding association with a transport host is more casual and often passive in nature. The two terms are sometimes used interchangeably with less precision.

d – Reservoir host: as the name suggests, this depicts a host population that acts as a source of infection for other animals.

e – Vector: this is a vague term for an insect, tick or other creature that carries (transmits) a disease-causing organism from one host to another.

Life-cycles are described as being:

a – Indirect (or heteroxenous): if an intermediate host is involved; or

b – Direct (or homoxenous): if there is no intermediate host.

Zoonoses

Parasitic zoonoses are diseases of mankind associated with animal parasites (see Section 9.3). They can be classified according to the various biological pathways that lead to human infection (see Figure 1.3):

a – Direct zoonoses: direct transfer from animal to human, e.g. *Cheyletiella* mites from an infested lap-dog.

b – Cyclozoonoses: where humans infect animals and vice versa in strict rotation, e.g. the beef tapeworm.

c – Metazoonoses: these involve a vector as intermediary, e.g. phlebotomine sandflies carrying *Leishmania* from dogs to humans.

d – Saprozoonoses: indirect transfer via the environment, e.g. children playing on ground contaminated with *Toxocara* eggs from a dog or fox.

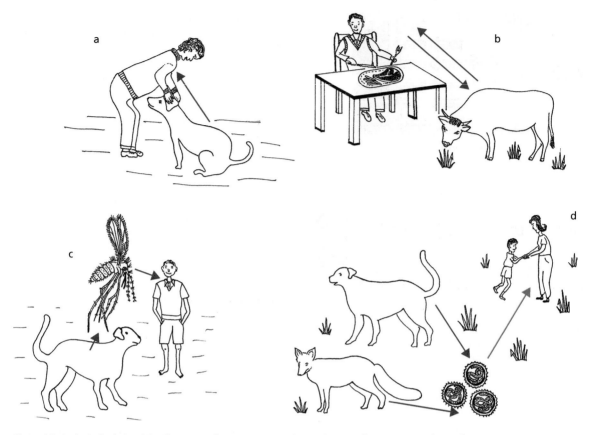

Figure 1.3 Ecological relationships that expose humans to zoonotic parasites: a – direct zoonoses; b – cyclozoonoses; c – metazoonoses; d – saprozoonoses (further explanation in text which uses same lettering as shown above). Sandfly redrawn after Mönnig from Lapage, 1962 with permission of Wolters Kluwer Health - Lippincott, Williams & Wilkins.

1.3 Host–parasite interactions

Hosts rarely gain any benefit from the presence of parasites and are often harmed by them. Defence mechanisms have therefore evolved which, if totally effective, would have extinguished parasitism as a lifestyle. But the continued existence of an abundance of parasites indicates that successful counter-strategies have arisen through natural selection. These in turn have driven the development of further protective measures and so the cycle known as the 'parasitic arms-race' continues. Coevolution has resulted in host–parasite interactions of such complexity that they can be reviewed only at a superficial level in an introductory text such as this.

1.3.1 Host defences

Hosts have evolved many behavioural and other strategies to reduce the risk of succumbing to parasitism. Herbivores, for example, will not eat the lush grass close to a faecal deposit where the greatest concentration of infective worm larvae occurs (the 'zone of repugnance'). The most powerful form of defence, however, is the immune system. This comprises a battery of chemical and cellular weaponry used to combat invasive organisms. Immune reactions may completely or partially disable the attacker or they may alleviate the clinical consequences of infection.

Ideally, immunity should protect against reinfection after the invading parasites have been eliminated. This is called 'sterile immunity'. It can last for a lifetime but often wanes with time. Sometimes, however, such protection persists only as long as a few parasites survive to continually boost the immune processes. This is known as 'premunity'.

In some cases, parasite evasion has gained an evolutionary advantage that renders host immunity relatively ineffective, so the host remains vulnerable despite being repeatedly exposed to infection (e.g. sheep with liver fluke). Some immune reactions directed at a parasite can produce collateral damage to host tissues. Hypersensitivity and allergy are well-known examples.

Innate and acquired immunity

Vertebrates have evolved two separate but closely linked systems to provide protection against invasive pathogens. These are known as innate and acquired immune responses.

Innate immunity

The innate (or nonspecific) immune response is the body's first line of defence. It functions similarly whatever the nature of the invader and whether or not the host has experienced similar attack before. It comprises a series of natural physical, chemical and cellular barriers that are either permanent features (such as the integrity of skin and mucosae or the acidity of the stomach) or that can be quickly mobilised. The latter include a variety of cell-types with different modes of attack as well as humoral factors such as complement. A spectrum of communication molecules (cytokines and chemokines) released by white blood cells (leukocytes) enables the innate immune system to interact with the acquired immune system.

Chemokines: a specific class of cytokines that attract cells towards each other (chemotaxis), e.g. immune cells to the site of infection.

Complement: a biochemical cascade of small plasma and membrane-bound protein molecules that assist in the destruction of some invading organisms. One such cascade is a nonspecific innate response (the 'alternative pathway') while another is antibody-dependent (the 'classical pathway').

Cytokines: signalling molecules that cells use to communicate with each other. The term includes the interleukins (with names such as IL-2 and IFN-γ) that serve to modulate immune responses.

Eosinophilia: an increase in the number of eosinophils (white blood cells with red-staining granules) in the blood.

Humoral: a word used to describe aspects of immunity mediated by macromolecules in the blood or other body fluids (as opposed to cell-mediated immunity).

Hyperplasia: greater than normal proliferation of a particular cell type or tissue.

Lymphocytes: mononuclear white blood cells. There are several types: NK (natural killer) cells involved in innate immunity; B cells that produce antibodies; T cells involved in cell-mediated immunity, including Th (helper cells) that produce cytokines and cytotoxic cells that can kill parasitized host cells. There are also memory cells which enable pathogens to be quickly recognised on reinfection.

MHC: Major Histocompatilibilty Complex. Molecules that carry parasite antigen to the surface of the host cell so that it can be recognised by antigen-processing cells.

Phagocyte: A cell that engulfs and ingests foreign particles.

Help box 1.4

Some key immunological and pathological terms

Antibodies: macromolecules (immunoglobulins) produced by the host adaptive immune system to recognise specific receptor sites on alien molecules (antigens) and to initiate or assist in their neutralisation or destruction. There are different classes of antibody that are labelled IgM, IgG, IgE etc.

Antigen: molecule presented to a host that invokes an adaptive immune response.

Apoptosis: controlled and purposeful cell death (as opposed to necrosis, which is cell death due to an acute insult or injury, and autophagy, which is related to recycling cell components).

Acquired immunity

Acquired (also called 'adaptive' or 'specific') immune responses come into action more slowly than innate reactions as they are tailor-made to combat the particular nature of each new challenge. A quicker response occurs when an animal is subsequently re-exposed to the same pathogen as the system is already primed for that specific reaction. Acquired immunity starts with the detection of foreign molecules (antigens) and the processing of these by antigen-presenting cells. This process generates two forms of adaptive response which are strongly linked to each other:

i)   a cellular response characterised by T-lymphocyte participation, and

ii) humoral immune reactions mediated by B-lymphocytes and antibody-producing plasma cells.

Extra information box 1.1

The Th1/Th2 dichotomy

Different Th-lymphocyte subpopulations have different cytokine profiles and therefore play different roles. As either the Th1 or the Th2 subpopulation tends to predominate in a particular parasitic infection, the 'Th1/Th2 dichotomy' is an important determinant in the pathogenesis of infection and in the design of vaccination strategies. Th1-mediated responses are concerned mainly with cellular immunity and lead to the activation of effector cells, such as macrophages and dendritic cells. Th2-mediated responses are primarily associated with humoral immunity, with cytokines that result in anti-inflammatory reactions accompanied by an increase of specific antibody production, in particular IgE. Mast cells and eosinophils are also activated. These contain granules which, when released onto the surface of larger organisms, are capable of initiating enzymatic digestion.

In general, antigen-presenting cells processing bacterial and protozoan antigens tend to produce IL-12 which leads to an expansion of the Th1 population, whereas antigens derived from helminths and arthropods trigger mainly IL-4 and IL-6 which stimulate Th2-cell proliferation.

Immunity to arthropods

Most parasitic arthropods are ectoparasites. The degree of contact they have with body tissues and the time they spend on the host vary greatly – from a mosquito's fleeting visit to mites that burrow into the superficial epidermis. A few, like warble fly larvae, are true endoparasites, penetrating much more deeply into the body. Thus, opportunity for host detection of arthropod antigens varies accordingly, influencing both the nature and effectiveness of the subsequent immune responses.

In cases where contact is intimate and prolonged, as with some mange mites, a cell-mediated and partially protective immunity often develops. But where the antigens presented to the host are confined to those in the saliva injected during transient feeding behaviour (e.g. biting insects), immune responses may be limited to a local hypersensitivity. Such reactions do little to discourage further flies from biting and can become very itchy (pruritic). This may be of benefit if it encourages animals to move away from infested land or to adopt a more effective grooming behaviour (e.g. in flea or louse infestations), but pruritus can also provoke excessive scratching, rubbing and biting.

Ixodid ticks are rather different as, although they are temporary parasites, they remain attached to their host for several days while taking a blood meal. This provides greater opportunity for immune attack and, over time, parasitized hosts can develop a partially effective species-specific immunity. This acts by interrupting bloodsucking processes, thereby reducing the well-being and reproductive capability of the tick.

Immunity to protozoa

Parasitic protozoa that establish in extracellular positions within the body are exposed to humoral immune responses and are thereby susceptible to destruction by membrane disruption or ingestion by phagocytes. Those that have adopted an intracellular lifestyle will be shielded from such attack (except when moving between host cells) and cellular immune mechanisms are then more likely to be effective.

Extra information box 1.2

Some immune effector mechanisms

Lysis: A complement-dependent process in which the alternative pathway is activated by parasite surface antigens leading to destruction of the parasite by membrane disruption.
Opsonisation: A process whereby a pathogen is 'labelled' with a molecule (e.g. complement factors or a specific antibody) that attracts destructive cells such as phagocytes.
Phagocytosis: Phagocytes such as neutrophils, macrophages, monocytes and dendritic cells will ingest opsonised protozoa or parasitized host cells and attempt to kill them with oxidants, nitrous oxide, etc. and to digest them with enzymes.

Immunity to helminths

In contrast to protozoa, helminths are multicellular, relatively large and have a less intimate relationship with host tissues. Generally, they are extracellular and do not multiply within the host. Consequently, it is more difficult for the host to respond effectively. This is especially true for the many helminths that live in the lumen of the gastrointestinal tract as they are not in direct contact with any body tissue (see Figure 1.1). Immune attack has to be multifaceted and is often aimed at securing the parasite's demise by long-term attrition rather than swift execution.

Expulsion of nematodes from the gastrointestinal tract is a complex two-stage process. Firstly, the mucosal lining has to become permeable to macromolecules so that specific antibodies (e.g. IgA) can 'leak' into the lumen at the site of parasitism. During this process goblet cell hyperplasia results in excess mucus formation. This helps to dislodge some helminths while others exploit it as their primary food-source, which illustrates the complexity and fascination of host–parasite relationships.

Extra information box 1.3

> **Immune effector mechanisms against helminths in the gastrointestinal tract**
>
> Immune protection against gastrointestinal helminths is largely orchestrated by Th2-cells situated in the Peyer's Patches (prominent thickenings of the gut wall). When activated by excretory/secretory (ES) helminth antigens, these cells produce a range of cytokines and chemokines which stimulate IgE production and eosinophilia, together with hyperplasia of mast and goblet cells. The IgE triggers mast cells to release granules containing vasoactive amines and histamine. These substances not only damage helminths directly but also increase gut permeability (permitting an outflow of specific antibodies). They also increase smooth muscle contractions in the gut wall (which helps to dislodge weakened parasites from their predilection sites).

Many gastrointestinal helminths migrate through body tissues en route to their predilection site and may consequently elicit different sets of immune responses during their parasitic life-cycle. They are likely to have reached the gut before acquired immunity to the tissue-stage becomes functional, but the activation of these adaptive responses will help protect the host against future invasion by the same species. Thus, there is an important difference between immunity that protects against reinfection and immunity that eliminates or ameliorates an existing infection.

Extra information box 1.4

> **Immune effector mechanisms against helminths within host tissues**
>
> Protection against tissue-dwelling helminths is predominantly of a cellular nature, reflecting their more intimate contact with their host. They are particularly prone to destruction by an antibody-dependent cell-mediated mechanism. IgE antibodies formed against surface antigens enable host cells such as eosinophils, neutrophils, macrophages and platelets to attach to the parasite and flatten out to ensure tight adhesion. The cells then secrete cationic proteins that are highly toxic to the helminth.

1.3.2 Parasite evasion of immunity

The survival of parasitic species is dependent on being able to escape the immune responses of its host. Such evasion strategies are multifaceted and can be divided into several main groups:

a – Sequestration: making it as difficult as possible for immune processes to reach the parasite. There are two main ways of doing this:

  i) by adopting a relatively inaccessible predilection site, e.g. within particular cell types or organs (such as the CNS or within the lumen of the gastrointestinal tract);

  ii) by generating a protective capsule, membrane or cyst wall.

b – Masking or changing surface antigens – examples include:

  i) incorporation of host molecules onto the surface of the parasite;

  ii) synthesis of parasite antigens which mimic host molecules;

  iii) antigen variance – periodic changes of surface antigens, thereby rendering previous host adaptive responses ineffective. Some parasites have stage specific antigens that serve the same purpose.

c – Disturbance of immunological effector mechanisms – examples include:

  i) surface shedding to remove adhering immune cells or specific antibodies bound to parasite antigen;

  ii) enzymatic digestion of antibodies;

  iii) inhibition of oxidative products synthesised by leukocytes;

  iv) reducing MHC-expression on the surface of infected cells, thereby inhibiting antigen presentation to the immune system.

d – Modulation of the host immune response – this can be achieved in various ways, for example:

  i) induction of multiple clones of T- and B-cells that produce nonspecific antibodies (polyclonal activation), thereby disabling the host's ability to manufacture in sufficient quantity the specific antibodies needed to combat the invading parasite;

  ii) induction of immune complexes in the blood and cleavage of antibody/ complement factors, both of which result in severe immune suppression.

e – Influencing apoptosis:

  i)   release of pro-apoptotic factors that shorten the life of leukocytes that might threaten the parasite;
  ii) synthesis of anti-apoptotic factors by an intracellular protozoan parasite to prolong the life-span of its host cell.

f – Arrested development and hypobiosis: Some parasites are able to pause their development at a strategic point in their parasitic life-cycle. This waiting phase (termed 'arrested development') is used to synchronise parasitic development with host or environmental events (e.g. parturition or the onset of a favourable season of the year). There are various biological advantages to be gained from this (see for example Section 6.3.1). During this process, parasites often 'hide' from targeted host immune responses by slowing or shutting down vulnerable metabolic processes ('hypobiosis').

1.4 Parasitic disease

1.4.1 The host–parasite balance
In nature, the coevolution of host defence mechanisms and parasite evasion strategies has resulted in an uneasy equilibrium whereby there is no undue threat to the continued existence of either at a population level, although the well-being or survival of individuals (host or parasite) may be compromised. The parasite needs to feed and reproduce, yet it faces extinction should infection jeopardise the survival of the host population. In a stable ecosystem, a well-adapted parasitic species is one that survives in the host long enough to replicate but provokes no more than tolerable damage to the host population.

Disease generally indicates a disturbance of this ecological balance. This may be caused by naturally occurring factors, such as unusual weather conditions, but is often due to human intervention. Compare, for example, zebra roaming the African savannah carrying large worm burdens seemingly without ill-effect, with the vulnerability of horses confined to small paddocks.

The host–parasite relationship can be perturbed in two ways:

a – Increased host susceptibility – for example, if animals are:

  i)   stressed, debilitated or immunocompromised;
  ii) exposed to parasites with which they have not coevolved (e.g. European cattle placed in a tropical environment);

  iii) not allowed to express natural behaviour (e.g. restrained so they cannot groom to remove ectoparasites);
  iv) selectively bred for production traits at the expense of natural ability to resist infection (innate or acquired);
  v)   inbred (e.g. some canine blood lines are particularly vulnerable to demodectic mange).

b – Increased parasite numbers – exposure to host-seeking (infective) life-cycle stages may increase, for example, if:

  i)   host stocking density is increased, thereby increasing the output of parasite eggs / larvae etc. per unit area (or per kg forage);
  ii) parasitized animals are introduced into a previously clean area (e.g. through livestock movements, global trade etc.), thereby infecting susceptible local livestock, potential wild-life reservoirs or vectors;
  iii) short-term weather patterns or longer-term trends such as global warming produce conditions more favourable for the development of preparasitic life-cycle stages;
  iv) there is a surge in the population of intermediate hosts or vectors, or an increase in the number infected or their accessibility;
  v)   the parasite population becomes resistant to anti-parasitic medication.

As host defences and parasite immune evasion are both contributory elements to a stable host–parasite relationship, the total elimination of a parasite from the host population can have unintended consequences. For example, without the immuno-modulatory effect of parasites, the human immune system can go into 'overdrive' in some individuals. This may, at least in part, account for the recent increase in allergies and immune-mediated diseases recorded in affluent societies (see Section 7.1.6).

1.4.2 Why parasites are important
Many microbial diseases sweep through populations as dramatic and sometimes devastating epidemics. While parasites can also kill or provoke acute disease, their greatest effect is in the form of chronic, low-grade and debilitating damage. Frequently, the deleterious consequences of parasitism are not readily apparent on clinical examination and so the term 'subclinical disease' is often employed. The various ways in which parasites impact veterinary medicine can be summarised as follows:

a – Animal welfare: many parasitic infections cause pain, discomfort or are otherwise distressing to the host.

b – Agriculture: as well as obvious losses due to death and disease, subclinical disease is of significance as it prevents farm animals from attaining their full genetic potential. The constant drain on bodily resources, imposed by the need to maintain the immunological battle against parasites and to repair the physiological and structural damage they cause, can lead to reduced weight-gain or an increased food conversion ratio, or to a reduction in meat, milk or fibre (e.g. wool) yield and quality. This obviously affects agricultural production and economics. In impoverished rural communities, it deprives the human population of much needed sustenance and diminishes the animal power available to work the land and carry produce to market.

c – Veterinary public health: many parasites of animals are transmissible to humans and capable of causing disease. Parasite vectors can also transfer microbial diseases from animals to humans, e.g. ticks carrying the Lyme disease bacterium. Veterinary input is important in food hygiene to ensure that zoonotic parasites, such as the nematode *Trichinella*, are excluded from the food chain (see Section 9.3.1).

d – Aesthetic considerations: animal owners and consumers often find the sight or thought of parasites repugnant, even though there may be no immediate danger to themselves or their pets, e.g. a cat passing a tapeworm segment, or foodstuffs harbouring an innocuous parasite. Affected meat may be condemned at the abattoir, even though the parasite concerned is neither capable of infecting humans nor of causing overt disease in animals, e.g. *Taenia ovis*.

1.4.3 Pathogenic mechanisms

There are many ways in which parasites can damage tissues or adversely influence bodily functions. These include traumatic outcomes and mechanical defects, parasite-induced cellular and pathophysiological changes, together with detrimental cellular and immunological 'own-goals'. Intracellular parasites not only use their host cell as a food source but may also reprogram its genomic expression to meet their physiological requirements. A selection of the most commonly encountered pathologies is listed in Table 1.1. These and other mechanisms are described in later chapters.

Table 1.1 Some examples of how parasites damage their hosts

Type of damage	An example	More information in Section:
Space occupying lesions	Hydatid disease	5.3.4
Intestinal obstruction/perforation	Ascarid infections	7.1.3
Mechanical damage	Blowfly myiasis	2.2.6
Cell damage/necrosis by intracellular parasites	Coccidiosis	4.6.2
Fibrosis	Liver fluke disease	5.6.2
Epithelial hyperplasia: protein-losing enteropathies	Parasitic gastroenteritis	6.3.2
Malabsorption: villous atrophy	Coccidiosis	4.6.2
Plug feeding	*Strongylus vulgaris*	6.3.3
Anaemia: blood sucking	Hookworms	6.3.4
Anaemia: haemolysis	Babesiosis	4.8.1
Thrombosis	*Strongylus vulgaris*	6.3.3
Lung damage	Bovine lungworm	6.3.5
Heart malfunction	Canine heartworm	7.1.5
Immunological damage	Leishmaniosis	4.5.1
Inflammatory damage	Sheep scab	3.3.3
Neurological damage	*Sarcocystis neurona*	4.7.1
Secretion of pharmacologically active substances	Canine heartworm	7.1.5
Secretion of toxins	Some ticks	3.2.1
Abortion	Toxoplasmosis	4.7.3
Dermatitis	Flea infestation	2.2.2
Tumour formation	*Spirocerca*	7.1.5
Transmission of other pathogens	Many dipteran flies	2.2.5

1.5 Diagnostic techniques

Accurate diagnosis is an essential prerequisite for effective treatment and control. Sometimes the cause of disease may be obvious from clinical signs and history. On many occasions, however, the root of the problem may be obscure or confirmation may be required in order to rule out other possibilities. Diagnosis involves demonstrating parasitic involvement, determining the identity of the organism and, if necessary, quantifying the intensity of infection. Detection of a causal agent can be by direct observation of life-cycle stages in faeces, blood etc. or by gathering indirect evidence, such as the occurrence of specific antigens, antibodies or DNA-sequences. Sometimes, particular biochemical changes are associated with a parasitic infection (e.g. elevated serum pepsinogen concentrations in bovine ostertagiosis). Similarly, quantification can be direct (e.g. worm counts at autopsy) or it may provide an indirect indication (e.g. eggs per gram of faeces or an antibody titre).

1.5.1 Direct detection methods

Some ectoparasites, such as blowfly maggots, are easily accessible and large enough to be collected manually for identification. Others, such as parasitic mites, are too small or too deeply embedded in the skin and so brushing or scraping techniques are needed, with collected material subsequently prepared for microscopic examination.

Haematogenous parasites (i.e. carried in the blood) can be demonstrated in blood samples, which can be prepared as wet or dry smears, centrifuged or filtered as appropriate. Other endoparasites may present a greater challenge, but biopsy may be an option in specific cases. If deaths have occurred, autopsy of representative animals provides an opportunity for investigating the whole body for parasites or parasitic damage.

With living animals, however, faecal examination ('coproscopy') is probably the commonest laboratory diagnostic procedure for demonstrating the presence of endoparasites. Many parasites living in the respiratory system, liver or gastrointestinal tract have life-cycle stages that leave the animal with digestive waste. Sometimes microscopic examination of a fresh faecal smear may suffice, particularly if motile forms are present in large numbers. More often, there are only a few parasitic structures in a large faecal volume. Concentration techniques are therefore needed to assist detection.

Flotation

An appropriate amount of faeces is mixed with a larger volume of an aqueous solution (such as saturated sodium chloride, sodium nitrate or sugar) with a specific gravity that allows lighter parasitic structures, such as eggs, cysts or oocysts, to float while heavier faecal debris sinks. If known weights and volumes are used, a quantitative estimate can be made, e.g. eggs or oocysts per gram of faeces (abbreviated to e.p.g. and o.p.g., respectively). A McMaster counting chamber is often used for this purpose (see Figure 1.4). A subsample (aliquot) of the faecal suspension is pipetted into each of the two chambers on the slide. Eggs that rise and come to rest within the boundaries of the marked grids are identified microscopically and counted. As the volume of fluid beneath each square is known (0.15 ml), the e.p.g. value can easily be calculated.

Sedimentation

Some parasitic structures (e.g. trematode eggs) are too heavy to rise reliably in commonly used flotation fluids and so, in these cases, the faecal sample is mixed with a large volume of water, sieved to remove larger particles, and allowed to stand in a tall vessel. The sediment is examined after an appropriate period.

There are also centrifugation techniques that increase the speed and sensitivity of flotation and sedimentation. Some parasitic structures are more delicate than others and a technique must be selected that does not distort or destroy the object being sought.

It is sometimes necessary to 'culture' faecal samples to encourage development to life-cycle stages that are easier to identify, e.g. by hatching strongyle eggs and

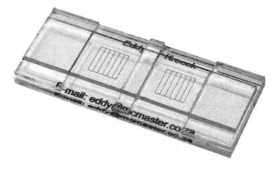

Figure 1.4 McMaster chamber (used for counting helminth eggs and/or coccidian oocysts in faecal samples). Reproduced with permission of T.E. Krecek.

allowing the emerging larvae to develop to the infective stage (see Figure 6.17) or by sporulating coccidian oocysts (see Figure 4.6). This is done by incubating the sample at an appropriate temperature in the presence of adequate air and humidity.

Practical tip box 1.1

Faecal samples

Faecal samples for parasitological examination should be freshly passed by the animal or, preferably, taken directly from the rectum. Faeces on the ground are quickly invaded by free-living nematodes and other organisms that can complicate interpretation. Samples should be examined as quickly as possible and kept refrigerated in the meantime. Even then there may be nonparasitic structures present that could confuse the unwary, e.g. pollen grains or fungal spores that have passed through the animal, or even small air bubbles introduced during preparation. Plant hairs can be easily mistaken for larvae. Such objects are sometimes called 'pseudoparasites'. It should also be remembered that herbivores harbour symbiotic protozoa in their digestive systems.

Nevertheless, most parasitic eggs, cysts and oocysts are easy to recognise with care and practice. Many of these are illustrated or briefly described in this book, as are some other parasitic life-cycle stages. However, reference to identification keys or other detailed publications will be needed for definitive identification.

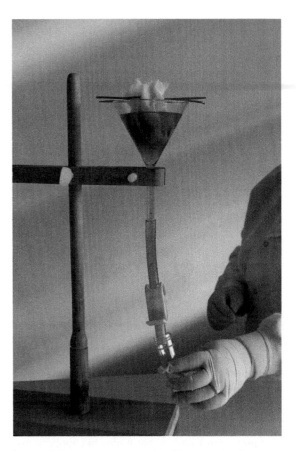

Figure 1.5 Baermann apparatus (used for recovering larvae from faecal samples).

Migration

Some motile parasitic life-cycle stages, e.g. nematode larvae, will migrate out of the faecal mass into water. This phenomenon is exploited in methods such as the Baermann technique in which a faecal sample is placed on a sieve or in a gauze bag in contact with water (see Figure 1.5). Any larvae that emerge are collected in a funnel. Such approaches are also useful for recovering nematode larvae from other materials, e.g. grass washings if the infectivity of a pasture is being investigated.

1.5.2 Indirect detection methods

Often, more information can be gained by searching for indirect evidence of infection than by looking for the parasite itself. Serological methods for detecting antibodies or antigens, and PCR techniques indicating the occurrence of unique genetic sequences are becoming more frequently used as diagnostic tools in Veterinary Parasitology.

Until recently, indirect diagnostic procedures were mostly the domain of laboratories with expensive equipment and highly trained personnel. But technology is advancing rapidly and easy-to-use diagnostic kits are increasingly becoming available for field use.

Immunological assays

Immunological diagnostic tests are designed to detect either antibodies generated in response to infection, or parasite antigen present in blood, tissue fluids or faeces. They are often known by acronyms such as IFAT, ELISA etc. This section outlines the principles that lay behind the commonest of the tests currently in use.

Indirect fluorescence antibody test (IFAT)

The IFAT (see Figure 1.6) is a means of making visible the occurrence of specific antigen on the surface

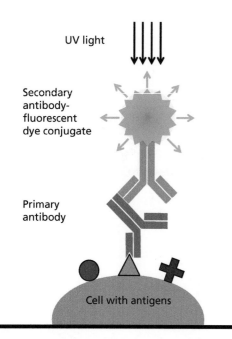

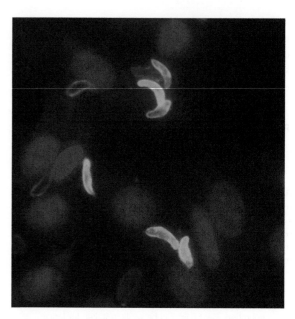

Figure 1.6 Diagram illustrating the principle of the IFAT. Redrawn after https://wiki.cites.illinois.edu/wiki/display/ BIOE414/Background with permission of University of Illinois at Urbana-Champagne.

Figure 1.7 IFAT: protozoan parasites (*Eimeria* merozoites) fluorescing green under UV light (with host cells stained blue). Reproduced with permission of D.J. Ferguson.

of a parasite (or within a cut section of the parasite). It is particularly useful for detecting and identifying some protozoan parasites, but it also has applications in other parasitic groups. The principle of the test is as follows:

a – The specimen is fixed on a microscope slide.

b – It is exposed to a reagent containing antibody specific for a particular parasite antigen (the primary antibody).

c – If the antibody meets matching antigen on the surface of the specimen, they will bind together; if there is no match, the antibody is removed when the slide is washed.

d – The next reagent is a secondary antibody designed to attach to any member of the antibody class (e.g. IgG or IgM) used in the first reagent.

e – The secondary antibody has previously been tagged ('conjugated') with a molecule that can be excited by UV-light.

f – Thus, the parasite antigen, if present, is indicated by luminescence when the slide is examined by fluorescent microscopy (see Figure 1.7).

Enzyme-linked immunosorbent assay (ELISA)

The ELISA is used to detect specific antibodies (e.g. in serum samples) or soluble antigen (e.g. in faecal samples). It is a highly sensitive method as antibody-antigen binding triggers a chain reaction which gives a measurable colour change. The tests are performed in a series of wells on a plastic microtitre plate (see Figure 1.8). This is often done manually but the process can be automated.

ELISAs can be performed in a number of ways for different purposes, one of which (the 'indirect' ELISA for detecting specific antibodies) is illustrated in Figure 1.9:

a – The wells of a microtitre plate are coated with purified antigen which binds to the plastic.

b – A series of dilutions of the test serum is prepared and pipetted into the wells. If specific antibodies are present they will bind to the antigen and remain when the plate is washed.

c – The next reagent contains a secondary antibody (as in the IFAT above) that is conjugated with an enzyme (such as alkaline phosphatase or horse radish peroxidise).

d – After further incubation and washing, a substrate is added that changes colour when digested. This will

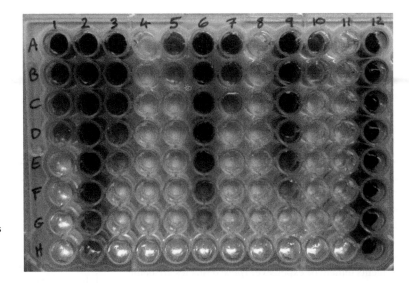

Figure 1.8 Microtitre plate displaying results of an ELISA assay: lanes 11 and 12 – negative and positive control sera, respectively; lanes 1 to 10 – test samples (two-fold dilutions from 1:20 from row A downwards). Reproduced with permission of B. Catchpole.

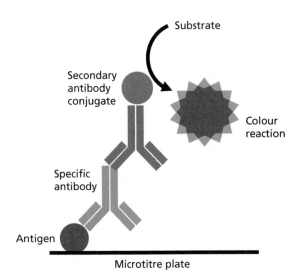

Figure 1.9 Diagram illustrating the principle of the indirect ELISA. Redrawn after http://www.abnova.com/support/resources/ELISA.asp with permission of Abnova Corporation.

happen only if the enzyme that triggers the reaction has been bound, via the two antibodies, to the antigen.

Complement fixation test (CFT)

The principle of this diagnostic test relies on the capacity of antibody-antigen-complexes to bind complement factors. In the CFT assay a specific parasite antigen is incubated with the test serum in the presence of complement. An indicator system is used, based on sensitised sheep erythrocytes. If the sample is positive, the antibody-antigen-complexes that form will bind to the complement and the erythrocytes will remain intact. On the other hand, if no specific antibodies are present in the test serum, haemolysis will occur since unbound complement factors will destroy the erythrocytes. The CFT is used routinely for detecting equine piroplasmosis, an important protozoan infection.

Western blotting

Antigens carry an electrical charge and so they can be spatially separated from other molecules, and from each other, by electrophoresis. They can then be transferred to a carrier membrane and incubated with a test serum. An enzyme-conjugated antibody (as in the ELISA above) is then used to indicate each site on the membrane where specific binding has taken place. A positive result will be depicted by a characteristic pattern.

The specificity of Western blotting is often higher than can be obtained with other techniques as electrophoresis generally separates out all the antigenic components in a sample, thereby isolating any cross-reacting molecules that might complicate interpretation in the other tests.

DNA techniques

As in all other branches of the life-sciences, DNA technology has opened up new possibilities for diagnosis and investigation. Specific primers are used in the polymerase chain reaction (PCR) to amplify unique segments of the parasite genome either for confirmation of identity or to provide fragments of DNA in sufficient quantity for sequencing. Such techniques have proved to be valuable tools for research, giving precise results from minute amounts of material, and have given many new insights into taxonomy and epidemiology. In particular, subtle but important variations can be detected between organisms that are morphologically identical. An important example is the recent differentiation of the protozoan species, *Giardia duodenalis*, into epidemiologically distinct 'genotypes' (see Section 4.5.2). To date, few of these tests are available for routine diagnosis as it can be difficult to extract standardised DNA-samples from field samples and the reagents tend to be expensive. These obstacles are being overcome and this technology will surely play an ever increasing role in the future, not only for identifying the cause of disease but for identifying other significant traits such as drug resistance.

1.5.3 Limitations

Diagnostic tests do not always give a reliable or definitive answer – results have to be interpreted with care. The limitations of each test have to be understood. This applies particularly with regard to sensitivity and specificity, which are rarely 100% even for the most sophisticated tests (except, perhaps, some DNA procedures):

a – Sensitivity: a measure of the proportion of infected animals in a population that will show up as positive using the test in question (e.g. if 100 animals in a flock or herd are infected and the test shows a positive result for 98 of them, then the sensitivity of the test is 98%).

b – Specificity: a measure of the proportion of uninfected animals that will actually register as 'negative' (the remainder being 'false positives'). Thus, if 1 of 100 uninfected animals gives a positive reaction, then the specificity of the test is 99%. False positives are usually caused by cross-reactivity with similar antigens expressed by other parasites or microbial organisms.

Finally, it has to be stressed that the demonstration of a parasitic infection does not necessarily mean that a diagnosis has been made, as the disease may be due to another concurrent aetiological factor.

1.6 Treatment and control

Veterinary Parasitology may be a fascinating topic for academic study but the primary purpose for its inclusion in the veterinary curriculum is to empower the practitioner with the knowledge and understanding needed to combat parasitic disease in an effective and sustainable way.

1.6.1 Key concepts

Although interrelated and often combined, treatment and control are distinct and separate concepts:

a – Treatment: Treatment is a short-term measure aimed at producing an immediate impact on the parasite population. The intended benefit could be alleviation of suffering, enhancement of productivity or prevention of further parasite replication. Additional supportive therapy is often given to help repair damage and restore health.

b – Control: Control has a longer-term perspective and is aimed at preventing future infection and minimising disease risk. It implies the development and implementation of a plan.

The aim of most control programmes is to prevent the parasitic population building up to pathogenic proportions, or to enhance the host's ability to withstand infection (e.g. by vaccination), or both. Such schemes often include strategically timed treatments, but nonchemical approaches can augment, reduce or even replace drug usage. For example, the coccidiosis risk in a poultry house can be lessened considerably by keeping the floor-litter dry so oocysts cannot develop to the infective stage.

Experience has shown that treatments rarely yield longer-term benefits if given in a haphazard or arbitrary way. On the other hand, over-reliance on routine treatments can give diminishing returns over time as parasite strains become resistant to the chemicals used (see Section 1.6.3). This is why control programmes require planned interventions based on epidemiological knowledge.

Very often the concepts of treatment and control are combined. When presented with an outbreak of parasitic disease, a veterinarian will first treat the animals to restore health and then give advice on how to prevent a recurrence of the problem.

1.6.2 Chemotherapy

Selective toxicity

Chemotherapeutic agents are medicinal compounds ('toxicants') that come as close as possible to the ideal of killing or disabling a target parasite without also poisoning the host. This differential effect is termed 'selective toxicity'. In some cases, it is achieved by exploiting differences in biochemical pathways between parasite and host. More often, a good margin of safety is assured because the drug molecule binds more readily or more enduringly to parasite receptors than it does to the host equivalent.

It has already been noted that the life-cycles of 'microparasites', such as protozoa and bacteria, are fundamentally different from those of 'macroparasites' such as helminths and arthropods (see Figure 1.2). Consequently, a different approach to chemotherapy is required in each case. The primary objective for antiprotozoal therapy is to curtail parasite replication within the host, ensuring that population growth does not reach a level that will overwhelm host immunity. Macroparasites (with some exceptions) do not multiply within the final host and the emphasis therefore is on disrupting the transmission of nervous impulses at synaptic and neuromuscular junctions. This action paralyses the parasite, thereby removing its ability to feed or maintain its favoured position ('predilection site') in or on the body. Some parasiticides achieve a similar end-result by impeding energy metabolism.

Formulation

Parasiticides can be administered in different ways depending on purpose and convenience. This may be by mouth, by injection or by skin exposure (dips, sprays, etc.). The term 'topical' is used to describe preparations applied externally with activity confined to the skin. Compounds that are carried to their site of action via the blood-stream are said to act 'systemically'.

In commercial products, the active ingredient is blended with inert materials to produce the required physical presentation, e.g. as a solution, suspension, shampoo, capsule, powder, granule, paste, pellet, etc. This process is known as 'formulation' and can also be used to modify biological and pharmacological properties (increasing potency or reducing toxicity, for example). Slow-release formulations emit their active compound continuously over a period of time (e.g. insecticidal collars, ear-tags, tail-bands etc.) thereby extending the duration of action. A similar effect can be obtained if the active compound is eliminated only slowly from the body, e.g. if a particular tissue such as fat acts as a reservoir. The dynamics of drug storage, metabolism and excretion are termed 'pharmacokinetics' and influence the way in which many parasiticidal drugs are used.

Help box 1.5

Some commonly used terms for antiparasitic drugs

Parasitic group	Collective term for drugs	Notes
Parasites	Parasiticides	
Ectoparasites	Ectoparasiticides	
Insects	Insecticides	This term often used to include ticks and mites as well
	Insect growth regulators	Do not kill adults but stop larval development
Acarina (ticks and mites)	Acaricides	
Protozoa	Antiprotozoals	
Coccidia	Coccidiocides/coccidiostats	These have slightly different meanings (Section 4.10.2)
Helminth	Anthelmintics	Note the correct spelling (left); 'antihelminthics' is sometimes seen but is wrong
Cestodes (tapeworms)	Cestocides	
Trematodes (flukes)	Flukicides	
Nematodes	Anthelmintics	This generic term is used as 'nematocide' is restricted by convention to chemicals used against plant-parasitic nematodes

Help box 1.6

Some pharmaceutical terms

Selective toxicity: the ability of a parasiticide to kill the target organism without harming the host.
Synergism: occurs when the biological activity resulting from the simultaneous application of two substances is greater than their additive effect.
Safety margin: The ratio between the recommended therapeutic and maximum safe doses of a drug formulation.

While prolonged activity may be of advantage in parasite control, residues of biologically active molecules when above defined safety levels render meat and milk products unfit for human consumption. Label instructions for farm animal medicinal products therefore stipulate a statutory interval between treatment and slaughter for meat, or release of milk for human consumption (the 'product withdrawal period').

Formulations providing prolonged delivery should be designed so that drug concentrations decline rapidly at the end of the therapeutic period. This is because a slow decline may expose some parasites to suboptimum doses which could encourage the onset of resistance (as explained in the next section).

1.6.3 Resistance to parasiticides

Many parasitic arthropod, protozoan and helminth species are capable of developing strains resistant to the effects of chemotherapeutic agents. This phenomenon is becoming an ever greater problem worldwide. Resistance not only restricts options for effective treatment but has already imposed severe constraints on agricultural practice in some parts of the world. For example, failing tick control in parts of the wet tropics prohibits the local use of susceptible European cattle (see Section 8.2.4), while sheep farming has been abandoned in parts of South Africa and Australia due to multiresistant stomach worms (see Section 8.2.1).

Most major classes of parasiticide have been in widespread use for several decades. Few chemical entities with a novel mode of action have been brought to the market in recent years. It is therefore important that control programmes do not encourage new resistant strains to develop.

Selection

'Resistance' is defined as the ability of a strain of an organism to tolerate doses of a chemotherapeutic agent that would prove lethal to a majority of individuals in a normal population.

Resistance has a genetic basis. If a treatment is, for example, 98% effective, it is likely that the proportion of individuals expressing genes for resistance will be higher in the 2% that survive than was the case in the whole population prior to exposure. Survivors will continue to produce offspring and the next generation will therefore have an increased prevalence of resistance genes. Thus, selection makes more common the resistance genes (either innate or the result of recent mutation) found originally in only a few individuals. Exposure of subsequent generations to the same or similar treatment will magnify this effect until a breakdown in control becomes clinically evident.

There is always a risk that newly acquired animals may be harbouring parasites carrying resistance genes. To avoid introducing these into the local gene-pool, such animals should be treated with an effective compound and quarantined until shown to be parasite-free.

Selection pressure

'Selection pressure' describes the intensity of the selection process and will be greatest when a high proportion of the parasite population (on a farm, for example) is exposed to the toxicant. The majority of the next generation will then be offspring of treatment survivors and the prevalence of resistance genes will be correspondingly higher. If only part of the parasite population is exposed, the untreated sector (which is said to be '*in refugia*') provides a reservoir of susceptibility genes that will dilute the prevalence of resistance genes in the general gene pool and thereby slow the development of resistance.

Rate of development

When a parasite population is regularly exposed to a particular chemical group, the onset of resistance can vary from a few months to several decades depending on:

a – Parasite factors: such as the nature of the resistance mechanism and its genetic basis; the initial prevalence of the resistance gene(s) in the population; and the biology of the parasite, particularly its biotic potential;

b – Management factors: such as husbandry, treatment strategies (e.g. timing and frequency of dosing), accuracy of dosing, opportunities for parasites to remain *in refugia* etc.;

c – Extraneous factors: such as climate – resistance is likely to occur sooner in warm humid regions where more intensive control measures are needed and parasite generation times are shorter.

Multiple resistance

A parasite population can become resistant to two or more parasiticides, including compounds to which it has never been exposed. This can happen in two ways:

a – Side-resistance: when resistance develops following exposure to a particular compound, it is likely that the parasite strain will also be resistant to other members of that same chemical class (since they will have a similar mode of action).

b – Cross-resistance: a strain resistant to one chemical group may also be resistant to a structurally unrelated class if both act on the same parasite target site (for example, descendents of a fly population resistant to DDT may be resistant to synthetic pyrethroids).

Reversion

Reversion to susceptibility can sometimes occur over time if a parasite population is no longer exposed to the chemical group that induced resistance, but unfortunately this does not always happen. Whether or not reversion occurs depends on:

a – Gene-flow dynamics: e.g. the rate of influx of susceptibility genes into the general gene-pool from parasites *in refugia* or in newly introduced hosts, or (in the case of mobile parasites such as insects) from neighbouring parasite populations;

b – Genetic mechanism of resistance: the genetic change responsible for resistance is sometimes irreversible (e.g. if a susceptibility gene has been deleted).

Treatment failures

It is easy to blame treatment failures onto resistance, but experience has shown that the majority of such events are due to other factors, such as:

i)   an inappropriate choice of parasiticide;
ii) an inadequate dose-rate;

iii) incompetent administration or faulty dosing equipment;
iv) posttreatment exposure to overwhelming parasitic challenge;
v)   hepatic damage (e.g. liver fluke infection) – some compounds need to be modified in the body (metabolised) before becoming active.

Evidence in the form of results from *in vivo* (animal) or *in vitro* (laboratory) tests is necessary before a suspicion of resistance can be confirmed.

1.6.4 Integrated parasite management

Integrated parasite management (IPM) is a concept that is increasingly being adopted in animal parasite control. It is based on the integrated pest management philosophy already well-established in agricultural and horticultural crop protection. IPM builds on acceptance of the view that total dependence on chemical control is no longer a sustainable option because:

a – Resistance: is limiting the use/ usefulness of many existing pesticides/ parasiticides;

b – Few replacement products: the rate of introduction of products active against resistant strains is restricted by the high cost of discovery, development, safety-testing, registration and marketing of novel chemical entities;

c – Meat and milk residues: are potential problems associated with chemotherapy if products are used inappropriately;

d – Ecological concerns: arise if significant quantities of biologically active materials are released into the environment.

The IPM model aims to manage pest or parasite populations, rather than eliminate them, by using chemicals intelligently as one component of a wider integrated control strategy based on epidemiological principles. This encompasses husbandry and hygiene measures, together with vaccines and other technological aids, if available. The use of parasiticides, when needed, is limited to sustainable strategic interventions.

1.6.5 Vaccination

Vaccination primes the host immune system so that it can react more quickly and effectively on encountering antigens associated with specific pathogens. Protozoan and metazoan parasites are structurally complex and have a broad range of strategies for avoiding or subverting host immune responses (see Section 1.3.2). Developing vaccines to protect against parasitic disease therefore presents formidable technological challenges and, consequently, relatively few such products are yet available for veterinary or medical use. Furthermore, their employment has to be economically justifiable within the constraints of veterinary and agricultural practice. Several innovative and technically effective vaccines have proved to be commercial failures in recent years. Nevertheless, vaccine technology is advancing and there is expectation that this situation will improve.

Vaccines tilt the host–parasite balance in favour of the host and this can be exploited in different ways. Most often, they are used to prevent parasite numbers building up in the host to pathogenic proportions, thereby protecting the vaccinated individual against disease. Not all vaccines block parasite establishment completely, however, and so vaccinated animals can still act as a source of infection for others (e.g. calves vaccinated against lungworm, see Section 8.2.2).

With some vaccines (e.g. the hidden antigen tick vaccine described below), parasites establishing on vaccinated animals may be weakened, but not necessarily killed. Their reproductive potential is greatly reduced with the result that fewer infective stages will accumulate on the pasture over the coming weeks and months. With this type of vaccine, therefore, the main beneficiary is not necessarily the vaccinated individual itself but the animals that subsequently graze the now-safer pasture (see Section 8.2.4). In such cases, vaccination is used for the future benefit of the herd or flock while not necessarily protecting the immediate health of the recipient of the vaccine dose – a concept that can be difficult for some farmers to accept.

Natural antigen vaccines

Vaccines can be prepared in a number of ways. The most obvious approach is to utilise antigens that stimulate immunity in natural infections. Sometimes a single antigen extracted from the parasite or its excretory/secretory products ('ES antigens') can induce a strong protective response. Molecular cloning techniques are used for large-scale manufacture of such molecules and the product is known as a 'recombinant vaccine'. One promising vaccine, currently being evaluated in the tropics, prevents pigs from becoming infected with a tapeworm cyst that is transmissible to humans (*Taenia solium*; see Section 9.3.1).

Hidden antigen vaccines

Many attempts at producing recombinant vaccines have yielded disappointing results as parasites generally only succumb when exposed to an array of antibody and cell-mediated attacks. This is partly because of their complexity but also due to their ability to evade or neutralise many specific host responses. An ingenious way has been found to circumvent this latter problem by exploiting molecules that are vital to the parasite's survival but are not detected ('seen') by the host immune system. Such molecules are called 'hidden' or 'concealed' antigens.

In nature, hidden antigens do not induce an immune response, and it follows that the parasite cannot have evolved any corresponding evasive strategy. The parasite is, therefore, highly vulnerable if a way can be found to promote host recognition of this antigen.

This concept is best illustrated with an example (see Figure 1.10). Troublesome ticks, such as *Boophilus*, have potentially antigenic molecules incorporated into their mid-gut wall but these are fixed and so 'hidden' from the host's immune system. After a tick attaches to the skin of its host to feed, it sucks a large quantity of blood into its mid-gut. If the host has been bitten previously by that tick species, the blood will contain antibodies to substances in tick saliva, but these do little harm to the tick and confer little protection to the host. If, however, the host has been vaccinated with a preparation made by cloning 'hidden antigen' isolated from the *Boophilus* mid-gut in the laboratory, then the feeding tick will ingest specific antibodies capable of attacking its gut lining with destructive effect.

One disadvantage of the hidden antigen approach is that the immunity of the vaccinated animal is not reinforced on exposure to natural reinfection (as no gut-surface antigens are presented to the host). This means that booster vaccine doses are needed at regular intervals to prevent immunity from waning.

Attenuated vaccines

One way of ensuring that the broadest spectrum of antigens is presented during the vaccination process is to expose the host to the living parasite. Of course, this has to be done without invoking the disease that we are trying to prevent. This can be achieved by using parasite strains of low virulence. These can be naturally occurring, or their pathogenicity can be diminished artificially, in which case the organism is said to

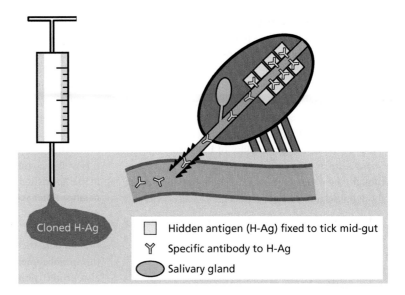

Figure 1.10 Diagram illustrating the principle of the hidden antigen tick-vaccine.

- ☐ Hidden antigen (H-Ag) fixed to tick mid-gut
- Ⴤ Specific antibody to H-Ag
- ⬭ Salivary gland

be 'attenuated'. For example, the blood parasite *Babesia* can be attenuated by infecting a splenectomised calf and using blood from this animal to infect another, and so on, until the desired effect is achieved. This process is known as 'passaging'. Such vaccines have been used with success in some tropical regions where babesiosis is a severe constraint on cattle production. With this approach, however, there is the theoretical possibility that, as the parasite can complete its life-cycle, it might revert to virulence and be transmitted to other animals.

Other attenuated vaccines have addressed this problem by using parasites that have been modified to such an extent that there is no possibility of onward-transmission. For example, the protozoan parasite *Toxoplasma gondii* normally enjoys a short period of uninhibited multiplication in a new host before encysting to hide from immune attack (see Section 4.7.3). The attenuated strain, which is the product of numerous rapid passages through laboratory mice, has lost the ability to encyst. When used as a vaccine, therefore, the resulting infection is self-limiting as the parasites are all killed by the protective immune responses that they themselves have engendered.

Another example is the cattle lungworm vaccine. This comprises living infective larvae that have been exposed to γ-radiation. When administered orally to calves, irradiated larvae migrate to the lungs in the usual way but die before they are able to do significant damage.

This vaccine has been successfully employed for over 40 years.

More recently, an effective vaccine for coccidiosis in poultry was created by passaging several species of the causal protozoan parasite, *Eimeria*, through chick embryos. The attenuated organism has a shortened ('precocious') parasitic cycle in which the most pathogenic of the several developmental stages has been lost and is skipped over. Once again, the host is exposed to the full array of antigens needed to induce a solid protective immunity but without risk of the live vaccine provoking disease.

Attenuated vaccines do have some limitations. As they consist of living organisms, they tend to have short shelf-lives and they require exacting conditions for transport and storage.

1.6.6 Alternative technologies

Concerns about the continued sustainability of some control methods, the current limitations of vaccines and the affordability of high-tech solutions for farmers in poorer countries, have lead to a great deal of research on alternative and low-input approaches to parasite control. The main aims are to maintain the health and productivity of livestock while reducing dependency on chemicals, and to maintain the susceptibility of parasite populations to parasiticides for as long as possible. In other words, to enhance host resistance to parasites while delaying the development of parasite resistance to parasiticides.

Enhancing host resistance

Genetic diversity within host populations influences the ability of individual animals to withstand parasitism. Typically, a few animals within a flock or herd will harbour large numbers of parasites while a greater number will have few or none. The usual spread of parasites through a host population is said to be 'overdispersed', i.e. it does not follow a normal distribution curve (see Figure 1.11).

This difference in vulnerability of individual animals to parasitism is often referred to as 'host resistance', although the phenomenon actually has two distinct, although interlinked, components:

a – Resistance: this is the ability of an animal to defend itself against parasitic attack by means of innate and acquired immune responses (see Section 1.3.1). The main methods of enhancing host resistance are by ensuring adequate nutrition and by vaccination.

b – Resilience: this is the ability of an animal to tolerate the presence of parasites. For example, two animals may harbour identical parasitic burdens yet only one may show signs of clinical disease. The healthier animal is better able to limit, or to compensate for, the damage caused by the parasites.

Breeding for resistance/resilience

Resilience is, to a greater or lesser degree, a heritable trait. In the case of gastrointestinal nematodes in some breeds of sheep, heritability is of the same magnitude as that for milk yield in dairy cows. Breeding programmes can therefore improve this trait if a suitable marker can be found for identifying the more resilient rams.

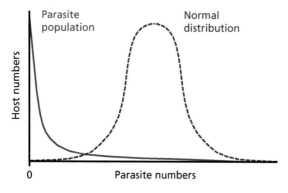

Figure 1.11 The typically skewed distribution of parasites within a host population compared with a 'normal' distribution curve (notional diagram).

Stock hybridisation is sometimes employed to achieve resistance or resilience. For example, *Bos indicus*-type cattle (humped tropical breeds) are much more tolerant of tick infestations than are European (*Bos taurus*) breeds. Cross-breeding can enable European cattle to survive in heavily tick-infested areas with fewer acaricidal treatments, albeit at a cost of reduced productivity.

Nutrition

It is well-recognised that parasitism is more pronounced in malnourished animals and that an adequate and well-balanced diet will boost both resistance and resilience. Some food-stuffs ('bioactive crops') can be particularly beneficial in this respect. For example, tannin-rich fodders such as lucerne (alfalfa) and clover reduce the establishment of infective nematode larvae. They also protect protein from microbial degradation in the rumen, thereby increasing the supply of plant protein to the abomasum. Many other plants, e.g. chicory, have antiparasitic properties that could theoretically be exploited, either as forages in a grazing programme or as feed supplements.

Delaying parasite resistance

It was noted in Section 1.6.3 that resistance to parasiticides is a selection process in which resistance genes become more prevalent in successive generations. Strategies to delay the onset of resistance must therefore block, dilute or reverse this trend. One approach is to combine or alternate the use of drugs with different modes of action, so that parasites surviving one treatment are killed by the next. There is, however, a risk that ill-considered dosing schedules could potentially lead to multiresistance.

Low-input approaches aim to keep a sufficient proportion of the parasite population *in refugia* to maintain the diversity of the gene pool (Section 1.6.3). To achieve this aim, interventions are designed to maintain the overall level of parasitism within tolerable limits, while allowing sufficient numbers of parasites not exposed to the drug to reproduce. This can be done in at least two ways:

a – Selective treatments: treatments are restricted to those animals in greatest clinical need, e.g. those exhibiting diarrhoea or anaemia;

b – Targeted treatments: these are given only to those individuals within the group that are contributing most to the infectivity of the environment.

Targeted treatments can be used, for example, in horse stables. Faecal egg-counts identify the few animals in a group that excrete large numbers of worm eggs and these are treated. This reduces pasture contamination substantially while the genetic diversity of the parasite population is maintained by the untreated members of the herd. The risk of future disease is not completely averted, however, and so good clinical judgement, careful management and regular monitoring are required.

Biological control

Biological control measures are widely used in horticulture, especially in greenhouses (e.g. parasitoid wasps to control aphids or nematodes for slugs). Similar approaches are being investigated for animal health application. For example, nematodes that kill flea larvae are commercially available for outdoor use in some countries.

A promising innovation that may have veterinary application in the future is the use of nematophagous fungi. A number of nematode-trapping species have been used successfully in field trials for reducing the numbers of infective gastrointestinal nematode larvae appearing on pasture. Fungal spores fed to ruminants pass through the animal and produce networks of hyphae throughout faecal deposits. These release compounds that attract nematodes, which are captured, killed and digested by a variety of means including adhesive nets (see Figure 1.12), nonadhesive constrictive rings or by deposition of droplets of paralytic toxin.

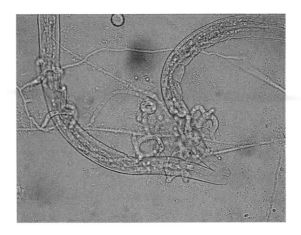

Figure 1.12 Nematode trapping fungi: two nematode larvae entrapped in an adhesive 3D network of hyphae. Reproduced with permission of N. Soto-Barrientos.

1.6.7 Concluding remarks

It will have become apparent during the course of this chapter that parasite control is not always straightforward but often requires a range of skills. It demands knowledge of the biology and epidemiology of each type of parasite, the ability to interpret laboratory findings and make an accurate diagnosis, an understanding of the rationale underlying different control methods, and an appreciation of the strengths and limitations of available parasiticides and vaccines. This is why the expertise of the animal health professional is so valuable to the animal owner.

CHAPTER 2
Arthropods part 1: introduction and insects

2.1 Introduction

Arthropods are invertebrates with jointed legs. Their bodies are bilaterally symmetrical and segmented. They are the most diverse of all animal life-forms. Two groups are of major veterinary importance: the insects with six legs and the arachnids with eight (see Figure 2.1). A third group, the Crustacea, contains just a couple of parasitic genera worthy of attention.

Most, but not all, arthropods of veterinary interest are associated in various ways with body surface tissues (see Figure 2.2). They commonly cause skin trauma and inflammatory or allergic reactions, often accompanied by pain or itching (pruritus). These infestations therefore play a prominent role in clinical dermatology.

This chapter focuses on the broad spectrum of the insect world, while the next covers parasitic acarina, crustacea and the drugs that are used to combat ectoparasites.

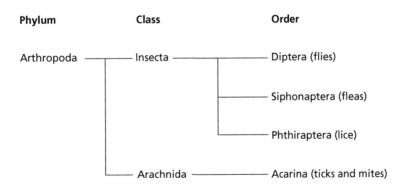

Figure 2.1 The major groups of parasitic arthropods.

Principles of Veterinary Parasitology, First Edition. By Dennis Jacobs, Mark Fox, Lynda Gibbons and Carlos Hermosilla.
© 2016 John Wiley & Sons, Ltd. Published 2016 by John Wiley & Sons, Ltd.
Companion website: www.wiley.com/go/jacobs/principles-veterinary-parasitology

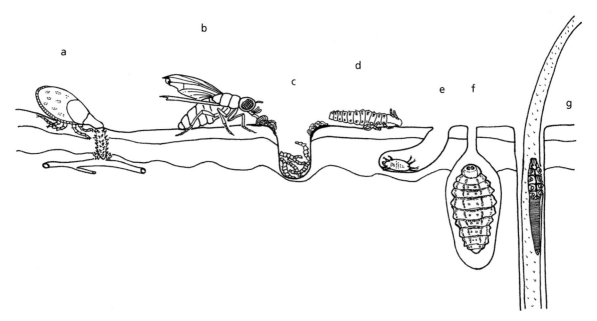

Figure 2.2 Some associations between arthropod parasites and skin: a - blood-sucking (tick); b - surface feeding on secretions and exudates (muscid fly); c - flesh-eating (cutaneous myiasis); d - surface feeding on skin debris (chewing louse); e - burrowing mite; f - warble fly developing under skin; g - mite in hair follicle. Based on Jacobs, 1986 with permission of Elsevier. Warble fly redrawn after Mönnig from Lapage, 1962 with permission of Wolters Kluwer Health - Lippincott, Williams & Wilkins. *Demodex* redrawn after James and Harwood, 1969 from Cheng, 1986 with permission of Elsevier.

2.2 Insects

The insects of greatest concern in clinical practice are fleas, lice and flies, although there are many others that can adversely affect animal and human health by means of bites, stings, blister-inducing venoms or irritating hairs, all of which can induce allergies and sometimes anaphylaxis. Insects also destroy and foul feedstuffs. Cockroaches are particularly adept at contaminating food and other surfaces by the mechanical transfer of pathogens. Along with many beetles, they can also act as transport or intermediate hosts for some helminth infections, e.g. the spiruroid stomach worms of dogs and pigs (see Table 7.2).

2.2.1 Key concepts

Body structure

A general appreciation of the body structure and function of insects and other parasites is needed at a practical level for two main reasons. Firstly, as an aid to diagnosis, since familiarity with the terminology used in

Help box 2.1

Technical names of insect groups

At first sight, the technical names given to the major groups of insects (see Figure 2.1) look daunting but they are easier to remember if their composition is understood. The key derivations are from ancient Greek: 'ptera' meaning 'wings', and 'a' which signifies 'no'. Thus, loosely translated:

Siphon/a/ptera – siphoning mouthparts/no/wings ('siphon' is actually Greek for 'tube').
Phthir/a/ptera – louse/no/wings ('phthir', pronounced *F-th-ire*, being Greek for 'louse').
Hemi/ptera – half/wings (refers to the top pair of wings being part thickened and part membranous).
Di/ptera – two/wings (an important diagnostic characteristic as all other flying insects have four wings).

books, on-line resources and identification keys facilitates the accurate recognition of pathogens. Secondly, to enhance understanding of key biological features that influence the epidemiology, pathogenesis or control of related disease processes.

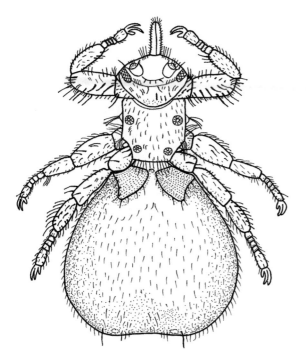

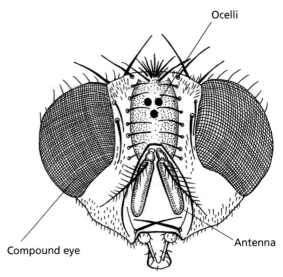

Figure 2.4 Head of the blowfly *Lucilia*. Adapted after Mönnig from Soulsby, 1982 with permission of Wolters Kluwer Health - Lippincott, Williams & Wilkins.

Figure 2.3 The sheep ked, *Melophagus ovinus*. Redrawn after Mönnig from Lapage, 1962 with permission of Wolters Kluwer Health - Lippincott, Williams & Wilkins.

The insect body is divided into three distinct regions: head, thorax and abdomen. These divisions are clearly seen in the sheep ked illustrated in Figure 2.3. The entire surface is covered by a hard protective noncellular exoskeleton, which is secreted by an underlying epidermis. The exoskeleton has three cuticular layers containing chitin (a long-chained polysaccharide) which provides mechanical support. The chitin molecules are sometimes cross-linked for extra strength. The outer layer often has a waxy surface.

The exoskeleton is composed of plates linked by flexible intersegmental membranes. These provide weak spots where contact insecticides can penetrate through to sensitive tissues beneath.

Head

The insect head is composed of a number of fused plates and acts as a support for eyes, mouthparts and a single pair of antennae covered with sensory hairs and bristles (see Figure 2.4).

The eyes vary greatly in complexity from simple 'ocelli', which monitor light intensity, to compound eyes made up of a honeycomb-like congregation of thousands of tubes, each covered by a cornea and containing sensory cells. These are sensitive to movement.

Insect mouthparts consist of several basic structures: upper and lower lips (the 'labrum' and the 'labium'), two pairs of jaws ('mandibles' and 'maxillae') and a protuberance like a drinking straw that channels saliva to where it is needed ('hypopharynx'). There may also be additional finger-like projections carrying sensory organs. The mouthparts differ in shape and size to suit the particular feeding habit of each type of insect. Two contrasting examples are shown in Figure 2.5. The mouthparts of the female mosquito on the left are long and slender, coming together to form a needle-like tube ideal for penetrating skin, probing for blood vessels and sucking blood, whereas the lower lip of *Musca*, on the right, is expanded into two retractable sponge-like structures ('labellae') which are used to mop up surface-lying pools of liquefied food.

Insects often have different feeding behaviours in their juvenile and adult stages with correspondingly dissimilar mouthparts. Compare, for example, the chitinous lacerating structures of blowfly larvae (see Figure 2.6) with the scraping and sponging mouthparts of the adult

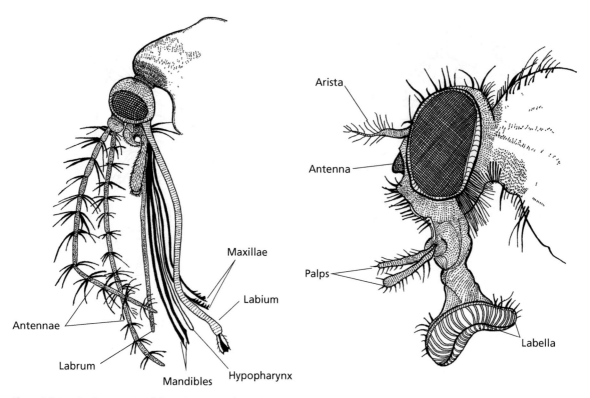

Figure 2.5 Heads of a mosquito (left) and *Musca* (right). Adapted from Urquhart *et al.*, 1996 with permission of John Wiley & Sons, Ltd.

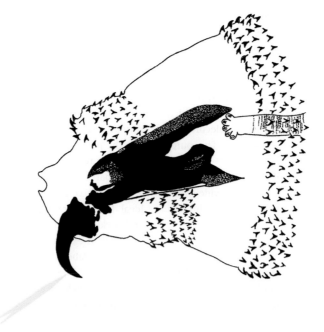

Figure 2.6 Head-end of a blowfly larva (maggot) showing the chitinous mouthparts (arrowed). Redrawn from Zumpt, 1965.

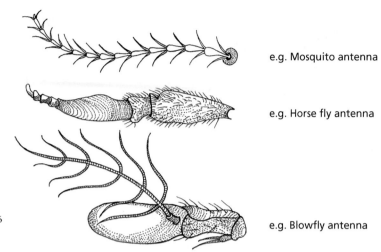

e.g. Mosquito antenna

e.g. Horse fly antenna

e.g. Blowfly antenna

Figure 2.7 Antennae of a mosquito (top); a horse fly (centre) and an adult blowfly (below). Adapted from Urquhart *et al.*, 1996 with permission of John Wiley & Sons, Ltd.

fly (similar to those of *Musca* illustrated in Figure 2.5). In many cases, the sexes utilise different food sources with males taking nectar from flowers while females also seek protein meals. This is often blood in the case of parasitic insects.

The form of the antenna varies greatly and is sometimes useful for identification (see Figure 2.7). Some antennae are long and segmented (e.g. mosquitoes) while others are short and squat (e.g. horse flies). Some are hairy, whilst others (e.g. houseflies and blowflies) carry special bristles ('aristae'). The antennae of males and females of some species are also different.

Thorax

The thorax is covered with fused plates supporting three pairs of jointed legs, each made up of several parts (see Figure 2.8). Insects that fly also have one or two pairs of wings mounted on the thorax.

The wing is a membranous outgrowth of the exoskeleton, supported and strengthened by a network of 'veins' which comprise breathing tubes ('tracheae') and blood vessels. The arrangement of the wing veins ('venation') is important in the identification of adult flies as illustrated in Figure 2.9 which compares the wing of a horse fly (which has a central 'discal cell') and a tsetse fly (which has a characteristic 'butcher's cleaver'-shaped cell).

One important group of flies, the Diptera, is easily recognised as they have only one pair of wings (see Figure 2.10). The posterior pair has evolved into small gyroscopic balancing organs ('halteres').

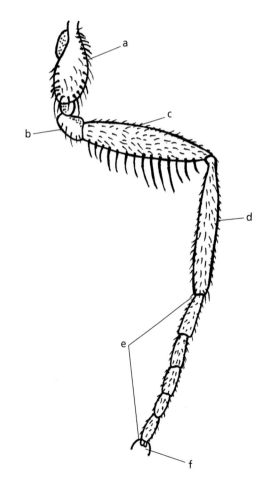

Figure 2.8 An insect leg: a – coxa; b – trochanter; c – femur; d – tibia; e – tarsus; f – claw. Redrawn after Cheng, 1986 with permission of Elsevier.

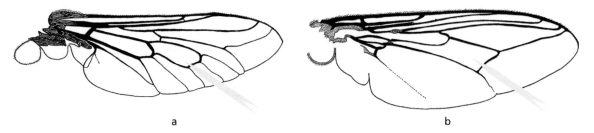

a   b

Figure 2.9 Wing of a horse fly (a) showing the 'discal cell' (arrowed) and a tsetse fly (b) showing the 'butcher's cleaver'-shaped cell (arrowed). Redrawn after Mönnig from Lapage, 1962 with permission of Wolters Kluwer Health - Lippincott, Williams & Wilkins.

Abdomen

The abdomen is usually a clearly segmented, soft structure. Various appendages may be present such as copulatory claspers, an ovipositor or external genitalia. The majority of body systems are located in the abdomen.

The respiratory system consists of a network of branching tubes ('tracheae'), which are strengthened by spiral thickenings. Airflow is regulated by muscular contractions of the body wall. The tracheae communicate with the atmosphere by means of chitinous surface openings ('spiracles') which can be opened and closed (see Figure 2.11). The shape of these and the plates upon which they are mounted ('stigmatic plates') are used for the identification of blowfly larvae in forensic medicine. (This, together with knowledge of the rates of development of individual species, can be used in investigations of human murder or animal abuse and neglect cases to deduce, for example, time of death and whether there had been prior trauma.)

The alimentary canal is divided into three main regions: a foregut which processes ingested food mechanically, a midgut for storage and enzyme secretion, and a hindgut for water resorption (see Figure 2.12). The midgut is also an outlet for the 'malpighian tubules', which are the insect equivalent of kidneys. The circulatory system comprises a dorsally-situated heart (essentially a thick-walled blood vessel with valves which permit the blood to flow

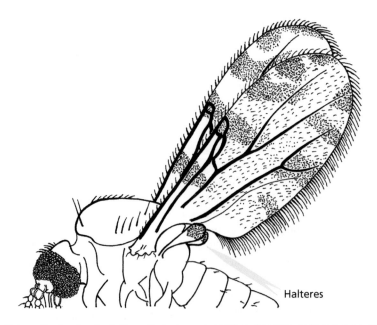

Halteres

Figure 2.10 Wing of a dipteran fly showing the halteres. Redrawn and modified after Mönnig from Lapage, 1962 with permission of Wolters Kluwer Health - Lippincott, Williams & Wilkins.

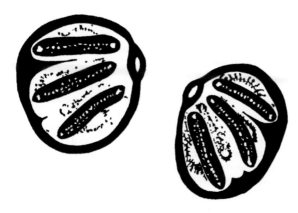

Figure 2.11 Spiracles of a blowfly larva. Redrawn after Zumpt, 1965.

only forwards) and branching blood vessels. There are no capillaries. Instead, the blood flows into the general body cavity ('haemocoele') which bathes the organs and tissues. It returns to the heart via openings in blood vessel walls.

The nervous system, which is the target for many insecticides, consists of a small brain, just above the pharynx, and a chain of fused ganglia, which lie on the floor of the thorax and abdomen and give off nerves to the various body parts.

The 'fat body' is a large structure made up of cells containing numerous fat vacuoles. Its form is variable but in many insects it lines the body cavity and all the internal organs (like the peritoneum in mammals). The fat body has many metabolic functions and acts as a food reserve for use during periods of hibernation or starvation. It also absorbs fat soluble insecticides, reducing their potency.

Reproduction

Most insect species have separate sexes. The reproductive tracts are directly analogous to those of vertebrates, i.e. testes, vas deferens and seminal vesicles (male) and ovaries, oviducts, common oviduct (or uterus) and vagina (female). Females also have an accessory organ, the spermatheca, which acts as a receptacle for spermatozoa after mating. This enables the female to fertilise subsequent batches of eggs in the absence of a male.

Most adult female insects are 'oviparous', i.e. they lay eggs which hatch after deposition. Some species are 'viviparous', i.e. the egg ruptures at some stage within the reproductive tract so the female gives birth to a juvenile.

There are two main types of insect life-cycle: simple and complex metamorphosis. In simple metamorphosis (see Figure 2.13), the insect which emerges from the

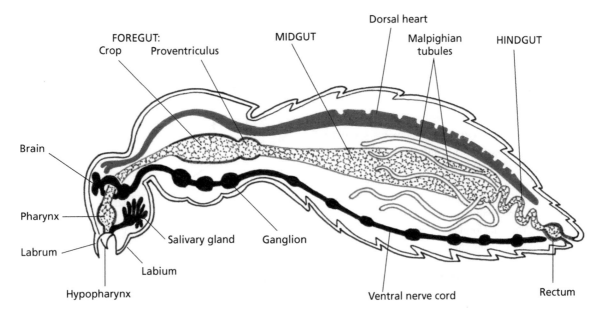

Figure 2.12 An insect in longitudinal section. Redrawn after Imms, 1957 and Urquhart *et al.*, 1996 with permission of John Wiley & Sons, Ltd.

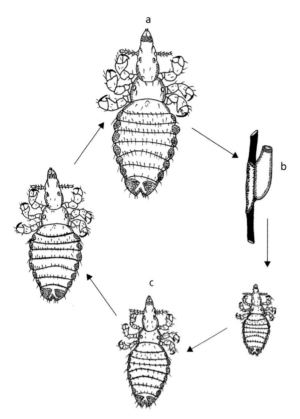

Figure 2.13 An example of simple metamorphosis (life-cycle of a louse): a – adult louse; b – egg; c – nymphal stages. Adult redrawn after Mönnig from Lapage, 1962 with permission of Wolters Kluwer Health - Lippincott, Williams & Wilkins, diagram partly based on Urquhart *et al.*, 1996 with permission of John Wiley & Sons, Ltd.

egg resembles the adult and is called a 'nymph'. This grows and undergoes several moults ('ecdyses') before attaining maturity.

In complex metamorphosis (see Figure 2.14), the young insect which emerges from the egg shows marked differences in morphology and structure from the adult and is called a 'larva'. After feeding, growing and moulting several times, the larva enters a quiescent phase and the outer cuticle hardens to form the 'pupa'. Some species spin a silk-like protective covering (the 'cocoon') before they pupate. The adult form develops inside the pupal case before the 'imago' finally emerges.

2.2.2 Fleas (Siphonaptera)

Adult fleas have an unmistakable appearance with a narrow mahogany-brown body that is superbly adapted for moving swiftly through fur or feathers (see Figure 2.15). They are wingless but their powerful

Help box 2.2

Definitions: 'larva', 'nymph' and related technical words

Nymph: a nymph looks like the adult it is going to grow into, but is smaller, sexually immature and (in the case of flying insects) with undeveloped wings.
Larva: a larva is markedly different in morphology and structure from the adult of the species. Colloquial names for different types of insect larva include maggot, grub and caterpillar.
Instar: insect nymphs and larvae are 'juvenile instars'. Instar is the technical word for an insect life-cycle stage that follows a moult (e.g. 'the third larval instar').
Imago: a technical name for the adult insect.
Parthenogenesis: the production of eggs or offspring by a female that has not been fertilised by a male.

hind legs enable them to jump many times their own height.

As blood-sucking ectoparasites, fleas are of considerable importance in small animal dermatology. Large numbers cause pruritus, considerable annoyance and

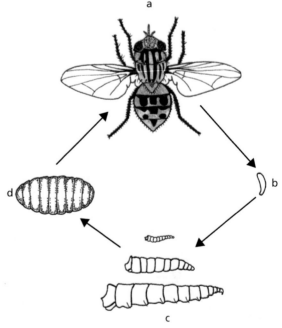

Figure 2.14 An example of complex metamorphosis – the life-cycle of a dipteran fly, *Stomoxys*: a – adult fly; b – egg; c – larval stages; d – pupa. Adult redrawn after Mönnig from Lapage, 1962 with permission of Wolters Kluwer Health - Lippincott, Williams & Wilkins. Diagram partly based on Urquhart *et al.*, 1996 with permission of John Wiley & Sons, Ltd.

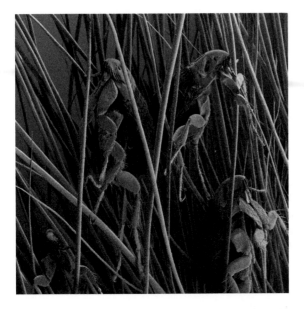

Figure 2.15 Fleas are well adapted to living in the hair-coat of their host (SEM). Reproduced with permission of Bayer plc.

sometimes anaemia. Moderate numbers are usually well tolerated and may not be noticed by the owner. Some animals, however, become allergic to substances in flea saliva. In highly vulnerable individuals, just a few bites will trigger hypersensitivity reactions.

In addition, fleas act as intermediate host for the tapeworm *Dipylidium* (see Section 5.3.5) and as vectors for microorganisms, such as those associated with cat scratch fever and bubonic plague in humans and myxomatosis in rabbits.

Important fleas

Most flea species have evolved as parasites of nest-building mammals and birds. Many have a preferred host but will feed on other animals. Primates and herbivores, therefore, tend to be incidental victims.

The most important fleas found on cats and dogs are listed in Table 2.1, although other species that feed mainly on wild-life may also be found occasionally on pet animals. In warmer regions, jiggers and stick-tight fleas can cause great distress to humans and pets as they burrow deeply into the skin.

General characteristics

Adult fleas are small (1.5–4 mm) but easily seen with the naked eye. They are flattened from side to side ('laterally compressed'). Each body segment has a row of backward pointing bristles ('setae') which ensure that they move through dense hair in one direction only – forwards (see Figure 2.16). This helps to protect them from host grooming activities. Identification requires some expertise but is aided by the rows of heavy chitinous spines ('combs' or 'ctenidia') that occur along the ventral ('genal') or posterior ('pronotal') aspects of the head (see Figure 2.17).

Life-cycle

Although all flea life-cycles follow the same general pattern, there is variation between species. Further discussion in this section is confined to the cat-flea, *Ctenocephalides felis* (see Figure 2.18). A full understanding of this species is required so that appropriate advice on flea control can be given to pet owners.

Table 2.1 Some important fleas found on dogs and cats

Common name	Species name	Distribution	Notes (More information)
Cat flea	*Ctenocephalides felis*	Cosmopolitan (different subspecies occur in some locations)	The most common flea on dogs as well as cats; also bites humans and other animals (see Section 9.2.3)
Dog flea	*Ctenocephalides canis*	Cosmopolitan	Less common than previously; fairly host specific
Poultry flea	*Ceratophyllus gallinae*	Cosmopolitan	Mainly poultry; also bites humans and other animals
Rabbit flea	*Spilopsyllus cuniculi*	Cosmopolitan	Mainly rabbits; also bites other animals
Human flea	*Pulex irritans*	Cosmopolitan; now rare in many affluent countries	Mainly pigs and humans; also bites other animals
Jigger flea	*Tunga penetrans*	Parts of Africa, Asia and the Americas	Mainly pigs and humans; also bites other animals. Females burrow into skin
Stick-tight flea	*Echidnophaga gallinacea*	Tropics and warmer regions	Mainly poultry; also bites humans and other animals. Females burrow into skin

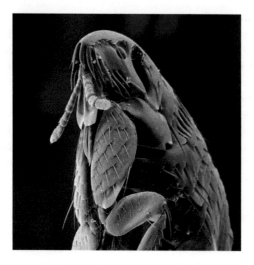

Figure 2.16 Head-end of flea (SEM). Reproduced with permission of Bayer plc.

a – Host-seeking adult *C. felis* use changes in light intensity, warmth and CO_2 to locate a host (cat, dog or other animal). Within minutes of jumping onto the host, they start to take frequent small blood meals. Females are larger than males and have a greater appetite. Seventy fleas can withdraw 1 ml of blood per day. They produce copious amounts of dark red faeces, known colloquially as 'flea dirt'.

The life-span of a cat-flea is determined by the grooming efficiency of the host, but is typically around 7–10 days. The cat flea is an 'almost permanent' parasite. There may be a small degree of transfer of fleas between animals in close contact, but the great majority are reluctant to leave once they have found a suitable host. After they start to feed, any cat-fleas that fall off an animal survive only a few hours.

HEAD WITHOUT COMBS

Head rounded anteriorly................*Pulex*

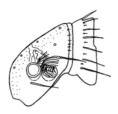

HEAD WITH COMBS

Pronotal comb only.................*Ceratophyllus*

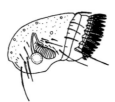

Both combs present..............*Ctenocephalides*
                                         Spilopsyllus

Genal comb mounted horizontally.........
                                         C.canis

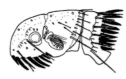

                        C. felis

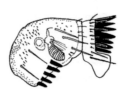

Genal comb mounted obliquely.........
                                Spilopsyllus

Figure 2.17 A chart for identifying the fleas most commonly found on dogs and cats. Fleas redrawn after Smart, 1943 with permission of The Natural History Museum, London, UK and Smit, 1957 with permission of the Royal Entomological Society, St Albans, UK.

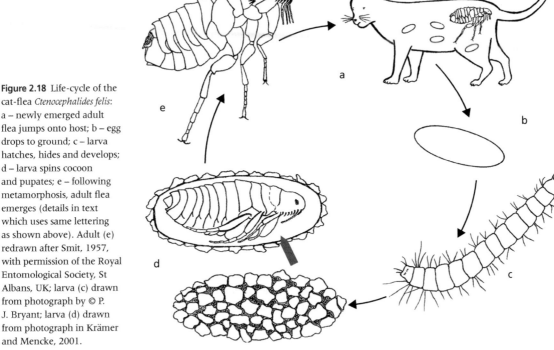

Figure 2.18 Life-cycle of the cat-flea *Ctenocephalides felis*: a – newly emerged adult flea jumps onto host; b – egg drops to ground; c – larva hatches, hides and develops; d – larva spins cocoon and pupates; e – following metamorphosis, adult flea emerges (details in text which uses same lettering as shown above). Adult (e) redrawn after Smit, 1957, with permission of the Royal Entomological Society, St Albans, UK; larva (c) drawn from photograph by © P. J. Bryant; larva (d) drawn from photograph in Krämer and Mencke, 2001.

b – Female fleas start to lay eggs 1–2 days after their first blood meal. Some 10–25 ivory-white oval eggs (0.5 mm long) are deposited into the pelage (coat) every day (see Figure 2.19). These are slippery and drop to the ground within a few hours.

c – The eggs start to hatch in 1–6 days (all off-host life-cycle phases are temperature dependent). The first larval instar is 2 mm long and after a period of growth moults to the second stage. The process is repeated until the third larval instar reaches about 5 mm in 1–7 weeks. The larvae (see Figure 2.20) are maggot-like and covered with bristles, which together with a pair of posterior protrusions ('anal struts') are used to assist rapid movement.

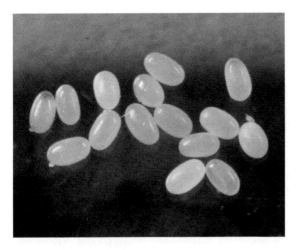

Figure 2.19 Flea eggs. Reproduced with permission of D.-H. Choe.

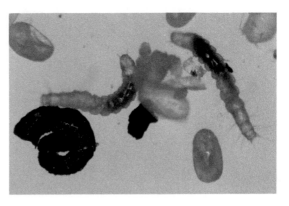

Figure 2.20 Flea larvae among hatched eggs and flea faeces. Reproduced with permission of D.-H. Choe.

They avoid light (i.e. they are 'negatively phototropic') and squirm deeply into the pile of carpets, under cushions and furniture and into dark crevasses. Their main source of nutrition is the flea dirt that falls off flea-infested animals, but they also eat shed skin flakes and other organic debris. They need high humidity to survive and are killed by near freezing temperatures.

d – Eventually, the third instar larva becomes quiescent and spins a silky cocoon. This is sticky and becomes camouflaged by picking up small particles from the surroundings (see Figure 2.21).

e – Pupation and metamorphosis take a week or more to complete. Newly developed adults do not all leave their cocoons immediately – some may wait several months before emerging. This protracted period is known as the 'pupal window'. Unfed host-seeking adults can live days or weeks without feeding.

The time for an egg to hatch and the larva to become a fully formed adult in the cocoon is typically 3–4 weeks in summer but this can be faster or slower depending on temperature and humidity. The complex development of the immature stages is coordinated by a juvenile hormone which activates genetic switches that determine the sequential development of organs and tissues. Chemicals that disrupt this hormonal activity, called Insect Growth Regulators (IGRs), can be used to break the flea life-cycle (see Section 3.5.3).

Flea habitats

The fleas on an animal are greatly outnumbered by the developing eggs, larvae, pupae and newly-emerged host-seeking adults in its environment. The largest accumulations of eggs and larvae tend to be where infested animals spend most time. These are known as 'hotspots'. They can be anywhere in the house, car or outbuildings and, in warmer climates, in humid, shady spots in the garden. Particularly high concentrations of eggs are found where pets sleep or where cats land after jumping.

Pathogenesis

All animals develop pruritic papules when bitten by fleas. In heavy infestations, excessive grooming can lead to self-trauma.

Some individuals become hypersensitive to flea bites, especially if exposure is long-term and intermittent. Several protein allergens occur in flea saliva, but not all are recognised by the immune systems of all cats or dogs. Responses therefore vary between individuals but often include IgE-mediated immediate hypersensitivity and delayed cell-mediated hypersensitivity reactions. In a small proportion of cases just a few flea bites can initiate extensive papular lesions with severe pruritus provoking self-harm through licking, scratching and biting. This disease process is known as 'flea allergic dermatitis', often abbreviated to FAD.

2.2.3 Lice (Phthiraptera)

Lice are dorsoventrally flattened, wingless insects with legs ending in claws. They are relatively small (just a few millimetres long), host-specific and spend the whole of their life-cycle on the same animal, causing a condition known as 'pediculosis'.

There are two types of louse: chewing lice (Mallophaga) and sucking lice (Anoplura). An ability to distinguish these is of clinical value as this influences chemotherapeutic choices, chewing lice being less vulnerable than sucking lice to systemic insecticides.

Chewing lice

Chewing lice are found on both mammals and birds. They have retained primitive insect mouthparts which are ideal for biting and rasping the surface of hair shafts, skin flakes and scabs, while those on birds also eat feathers and down. To accommodate this style of feeding, they have a broad head which is often wider than the thorax (see Figure 2.22). Their claws are relatively small (compared to those on sucking lice) and are single on mammalian parasites and double on avian species.

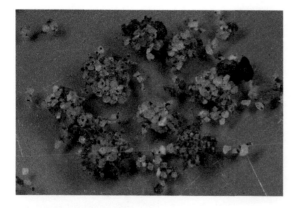

Figure 2.21 Flea cocoons covered in sand particles. Reproduced with permission of D.-H. Choe.

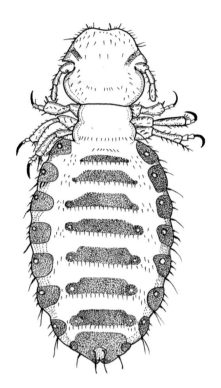

Figure 2.22 A chewing louse. Redrawn after Mönnig from Lapage, 1962 with permission of Wolters Kluwer Health - Lippincott, Williams & Wilkins.

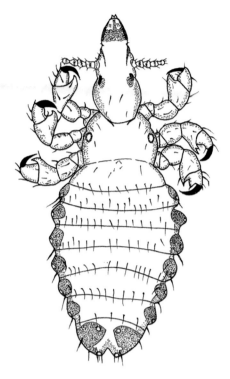

Figure 2.23 A sucking louse. Redrawn after Mönnig from Lapage, 1962 with permission of Wolters Kluwer Health - Lippincott, Williams & Wilkins.

Sucking lice

Sucking lice occur only on mammals. They have evolved highly specialised mouthparts for piercing skin and drawing up blood and tissue fluids. The head is adapted for exerting downward pressure and so is narrower than the thorax (Figure 2.23). In order to maintain a correct body position while feeding, they have powerful legs with big claws for holding onto hairs. When closed, each claw meets a thumb-like projection and pad on the leg to form a ring perfectly matching the circumference of their particular host's hair shaft.

Life-cycle

Louse eggs, known as 'nits', are cemented individually onto hairs (see Figure 2.24). A nymph hatches from the egg (there is no larval stage) and moults three times before becoming an adult (see Figure 2.13). Parthenogenesis can take place in some species. The whole life-cycle occurs on the animal and takes 2–3 weeks.

Pediculosis

Heavy infestations with lice irritate the skin. Host scratching and licking exacerbate the condition as allergenic substances in louse saliva and faeces are rubbed into the bite wounds. Pediculosis is therefore characterised by skin damage and loss of hair or feathers. It can result in reduced productivity in farm livestock. Sucking lice can also cause anaemia if present in large numbers.

Transmission from host to host occurs only during close contact. Lice cannot survive more than a few days if accidentally separated from their host. Pediculosis in farm animals is usually seen in the winter when their coat is thickest. This creates a particularly favourable microclimate for parasitic development. Sick or debilitated animals often carry large numbers of lice as they do not groom efficiently.

Cattle

Cattle have one species of chewing louse and several sucking lice (see Table 2.2). Each has its own predilection

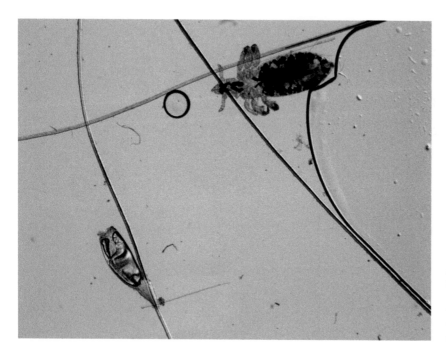

Figure 2.24 A louse egg attached to a hair (below-left) and a sucking louse (above-right). Reproduced with permission of AHVLA, Carmarthen, © Crown copyright 2013.

site on the body and some tend to cluster. They are seen mostly in housed cattle in winter. Heavy infestations cause ill-thrift, anaemia and lead to downgraded leather.

Sheep

Sheep have one chewing louse and two sucking lice (the 'foot louse' and the 'face louse') which can result in damage to the fleece. They became rare in countries with compulsory dipping programmes (e.g. for sheep scab control – see Section 3.3.3), but their population numbers are rising again. This may be an unintended consequence of regulatory restrictions placed on the use of insecticides.

Pigs

Pigs have just one large (5 mm) sucking louse which is easily seen on the sparsely haired skin. It is very common, particularly on adult pigs. It can act as a vector for African swine fever and some other viruses and rickettsiae.

Horses

Horses have one chewing louse and one sucking louse. The former favours skin with finer hair while the latter is seen mainly in the mane and tail, but they can spread over the whole body.

Table 2.2 Some important lice of domesticated animals and poultry

Host	Chewing lice	Sucking lice	More information in Section:
Cattle	*Bovicola* * *bovis*	*Linognathus vituli, Haematopinus* spp. etc.	
Sheep	*Bovicola* * *ovis*	*Linognathus* spp.	
Pig	None	*Haematopinus suis*	
Horse	*Bovicola* * *equi*	*Haematopinus asini*	9.1.3
Dog	*Trichodectes canis*	*Linognathus setosus*	9.2.3
Cat	*Felicola subrostratus*	None	
Poultry	Many	None	8.4.2

* *Bovicola* is also known as *Damalinia*.

Dogs and cats

Dogs have both a chewing louse and a sucking species, while cats have only a chewing louse. Heavy infestations are often, but not always, associated with neglect.

Poultry

Birds have many species of chewing lice, but no sucking lice. The most pathogenic belong to the genera *Lipeurus* (including the 'wing louse' and 'head louse') and *Menacanthus* (the 'body louse').

Help box 2.3

Fleas and lice compared

Fleas and lice are both wingless insects that live in hair, fur or feathers. Key differences include:

	Fleas	Lice
Body	Laterally compressed	Dorso-ventrally flattened
Legs adapted for	Jumping and running	Grasping and walking
Host specificity	Broad	Narrow
Parasitic as	Adult only	All stages
Eggs	Fall off host	Stuck to hairs
Immature stages	Larvae	Nymphs
Metamorphosis	Complex	Simple

2.2.4 Bugs (Hemiptera)

The Hemiptera (known colloquially as 'bugs') are specialists in sucking juices from the stems of plants and are important pests in horticulture and arable farming. Two members of the group, however, have switched from a vegetarian diet to a vampire existence, becoming nocturnal blood feeders. These are the assassin bugs (also called by their anglicised family name 'reduviid' or subfamily name 'triatomine') and the bed bugs (*Cimex* spp.).

Assassin bugs

True to their name, assassin bugs (reduviids) are potential killers as they are the vector of *Trypanosoma cruzi*, a protozoan parasite responsible for a debilitating and sometimes fatal condition known as Chagas disease in humans. This occurs throughout large areas of Central and South America (see Sections 4.5.1 and 9.3.2). Reduviids are also found in some other tropical regions as well as parts of the USA.

Reduviids are dark-coloured, up to 3 cm long and 1 cm wide, and have a narrow head with lateral compound eyes (see Figure 2.25). A long proboscis with probing and piercing components is folded underneath out of sight. The anterior wings are partly hardened and cover the broad abdomen when at rest. The body is flat but swells up during feeding as they take in 1.5 times their own weight of capillary blood.

Assassin bugs live close to their preferred food-source within buildings or in the crowns of trees. There are

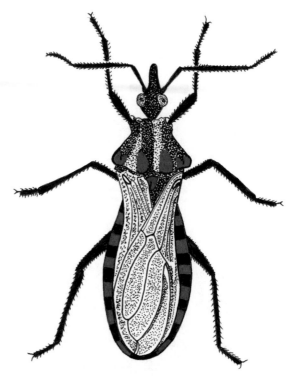

Figure 2.25 An assassin (reduviid) bug. Redrawn after Hegner *et al.*, 1929 from Cheng, 1986 with permission of Elsevier.

many species feeding on a wide variety of animals and birds. Those in domestic homes will parasitize dogs, cats, farm livestock and rodents as well as humans. Eggs are laid in cracks and crevices. There are five nymphal stages, each of which requires a blood-meal.

Feeding on exposed skin takes up to 30 minutes and the insect defecates when replete. The bites are painless and reduviids are often seen on the faces of unsuspecting victims while asleep. This explains the derivation of another colloquial name: 'kissing bug'. The penetration wound, however, subsequently starts to itch and the Chagas disease organism is transmitted when faeces from an infected bug is rubbed into the lesion.

Bed bugs

Bed bugs are much smaller than the reduviids, measuring less than 0.5 cm (see Figure 2.26). They are dark brown in colour and negatively phototropic, so they hide during the day in deep recesses. They move very fast when disturbed so are difficult to find. Their presence in an infested room is often indicated by a characteristic smell (an alarm pheromone) as well as small smudges

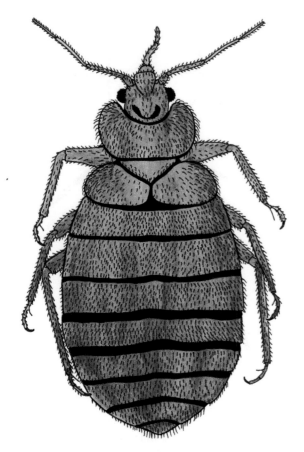

Figure 2.26 A bed bug (*Cimex*). Redrawn after Mönnig from Lapage, 1962 with permission of Wolters Kluwer Health - Lippincott, Williams & Wilkins.

of faecal material on bedding, furniture and walls. They produce multiple skin punctures when feeding and can be very debilitating. Although domestic species feed primarily on humans, they also bite cats and dogs.

2.2.5 Biting and nuisance flies (Diptera)

Most flying insects, such as mayflies, dragonflies, butterflies, cockroaches, beetles, bees and wasps, have two pairs of wings, but dipteran flies have just one. Almost all flies of veterinary importance belong to the Diptera. Their medical significance is often attributable to adult females seeking a protein-rich meal prior to egg-laying. Painful bites can induce behavioural responses such as tail switching, biting, kicking, restlessness and interruption of grazing. Rubbing and scratching can lead to secondary bacterial infection. Bites can also result in allergic responses which provoke yet more self-inflicted skin damage.

Some nonbiting dipterans also cause considerable nuisance, discomfort and reduced productivity by swarming around animals to feed on secretions from eyes, mouth and genitalia or on exudations from wounds. Both biting and nuisance flies are responsible for disease transmission, either as vector hosts or passive (mechanical) carriers of pathogenic organisms.

In some cases it is not the adult fly but larval instars that are parasitic. Such infestations are known as 'myiasis' and can cause substantial damage. They are considered separately in Section 2.2.6.

Dipteran flies are divided into three major groups based on their morphology:

a – Nematocera: small, delicate flies with long multi-articulated antennae; the larvae have a large, well-developed head.

b – Brachycera: large, heavy flies with short three-part antennae.

c – Cyclorrhapha: middle-sized flies; the last section of their three-part antenna has a feathery appendage (the 'arista'). The larval head is very small compared with total body size.

From a veterinary perspective, however, it is more convenient to study the Diptera at family level (see Figure 2.27) as each has its own particular clinical significance.

For descriptive purposes, adult flies can be crudely defined as: 'large' (length over 1 cm); medium (0.5–1.0 cm) and small (less than 0.5 cm long).

Biting midges and blackflies

Biting midges and blackflies are both small flies (2–5 mm long) with a hump-back appearance. Despite their diminutive size, each has a painful bite and can inflict severe injury if large swarms are feeding. They are cosmopolitan but with a different range of species in each geographical region. Both are important vectors of other pathogens, particularly arboviruses.

Biting midges

Most biting midges of veterinary importance belong to the genus *Culicoides*. These miniscule flies have mottled wings and long antennae (see Figure 2.28). There are many species, each with its own feeding preferences with regard to host, anatomical site and time of day. They are mostly on the wing when conditions are still and humid, especially around dusk. Midges are not strong fliers and so are found in greatest numbers close

Order	**Suborder**	**Family**
DIPTERA	NEMATOCERA	Ceratopogonidae (midges)
		Simuliidae (black flies)
		Culicidae (mosquitoes)
		Psychodidae (sandflies)
	BRACHYCERA	Tabanidae (horse flies)
	CYCLORRHAPHA	Muscidae (nuisance and biting flies)
		Glossinidae (tsetse flies)
		Hippoboscidae (forest flies and keds)
		Calliphoridae (blowflies and screwworm flies)
		Sarcophagidae (flesh flies)
		Oestridae (bot and warble flies)

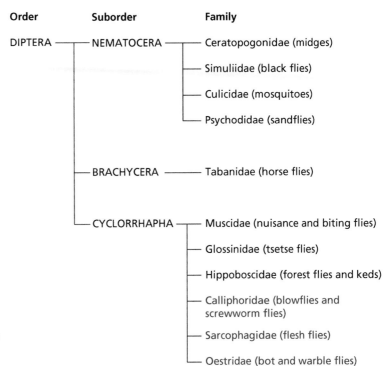

Figure 2.27 Dipteran families of veterinary importance (biting and nuisance flies in black; myiasis flies in purple).

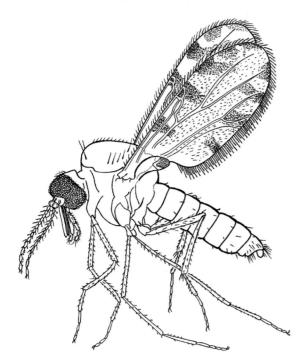

Figure 2.28 A *Culicoides* midge. Redrawn after Mönnig from Lapage, 1962 with permission of Wolters Kluwer Health - Lippincott, Williams & Wilkins.

to their breeding sites. They can, however, be dispersed over great distances by strong winds (an important factor in the epidemiology of some viral diseases).

Favoured breeding sites vary with species but are generally muddy places with still water. There can be up to three generations per year in cooler temperate regions, depending on ambient temperatures, but adults can be present all year round in the tropics and subtropics. *Culicoides* mainly overwinters as the egg in harsher climates. A detailed knowledge of the biology of each disease-carrying species is needed by scientists developing predictive models of epidemic diseases such as those caused by the blue-tongue and Schmallenberg viruses in sheep and cattle. Species of *Culicoides* also act as vector for other important viral conditions including African horse sickness, bovine ephemeral fever and eastern equine encephalitis, as well as some species of the filarial worm, *Onchocerca*.

The bites of some *Culicoides* species provoke a seasonally-occurring allergic dermatitis in susceptible horses. This common and distressingly pruritic condition, generally known as 'sweet itch', is the result of an immediate-type hypersensitivity reaction. It principally affects the withers and tail-base (see Section 9.1.3).

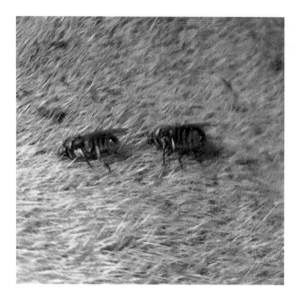

Figure 2.29 *Simulium* feeding. Reproduced with permission of D.C. Knottenbelt.

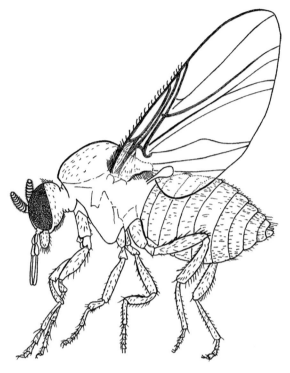

Figure 2.30 A *Simulium* blackfly. Redrawn after Mönnig from Lapage, 1962 with permission of Wolters Kluwer Health - Lippincott, Williams & Wilkins.

Blackflies

Most blackflies of veterinary importance belong to the genus *Simulium*. In some countries they are known as 'buffalo gnats'. Many species are indiscriminate in their choice of host but they have preferential feeding sites. Some, for example, cluster inside a nostril or the pinna of an ear. They are more obvious than midges, appearing darker and more bulky (see Figure 2.29). They have clear wings and short antennae (see Figure 2.30). They are strong fliers, easily covering several km without wind-assistance, and are most active during the morning and evening on warm, cloudy days. Eggs are laid on plants or stones under rapidly-flowing water. Development times are dependent on water temperature and adult flies tend to emerge *en masse*.

Swarms of *Simulium* interrupt grazing, cause stampedes and reduce productivity. In addition to local reactions, more general effects, such as capillary permeability, are thought to be due to a salivary toxin. Animals as large as camels, horses and cattle can die if exposed to great numbers of bites. In badly affected regions, animals must be withheld from high risk pastures during potential danger periods. Blackflies are also vectors of the eastern equine encephalitis and vesicular stomatitis viruses, as well as some *Onchocerca* species (including *O. volvulus*, the cause of 'river blindness' in humans) and *Leucocytozoon* (an avian protozoan parasite).

Mosquitoes and sandflies

Mosquitoes need no introduction, being a well-known and ubiquitous hazard for humans and animals alike. Sandflies resemble miniature mosquitoes and are more localised in distribution. The term 'phlebotomine sandfly' is often used in technical literature as the word 'sandfly' can refer to biting midges in the common parlance of some countries (e.g. New Zealand and the Caribbean).

Mosquitoes

Mosquitoes are up to 1 cm long with a slender body and long legs (see Figure 2.31 and Figure 2.32). They have a needle-like forward-pointing proboscis and long antennae. The wings are narrow and covered in scales with a fringe along the posterior margin. They are crossed over the abdomen at rest. The most important genera are *Culex*, *Anopheles* and *Aedes*.

The eggs are laid on water in 'rafts' or singly, depending on genus. Larval and pupal stages are both aquatic and may be seen hanging from the water surface or lying horizontally beneath it. The whole life-cycle takes two weeks to several months to complete depending on temperature.

Mosquitoes are most active at night. Reaction to their bites can vary from mild irritation to severe local hypersensitivity. They transmit numerous human diseases including malaria, yellow fever, Dengue fever, elephantiasis etc. Animal pathogens include many viruses (e.g. equine encephalitis and equine infectious anaemia); filarial nematodes such as *Dirofilaria immitis*, the cause of canine heartworm disease (see Sections 7.1.5 and 9.2.2); and the protozoon responsible for avian malaria.

Phlebotomine sandflies

Phlebotomine sandflies are smaller than mosquitoes and have a more furry appearance (see Figure 2.33). Their mouthparts are shorter. The wings are covered in hairs and are held erect when the fly is resting. They are found in many warmer parts of the globe including the Mediterranean area. Two genera are of major veterinary importance, *Phlebotomus* in the Old World and *Lutzomyia* in the New World.

Eggs are laid in humid holes or crevices outdoors and indoors. The life-cycle takes a minimum of a month to complete. Adult sandflies tend to bite exposed skin, such as ears, nose, eyelids, feet and tail. They transmit *Leishmania* which is the protozoan parasite responsible for leishmaniosis, a serious disease of dogs and humans (see Sections 4.5.1, 9.2.3 and 9.3.2).

Horse flies (tabanids)

Anyone who has been bitten by a horse fly will know how painful this experience can be. They feed on a variety of large animals (see Figure 2.34) by violently abrading the skin to create a pool of blood, which is then sponged up. This activity often upsets the victim with the result that the fly is dislodged. When this happens, it immediately seeks another animal so it can satiate its hunger. Horse flies are thereby highly efficient mechanical transmitters of blood-borne pathogens from host to host (e.g. *Trypanosoma evansi* – see Section 4.5.1).

Tabanids are large sturdy flies up to 2.5 cm long (see Figure 2.35). They have a large head with short, downward pointed mouthparts and a characteristic wing venation (see Figure 2.9). There are three genera of veterinary importance: *Tabanus*, *Chrysops* and *Haematopota* which can be distinguished by wing colouration (transparent, banded and mottled, respectively) and by the shape of their antennae.

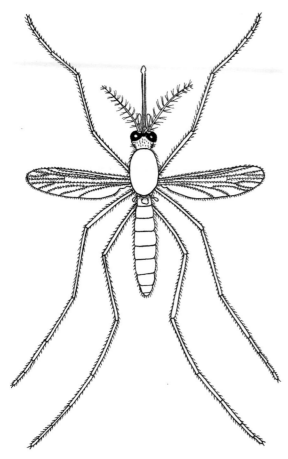

Figure 2.31 A female mosquito. Redrawn after Bedford, 1928 from Lapage, 1962 with permission of Wolters Kluwer Health - Lippincott, Williams & Wilkins.

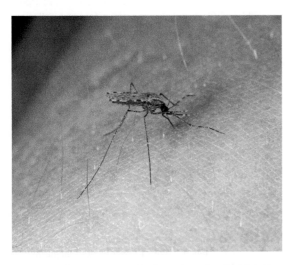

Figure 2.32 Mosquito (*Aedes*) feeding. Reproduced with permission of J.G. Logan.

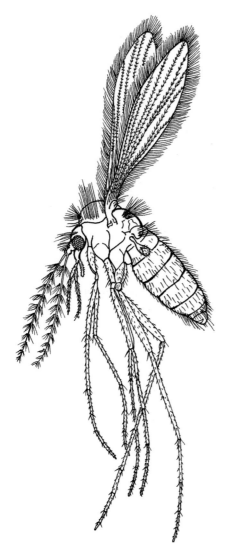

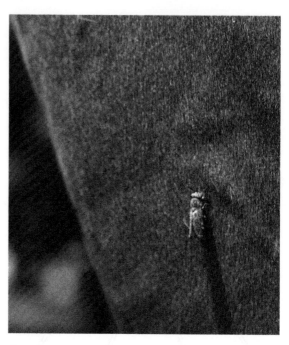

Figure 2.34 A tabanid fly biting a horse.

Nonbiting muscids

The family Muscidae contains many medium-sized non-biting ('nuisance') and some blood-sucking ('biting') flies. Together, they are responsible for 'fly worry' (see Section 9.1.3) and they act also as vectors and/or passive carriers of pathogenic organisms. Their immature stages develop in fermenting organic material such as herbivore dung. Nuisance flies of veterinary importance include *Musca* (face flies and houseflies) and *Hydrotaea* (the sheep head-fly).

Figure 2.33 A female phlebotomine sandfly. Redrawn after Mönnig from Lapage, 1962 with permission of Wolters Kluwer Health - Lippincott, Williams & Wilkins.

Tabanids are most active on hot, sunny days. Eggs are laid on leaves overhanging wet areas. Newly-hatched larvae drop into water or mud, later returning to dry land to pupate. The whole life-cycle takes several months, or more if the larvae have to overwinter.

Horse flies are vectors for diseases caused by bacteria (anthrax, pasteurellosis), viruses (equine infectious anaemia, African horse sickness), rickettsiae (anaplasmosis); and protozoa (such as *Trypanosoma evansi* – see Section 4.5.1).

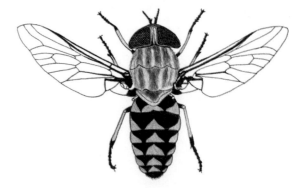

Figure 2.35 A tabanid (horse fly). Redrawn from Lapage, 1962 with permission of Wolters Kluwer Health - Lippincott, Williams & Wilkins and photograph by © D. Geystor.

Musca spp.

The most widespread members of the genus *Musca* are *M. autumnalis* (the face fly) and *M. domestica* (the housefly). There are also other species of more limited distribution. The face fly is the most numerous of the flies that worry cattle outdoors. As its common name suggests, it swarms around the head and upper parts of the body, feeding on secretions, exudates and blood seeping from wounds induced by injury or biting flies. The housefly occurs both inside and outside animal buildings, often in enormous numbers. It is not a parasite as it feeds only on nonliving organic materials such as foodstuffs, decaying waste materials and faeces, but it is nevertheless an important disseminator of disease.

Everyone is familiar with the ubiquitous housefly (see Figure 2.36). The face fly is almost identical in appearance. It is a little over 0.5 cm long and has a grey thorax with longitudinal stripes and a yellowish abdomen with a single black streak. It has sponging mouthparts which point downwards.

Adult *Musca* spp. are active only during the day, *M. autumnalis* preferring sunlight and *M. domestica* shade. They both overwinter as hibernating adults, sheltering inside buildings. *M. autumnalis* lays eggs in fresh cattle dung, while the housefly will choose any fresh or rotting organic material. The life-cycle is completed in a minimum of two weeks, so several generations can procreate during the summer.

Cattle exposed to large numbers of *M. autumnalis* become restless and spend less time grazing, which reduces growth-rate and milk-yield.

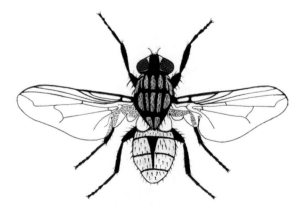

Figure 2.36 The common housefly, *Musca domestica*. Redrawn and modified after Hewitt, 1914. Reproduced with permission of Cambridge University Press.

Musca spp. transmit disease in a number of ways:

a – Mechanical transfer: pathogens (viruses, bacteria, helminth eggs, protozoan cysts etc.) can be carried passively on feet, hairs or mouthparts and deposited on surfaces such as skin, eyes, wounds and feedstuffs. Of particular note is a damaging eye condition (infectious bovine keratoconjunctivitis or 'pink eye') caused by a bacterium, *Moraxella bovis*.

b – Regurgitation: *Musca* spp. deposit saliva and regurgitate remnants of their last meal, possibly containing viable pathogens, onto animal skin and other surfaces as part of their normal feeding process.

c – As a true vector: *Musca* spp. act as intermediate hosts for some nematode parasites, including *Thelazia*, *Habronema* and *Parafilaria* (see Section 7.1.5), and some poultry cestodes (see Section 5.3.5).

Hydrotaea

Hydrotaea irritans is troublesome to sheep, cattle and horses in Northern Europe. It is similar to *Musca* but has an olive-green abdomen. It, too, is a sponge-feeder but, unlike *Musca*, it actively encourages tears and secretions, as well as blood seepage from wounds and abrasions, by rasping exposed surfaces. Animals find this very irritating. Fighting rams are particularly vulnerable as clusters of flies attack wounds at the base of the horns – hence the name 'sheep head-fly'. Attempts to dislodge the flies by head-butting lead to further damage, secondary infection and blowfly strike (see Section 2.2.6). *H. irritans* is also a common visiting fly on cattle and horses. On these hosts, it tends to congregate on the underside of the body, including the udder and teats, and has been implicated in the spread of bovine summer mastitis.

There is only one generation of adult flies each year. They are most numerous in mid-summer on pastures close to woodland. Eggs are laid in decaying organic material and it is the hatched larva that overwinters.

Extra information box 2.1

'H. irritans'

Care! Confusingly, *Hydrotaea irritans* and *Haemotobia irritans* are both abbreviated to '*H. irritans*', although which is intended should be clear from the context. To avoid this ambiguity, some texts use the genus name *Lyperosia* in place of *Haemotobia*.

Biting muscids

Biting muscid flies include *Stomoxys calcitrans* (the stable fly) and several species of *Haematobia* (for example, the horn fly, *H. irritans*, and the buffalo fly, *H. exigua*). They can be distinguished from nonbiting muscids, which they otherwise resemble, as their skin-penetrating mouthparts are obvious and forward-pointing (see Figure 2.37). *Stomoxys* is a little larger than *Musca* and has spots rather than stripes on the abdomen, but *Haematobia* is smaller (3–7 mm). Unlike most other biting flies, males as well as females are blood-sucking.

Stomoxys

S. calcitrans is found worldwide. It attacks most animals, including humans, favouring the legs and lower body. It is a 'visiting' fly (i.e. it settles on an animal to feed but otherwise spends most of its time off the host, either in flight or resting on buildings, foliage and fences). It is most active on sunny days and can travel 5 km (and considerably more when carried by strong winds). The bites are painful and troubled animals may suffer reduced weight gains or significant milk yield losses. It takes several minutes for the fly to complete a blood meal and the process is frequently interrupted. Females need several feeds before egg-laying. Stable flies are therefore efficient mechanical transmitters of blood parasites such as trypanosomes (see Section 4.5.1) as well as many microbial diseases. *S. calcitrans* is also intermediate host for the equine nematode, *Habronema* (see Sections 7.1.5 and 9.1.3).

Eggs are laid on rotting hay and straw, particularly if soiled with faeces and urine. The life-cycle (see Figure 2.14) is completed in about a month and adult flies can survive for a further month, or longer at cooler times of year.

Haematobia

Haematobia spp. feed mostly on cattle and buffalo. They are 'resident' flies, i.e. they spend almost all their time feeding or resting on the host (as opposed to 'visiting flies' that come just to feed or lay eggs). They rest along the back, shoulders and flanks of their host. Hundreds or even thousands can cluster on an animal (see Figure 2.38). They are particularly irritating to their host as they take frequent small meals. Blood losses and adverse impacts on welfare and production can be significant.

Females ready to lay eggs take to the wing when their host defecates, ovipositing in the freshly deposited dung. Larvae pupate in the soil beneath the dungpat to emerge as adult flies one week later or after overwintering.

Haematobia acts as intermediate host for the skin nematode, *Stephanofilaria* (see Section 7.1.5).

Tsetse flies

Although confined to the central belt of Africa, the tsetse fly (*Glossina* spp.) plays a devastating role in human and animal welfare as it is the principal vector of the protozoan parasites responsible for sleeping sickness in people as well as the several forms of animal trypanosomosis (see Sections 4.5.1, 8.2.3 and 9.3.2).

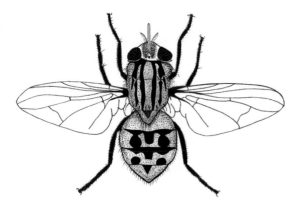

Figure 2.37 The stable fly, *Stomoxys*. Redrawn after Mönnig from Lapage, 1962 with permission of Wolters Kluwer Health – Lippincott, Williams & Wilkins.

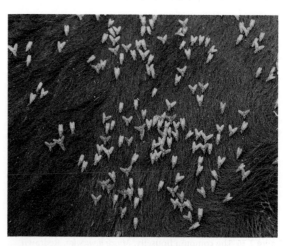

Figure 2.38 Horn flies (*Haematobia*) clustered on a cow. Reproduced with permission of D.E. Snyder.

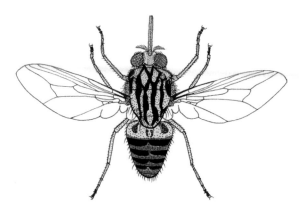

Figure 2.39 A tsetse fly. Redrawn after Mönnig from Lapage, 1962 with permission of Wolters Kluwer Health - Lippincott, Williams & Wilkins.

Tsetse flies are easily recognised (see Figure 2.39). They are narrow, brown, medium-sized flies that rest with wings overlapping like closed scissors. To confirm identification, should there be any doubt, the wing venation has a characteristic closed 'butcher's cleaver cell' (see Figure 2.9).

Both males and females are blood-sucking and have a long forward-pointing proboscis. They feed on a wide variety of animals and need a blood meal every 2–3 days. They cannot fly very far without resting, but they are able to home in on a victim from a distance by using a combination of odour and visual stimuli. These have been exploited in the design and construction of highly effective insecticide-baited lures and traps.

Tsetse flies are active during the day, particularly in the morning and evening. They occur all year round but are most numerous in the rainy season. Their reproductive rate is very slow since the female gives birth to just a single larva at 10-day intervals. The larva, laid at the base of vegetation, immediately wriggles into the soil to pupate. The adult fly emerges after a month but needs another 1–2 weeks to develop and harden its exoskeleton. The whole life-cycle takes around two months.

There are a number of tsetse species but they can be split into three main groups according to their ecology: riverine, savannah and rainforest species. This determines the epidemiology of the various forms of trypanosomosis, since different *Trypanosoma* species utilise different *Glossina* species as vector.

Hippoboscids

While the great majority of dipteran flies visit an animal only to obtain a protein meal, the hippoboscids are true parasites. They are sometimes called 'louse flies' because their leathery, dorso-ventrally flattened bodies with clawed feet (see Figure 2.3) are reminiscent of lice (see Figure 2.23) – although they are much bigger (0.5–1 cm). They are found mainly on wild birds (although not on domesticated poultry), but a few species occur on mammals. Like tsetse flies, female hippoboscids give birth to larvae.

The group presents a nice demonstration of the evolutionary process. Adults of the genus *Hippobosca* are not strong fliers and are very reluctant to leave their host until they are ready to deposit a larva in soil, damp humus or animal housing. Newly emerged deer keds use their wings to find a host, but these then become redundant and are shed. Their larvae are left to fend for themselves by falling off the host and finding a suitable pupation site. Finally, the sheep ked is completely wingless for its whole life-cycle, all of which takes place on the host.

Hippobosca

Members of this genus are found only in the Old World, with species parasitizing horses, cattle, camels and dogs. They are about 1 cm long and reddish-brown with yellow spots (see Figure 2.40). The wing veins are crowded towards the anterior margin. The biting mouthparts are not visible if the fly is not feeding. Males and females are both parasitic, feeding several times a day and mating on the host. The forest fly, *H. equina*, tends to aggregate on the thinner skin beneath the tail of horses and around the perineum and udder of cattle, causing annoyance. Adults can persist on the animal through the winter.

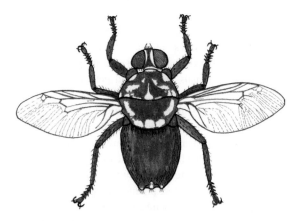

Figure 2.40 A hippoboscid fly. Redrawn after Bedford, 1932 and Mönnig from Lapage, 1962 with permission of Wolters Kluwer Health - Lippincott, Williams & Wilkins.

Sheep ked

The sheep ked (*Melophagus ovinus*) is a brown, wingless, blood-sucking fly. It occurs in all sheep-rearing regions, but most commonly in temperate climates. It is seen occasionally on goats. Its biting mouthparts project forwards from a short head recessed into the thorax (see Figure 2.3). Over a life-span of up to 5 months, female keds produce a total of about 15 larvae. These attach themselves to the fleece and immediately pupate. The life-cycle extends over a minimum period of 5 weeks. The numbers of keds on a host depends on the thickness of the wool and so populations are greater in autumn and winter than in summer. For the same reason, long-wooled breeds of sheep are more susceptible to infestation. Adult keds come to the surface of the fleece when ambient temperatures are warm and can then transfer to other sheep during close contact. They are, however, vulnerable at this time to being nibbled and swallowed by the host, which makes them an effective vector for the nonpathogenic protozoan, *Trypanosoma melophagium*.

If uncontrolled, sheep ked infestation can be economically damaging. The pruritus associated with heavy infestations leads to self-inflicted damage to the fleece and the wool becomes discoloured by ked faeces, leading to down-grading of the market value. Disturbed grazing and secondary infections can further undermine growth and productivity.

2.2.6 Myiasis-producing dipterans

The previous section described dipterans that seek protein meals from living animals only as adult flies. This section focuses on those dipterans that have larval instars capable of feeding on the tissues of living hosts, a phenomenon known as 'myiasis'. This condition can be distressingly destructive and poses serious welfare problems for farm animals, wildlife and pets in all but the driest or coldest climates.

Myiasis-producing dipterans fall into two broad categories depending on how the adult flies derive their nutrition. The first group encompasses blowflies, screwworms and flesh flies. Their adults have functional mouthparts as the female needs a protein meal (although not necessarily from a living animal) before producing eggs or larvae. The second group comprises members of the family Oestridae (see Figure 2.27). These have vestigial mouthparts in the adult stage and do not feed. All the energy and protein needed for flight and reproduction is accumulated and stored during larval development.

Help box 2.4

Definition of 'myiasis'

Myiasis is defined as: 'parasitism of living animals by dipteran larvae'.
In this section of the book, myiasis is categorised from a biological perspective as this understanding is helpful in the design of control programmes. An alternative approach is to differentiate on the basis of host tissues affected. For example:
Cutaneous myiasis e.g. blowflies and screwworms;
Nasal myiasis e.g. sheep nasal fly;
Somatic myiasis e.g. warble fly.

There are also colourful local clinical descriptors such as 'pizzle-rot' in Australasia.

Blowflies, screwworms and flesh flies

The most important blowflies, screwworms and flesh flies are listed in Table 2.3. They are not all equally dependent on a parasitic lifestyle, but may be divided into:

a – facultative myiasis-flies: those that are capable of depositing eggs or larvae on living animals, but which may also select nonliving feeding sites for their offspring, such as carrion or other protein-rich organic substrates;

b – obligate myiasis-flies: those that have no option but to use living animals for larval development.

Myiasis flies are further categorised according to their egg-laying behaviour:

a – primary myiasis flies: these are parasitic species which usually lay their eggs on animals, although the life-cycle can be completed on nonliving decaying organic materials; the larvae can feed on intact skin and penetrate through to underlying tissues;

b – secondary myiasis flies: these are species that normally employ nonliving decaying organic material for larval development, but which will utilise a living animal if the opportunity arises; they cannot initiate a lesion; eggs are therefore laid beside an open wound or body orifice and the larvae extend and deepen any pre-existing abrasion;

c – tertiary myiasis flies: these usually place their eggs or larvae on dead animals (carrion) but may on occasion exploit skin lesions, especially on moribund animals.

Table 2.3 Some important non-oestrid myiasis flies

Common name	Latin name	Distribution	Egg laying behaviour	Parasitic status of larvae
Greenbottles	*Lucilia sericata*[1]	Cooler regions esp. northern hemisphere	1° fly	Mostly parasitic
	L. cuprina[1]	Warmer regions esp. South Africa, Australia	1° fly	Mostly parasitic
Blackbottles	*Phormia*	Cosmopolitan	2° fly	Facultative
Bluebottles	*Calliphora*	Cosmopolitan	Most spp.: 2° Some spp.: 1°	Facultative
Screwworms	*Cochliomyia*[2]	New World tropics	2° fly	Obligate
	Chrysomia	Mainly Old World tropics (some spp. Australia and elsewhere)	2° fly	Obligate
Flesh flies	*Wohlfartia*	Different spp. in Americas and Europe/North Africa	2° fly	Some spp. obligate; others facultative
	Sarcophaga	Cosmopolitan	2° or 3° flies	Facultative

[1] Further information – see Section 8.2.4. [2] Sometimes called *Callitroga*.

When a blowfly lays its eggs on a host, the animal is said to have become 'blown'; subsequent maggot damage is called 'strike' and affected animals are 'struck'.

Blowflies and screwworm flies belong to closely related families (see Figure 2.27). The adults are about 1 cm long and are conspicuous as the abdomen has a bright metallic sheen (as seen, for example, on the familiar bluebottle flies that try to come into the kitchen and the green-coloured *Lucilia* illustrated in Figure 2.41).

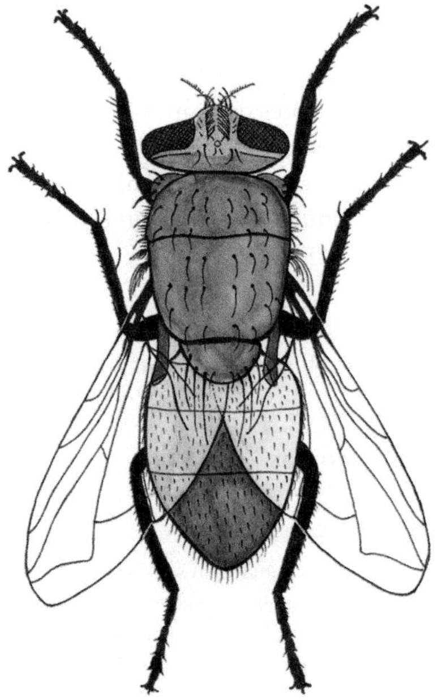

The larval stages, however, differ markedly in appearance and behaviour. Blowfly larvae are smooth-skinned, whereas screwworm larvae have rings of hooks around the body (Figure 2.42). Blowfly larvae are mostly carrion feeders, with only a few genera attacking living animals, while all screwworms are obligate parasites (see Table 2.3). Finally, blowflies are surface-feeding maggots, while screwworms bury themselves in host

Figure 2.41 An adult blowfly (the greenbottle, *Lucilia*). Redrawn and adapted from a photograph by Smit from Lapage, 1962.

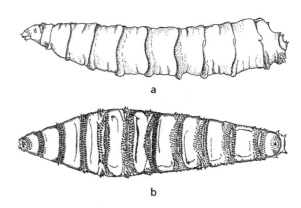

a

b

Figure 2.42 Lateral view of a blowfly larva (a); ventral view of a screwworm larva (b). Redrawn after C.G. Walker from Lapage, 1962 with permission of Wolters Kluwer Health - Lippincott, Williams & Wilkins and Zumpt, 1965.

tissue so only the respiratory spiracles on their tail are exposed to the air.

To avoid ambiguity the term 'calliphorine blowfly' is often used in technical dialogue as the word 'blowfly' sometimes includes screwworms in common usage.

Calliphorine myiasis

Female *Lucilia* lay clusters of 100–200 yellow-cream eggs on hair or around wounds. Larvae hatch within 24 hours and feed on surface tissues and exudates. They lacerate superficial skin layers with their chitinous oral hooks (see Figure 2.6) and liquefy host tissue by secreting proteolytic enzymes. Young larvae are susceptible to desiccation and so a humid microclimate, as occurs in the fleece after prolonged rainfall, provides optimal conditions for development. A length of 1–1.5 cm is attained after two moults in 1–2 weeks. Fully developed larvae fall to the ground to pupate. The adult fly emerges in less than a week and survives for about a month. Females need a protein meal to reach sexual maturity. This is usually derived from decaying organic material although they may visit animals to feed on oro-nasal secretions and seeping wounds. As many as ten generations per year can occur in warmer regions and up to four in temperate zones. The last generation each year survives the winter as pupae.

Animals with a dense coat, like sheep and rabbits, are most likely to be struck, but all are potentially vulnerable. Blowflies can travel long distances and are most active on warm, still days with high relative humidity. Egg-laying females are attracted by odour from a distance of 10–20 m and so host vulnerability is greatest when fur or wool is soiled with urine or diarrhoea, or when the skin is damaged by shearing, fighting, barbed wire, foot-rot, insect or tick bites, etc. Similarly, material collecting in the penile sheath can provide a magnet for blowfly strike.

Screwworm myiasis

The name 'screwworm' is derived from the bands of spines around the larva which are reminiscent of the thread on a screw (see Figure 2.42). There are two major genera, both occurring in the tropics: *Cochliomyia* in the New World and *Chrysomya* in the Old. Both attack a range of animals including humans.

They are medium to large obligate parasites, similar in appearance to bluebottles. Eggs are laid on the edge of wounds and the navels of new-born animals. The emergent larvae burrow into the flesh where they liquefy the surrounding host tissues. They tend to feed as a group creating a large foul-smelling pocket under the skin. This often has a narrow entrance marked by a serosanguineous (bloody) exudate around the exposed tail-ends of the parasites.

Cochliomyia has been eradicated from the USA and parts of Central America. This was achieved by employing the 'sterile male technique', an approach utilising laboratory bred males subjected to a level of irradiation that induces sterility without impairing the ability to compete for females. Irradiated males are released in enormous numbers at appropriate intervals from aircraft over endemic areas. This has a dramatic effect on the reproductive capability of the fly population as a female *Cochliomyia* mates only once in her lifetime. The progressively expanding eradication programme was rolled out over a period spanning more than two decades and still continues along its southern buffer zone.

Flesh flies

Flesh flies are mainly tertiary myiasis flies. One genus, *Wohlfahrtia*, is an obligate secondary fly with various

---

Extra information box 2.2

Maggot debridement therapy

In human and veterinary medicine, specially bred pathogen-free *Lucilia sericata* maggots are used to treat infected and/or necrotic wounds that do not respond quickly to more conventional treatments. If a suitable number of larvae are applied for an appropriate time, dead tissues are rapidly removed leaving a clean and healthy lesion that is able to heal.

Extra information box 2.3

The Tumbu fly, *Cordylobia*

Dogs, and sometimes humans, in sub-Saharan Africa can develop a 1 cm subcutaneous swelling with a small hole displaying the spiracles of a single dipteran maggot. This is not a screwworm but the Tumbu fly, which is more closely related to the calliphorine blowflies. Eggs are laid singly in shady, dry, sandy places and larvae quickly burrow through skin on contact.

species in the Americas and parts of the Old World. They are large grey flies with black patterning on the abdomen. They deposit either larvae or eggs that hatch immediately on dry skin close to a wound or orifice. The larvae create a deep crater which attracts other gravid *Wohlfahrtia* females (see Figure 2.43). In North America, *W. vigil* is associated mainly with mink, but occasionally attacks young pets and human babies. The larvae can penetrate soft skin to create boil-like subcutaneous swellings.

Oestrid flies

The Oestridae are a family of large bee-like flies with nonfunctional mouthparts (see Figure 2.44). The three larval instars are invasive obligatory parasites. The main genera of veterinary significance are: *Hypoderma* (warble fly), *Oestrus* (nasal bot fly) and *Gasterophilus* (stomach bot fly). They are found mostly in the northern hemisphere, although their range has extended to some other regions via livestock importations. A fourth genus, *Dermatobia* (human bot fly), afflicts animals and humans in parts of Central and South America (see Section 9.3.2).

Help box 2.5

Dipteran flies: recognition

Insects typically have two pairs of wings. In dipteran flies, however, the posterior pair is reduced to gyroscopic pegs ('halteres') that provide extra stability in flight (see Figure 2.10). Oestrid flies may superficially resemble bees to a greater or lesser extent, but they have just one pair of wings while real bees have two pairs. Bees also have a highly developed proboscis for collecting pollen and nectar, while oestrid flies have rudimentary nonfunctional mouthparts (see Figure 2.44).

Warble flies *(Hypoderma)*

Hypoderma spp. are of animal welfare and economic significance because their larval instars migrate through body tissues and later cause large subcutaneous cysts ('warbles'). Two major species parasitize cattle: *Hypoderma lineatum* and *H. bovis*. Other species parasitize deer and reindeer. Warbles occasionally cause problems in abnormal hosts, e.g. when a deer warble appears in the saddle area of a horse, but they do not reach maturity.

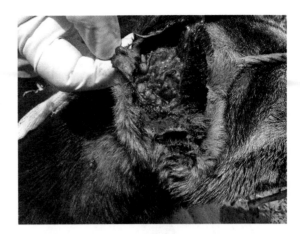

Figure 2.43 *Wohlfahrtia* larvae in wound on a dog's ear. Reproduced with permission of The Natural History Museum.

Adult warble flies emerge from pupae on warm sunny days from June to September. *H. lineatum* is first, with *H. bovis* following a few weeks later. The flies are up to 1.5 cm long and resemble hairy bumble bees. The abdomen is yellowish orange with a broad black band (see Figure 2.45).

Eggs are cemented with a small terminal clasp onto hairs covering the host's belly or legs. *H. lineatum* approaches its victim stealthily and usually has ample time to deposit a row of eggs along a single hair

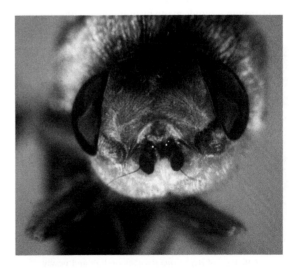

Figure 2.44 Head of an oestrid fly (*Gasterophilus*). From Jacobs, 1986 with permission of Elsevier.

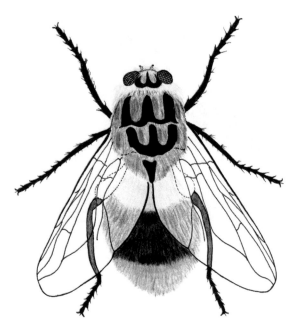

Figure 2.45 A warble fly (*Hypoderma*). Redrawn after Urquhart *et al.*, 1996 with permission of John Wiley & Sons, Ltd.

(see Figure 2.46). In contrast, *H. bovis* makes a loud humming noise which agitates cattle and may cause panic ('gadding'). Consequently, *H. bovis* deposits only a single egg at a time.

Larvae only 1 mm long hatch after a few days, crawl down the hairs and enter hair follicles or penetrate the skin through wounds made by biting flies. They migrate

through body tissues for about three months to reach their winter resting sites. *H. lineatum* passes through connective tissues to the oesophageal wall; while *H. bovis* follows nerves to access epidural fat within the spinal canal. Here they remain until they resume their migration in early spring.

Warble fly larvae eventually come to a halt in the subcutis close to the midline of the back and each bores a breathing hole through the skin (see Figure 2.47). Here, the barrel-shaped pale larva grows from 1.5 to 3 cm in length. It is initially creamy-yellow but darkens to brown as it matures. It is obviously segmented and has rows of small spines. A palpable cyst forms that is visible as a lump under the skin. In early summer, the larva forces itself through the breathing hole (see Figure 2.48), drops to the ground, darkens still more in colour and pupates under loose vegetation.

There is only one generation per year and the entire warble fly population is resident within the host over the winter. This makes infestation relatively easy to control with appropriately timed applications of systemic insecticide (see Section 8.2.4). Warble flies have been eradicated from some countries, including Great Britain and Ireland, Denmark and the Netherlands.

Stomach bots *(Gasterophilus)*
Once seen, the large bright red larvae of *Gasterophilus* ('bots') are never forgotten, especially at autopsy if large numbers are attached to the stomach mucosa

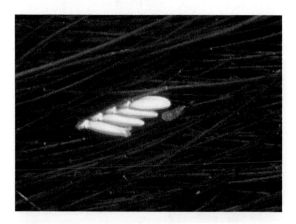

Figure 2.46 Eggs of *Hypoderma lineatum* on hair and newly hatched larva. Reproduced with permission of Agriculture and Agri-Food Canada Lethbridge Research Centre.

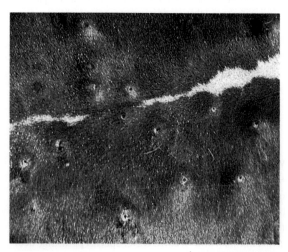

Figure 2.47 Calf badly infested with warbles. Reproduced with permission of Agriculture and Agri-Food Canada, Lethbridge Research Centre.

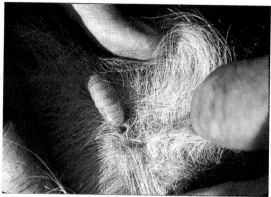

Figure 2.48 A fully grown warble larva. Reproduced with permission of Agriculture and Agri-Food Canada, Lethbridge Research Centre.

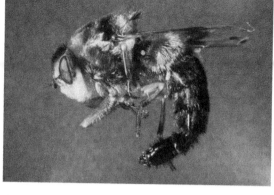

Figure 2.50 *Gasterophilus* adult. From Jacobs, 1986. Reproduced with permission of Elsevier.

(see Figure 2.49). The most widely distributed species are *G. intestinalis*, *G. nasalis* and *G. haemorrhoidalis*.

Adult *Gasterophilus* are 1–1.5 cm long with an appearance reminiscent of a worker bee (see Figure 2.50). The female has a prominent ovipositor which curves under the abdomen. She does not land to deposit eggs but hovers close to the skin (see Figure 2.51). This behaviour upsets horses when the adult flies are active in late summer.

The eggs are 1–2 mm long, creamy-white and familiar to most horse owners. Each is fixed to a hair with two flanges. Details of the life-cycle vary with species (see Table 2.4).

Eggs hatch spontaneously or are stimulated to do so by licking. Larvae enter the horse's mouth during grooming and spend several weeks tunnelling in the tongue or buccal mucosa before passing down to the stomach. The commonest species, *G. intestinalis*, adheres to the pharynx for a few days *en route* before

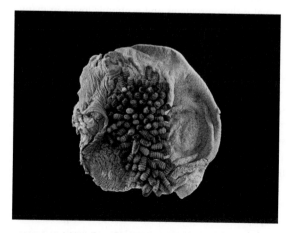

Figure 2.49 Museum specimen: *Gasterophilus* lavae attached to stomach wall. Reproduced with permission of The Royal Veterinary College.

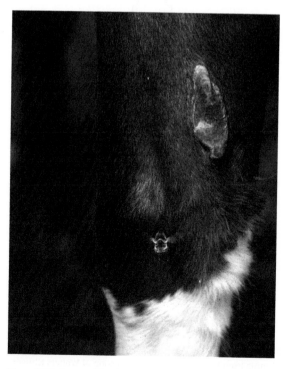

Figure 2.51 *Gasterophilus* fly laying an egg on a horse's leg.

Table 2.4 Some differences between horse bot flies

	Eggs deposited:	Initial infestation site:	Later attachment sites:
G. intestinalis	Fore legs and shoulders	Tongue, buccal mucosa	Pharynx then stomach
G. nasalis	Intermandibular area	Between teeth and gums	Pylorus/ duodenum
G. haemorrhoidalis	Around the lips	First lips, then tongue/ buccal mucosa	Stomach then rectum

attaching to the nonglandular (oesophageal) part of the stomach. The others fasten onto the glandular epithelium. All species stay in the host for up to a year before being passed in faeces. *G. haemorrhoidalis* pauses in the rectum for a few days on the way out. The larvae pupate on the ground and the imago fly emerges 1–2 months later.

Bot larvae in the stomach grow to 2 cm long (see Figure 2.52). They are plump and have prominent spines

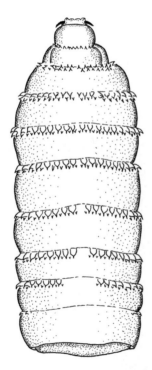

Figure 2.52 A *Gasterophilus* (stomach bot) larva. Redrawn after Mönnig from Lapage, 1962 with permission of Wolters Kluwer Health - Lippincott, Williams & Wilkins.

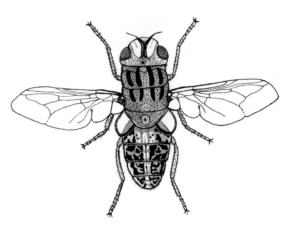

Figure 2.53 The nasal bot fly (*Oestrus ovis*). After Wall and Shearer, 1997, Urquhart *et al.*, 1996 with permission of John Wiley & Sons, Ltd and Chinery, 1977.

encircling the segments. Although they are reddish-brown and have well-developed mouth hooks, they feed on tissue exudates, not blood. *G. intestinalis* larvae thrust their heads deep into the stomach wall stimulating hyperplasia of the adjacent squamous epithelium to form a crater-like rim. Surprisingly, bots seem to be of little clinical consequence, unless large numbers interfere with the passage of food or action of sphincters.

Nasal bot fly *(Oestrus ovis)*
Oestrus ovis is a medium-sized grey coloured fly with yellowish hairs on the thorax and black spots on the abdomen (see Figure 2.53). The larvae are parasitic in the nasal chambers of sheep and goats. They provoke animal welfare problems and economic losses in many sheep-rearing localities.

Female flies squirt a jet of liquid containing up to 25 first instar larvae into the nostrils of the host. The larvae crawl up the nasal passages into the frontal sinuses where they feed on the mucosa. Larvae deposited in the spring are ready to leave as third-stage larvae within a month or two, whereas those deposited later in the summer may become arrested in their development. These overwinter as first-stage larvae and resume their life-cycle the following spring.

Mature larvae, with a characteristic black band on each body segment (see Figure 2.54), are sneezed out and pupate on the ground. The adult fly emerges about a month later. Two or three generations can occur in a year.

The adult flies cause considerable annoyance making sheep very nervous, although goats seem more tolerant.

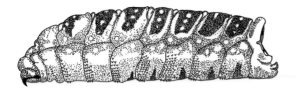

Figure 2.54 *Oestrus ovis* larva. Redrawn after Mönnig from Lapage, 1962 with permission of Wolters Kluwer Health - Lippincott, Williams & Wilkins.

The larvae irritate the nasal mucosa with their oral hooks and spines, provoking secretion of a viscid mucous exudate upon which they feed. Heavy infestations may erode bones in the sinuses, sometimes penetrating through to the brain provoking neurological signs. This is called 'false gid' to differentiate the condition from the similarly presenting 'true gid' caused by the larva of a tapeworm, *Taenia multiceps* (see Section 5.3.3).

CHAPTER 3

Arthropods part 2: ticks, mites and ectoparasiticides

3.1 Introduction

The arthropod groups featured in this chapter are those that have more than six legs as adults: the Arachnida with eight and the Crustacea with even more. Apart from scorpions and venomous spiders, the eight-legged creatures of veterinary interest are all ticks or mites. These belong to a zoological group known variously as the 'Acarina' or 'Acari' (see Figure 2.1). This explains why drugs used to combat ticks and mites are called 'acaricides'.

3.2 Ticks

Ticks are blood-sucking ectoparasites of worldwide veterinary significance. Although some are found in dry habitats, ticks are particularly important in warmer, wetter regions where they can be a serious constraint on agricultural production if not adequately controlled.

3.2.1 Key concepts

Body structure

Ticks have no obvious body segmentation (see Figure 3.1). Adult females engorged with blood resemble beans with projecting legs and mouthparts (see Figure 3.2). They vary in size according to species, life-cycle phase and stage of engorgement, but unfed adult females are typically some 0.5 cm in length.

Tick genera fall into two categories:

a – Ixodidae (hard ticks): which have a chitinous dorsal plate (the 'scutum') and visible mouthparts;

Principles of Veterinary Parasitology, First Edition. By Dennis Jacobs, Mark Fox, Lynda Gibbons and Carlos Hermosilla.
© 2016 John Wiley & Sons, Ltd. Published 2016 by John Wiley & Sons, Ltd.
Companion website: www.wiley.com/go/jacobs/principles-veterinary-parasitology

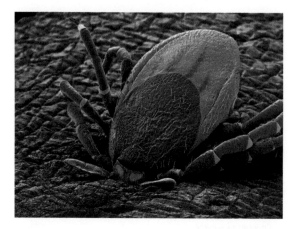

Figure 3.1 Adult tick feeding (an unengorged female *Ixodes*). Reproduced with permission of Bayer plc.

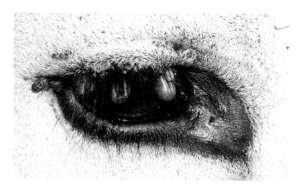

Figure 3.2 Ticks (*Boophilus microplus*) in various stages of development and engorgement feeding around the eye of a bovine (*Bos indicus*). Reproduced with permission of C.C. Constantinoiu.

b – Argasidae (soft ticks): which do not have a scutum. Their mouthparts are hidden from view beneath the body.

The scutum covers the whole dorsal surface of the male ixodid tick (see Figure 3.3). It is, however, restricted to a small area immediately behind the mouthparts in females. This arrangement leaves her body free to swell grotesquely as she feeds. Ixodid ticks are said to be 'ornate' if their scutum has coloured patches (and 'inornate' if they do not). In some cases, the posterior margin of the body is sculpted by a series of notches to form 'festoons'. Some genera have eyes at the side of the scutum. On the ventral aspect of the body, grooves around the anus and genital opening are sometimes useful for purposes of identification.

Soft ticks have a wrinkled leathery body (see Figure 3.4) which does not distend to any great degree when they feed.

Mouthparts and feeding

The deleterious effects of ticks on their host are all associated directly or indirectly with their feeding activity. Each stage in the ixodid life-cycle takes a single blood meal over a period of several days. The volume taken is relatively small except in the case of the adult female, those of some species imbibing 300 times their own body-weight. Even after surplus water has been pumped back into the host as saliva, she is typically 2–3 times her unfed size. This large meal provides the protein needed for the production of a single clutch of between 2000 and 20 000 eggs.

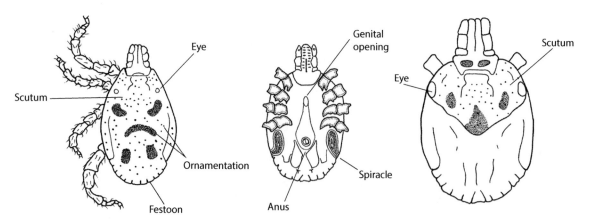

Figure 3.3 Ixodid (hard) tick – from left: dorsal view of male; ventral view; dorsal view of female (legs shown in full only on left side of first drawing). Redrawn from MAFF 1986 with permission © Crown copyright 1986.

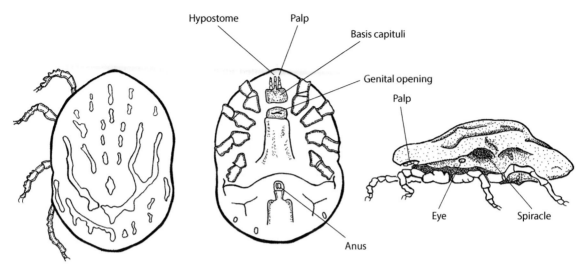

Figure 3.4 Argasid (soft) tick – from left: dorsal, ventral and side views. Redrawn from MAFF 1986 with permission © Crown copyright 1986.

In contrast, argasid ticks take multiple small feeds and excess water is expelled through a gland behind the first pair of legs. The female argasid produces a small batch of eggs after each meal.

The tick feeding apparatus has the following components (see Figure 3.5):

a – Basis capituli: a platform supporting the functional mouthparts.

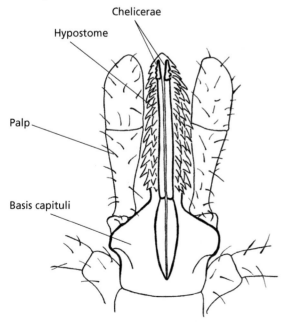

Figure 3.5 Tick mouthparts. Redrawn after various sources.

b – Palps: a pair of sensory organs used for locating a suitable feeding site. Ticks are fussy eaters and spend a lot of time finding just the right spot for attachment.

c – Chelicerae: the tips work in a scissor-like fashion to cut a hole through the skin.

d – Hypostome: this is pushed through the wound made by the chelicerae. Backward-pointing barbs lock it in position. This is why ticks are so difficult to remove.

After the hypostome has been inserted into the skin (see Figure 3.6), most tick species secrete a fluid which hardens to form a cement cone. A dorsal groove along the hypostome permits an alternating flow of tick saliva

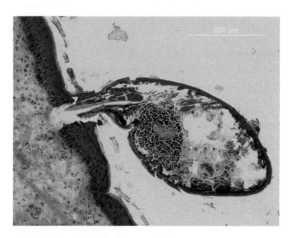

Figure 3.6 Section through a larval tick feeding on a cow. Reproduced with permission of C.C. Constantinoiu.

in one direction and host blood and tissue fluids in the other. Initially, the feeding process is slow but it culminates in a phase of rapid engorgement. The cement liquefies when feeding is complete allowing the tick to detach.

Ixodid life-cycles

Hard ticks have three developmental stages: larva, nymph and adult. Apart from size and sexual maturity, they are similar except that the larva has six legs and no spiracles. When not on the host, most are hidden in the debris that collects at the base of thick vegetation. This provides the humid microclimate essential for their survival, as well as protection from predators. Ticks tend to have very specific environmental requirements and these determine the geographical distribution and seasonal abundance of each species. In temperate and cold climates, tick development is halted during winter. In warmer climates, no break occurs if year-round rainfall maintains a favourable microclimate. If rainfall is seasonal, tick activity will be governed by plant transpiration rates and their effect on relative humidity within the vegetation mat.

When ticks seek a host, they climb to the top of nearby foliage. A motionless posture is adopted with the front legs, which carry sensitive sensory organs, testing the air for chemical signals that might indicate the proximity of a potential host. This ensures they are ready to scramble onto a passing animal as soon as it comes in contact. This behaviour is called 'questing'.

Ixodid species are categorised as three-, two- or one-host ticks, depending on the number of animals used by an individual tick of that species during its life-cycle. Note that this refers to the number of host individuals each tick feeds on – not the number of host species involved.

Three-host ticks

The three-host life-cycle is the most common (see Figure 3.7):

a – When fully engorged, the adult female tick detaches from her host and slithers off to the ground.

b – She finds a suitable site for egg-deposition and dies. Larvae are 1–2 mm long when they hatch and, because of their size and appearance, they are known as 'seed ticks'. They climb vegetation and quest.

c – Having found a host, the larva attaches and feeds.

d – When replete, it drops to the ground, digests its blood-meal and moults to become a nymph.

e – Unfed nymphs quest, find a host and feed.

f – They drop to the ground, digest their meal and moult to become an adult.

g – Unfed adults quest and find a host. Females attach to the skin but do not feed until they have been fertilised by a male.

Two- and one-host ticks

The life-cycle of a two-host tick is similar to that described above, except that the fed larva remains on its first host where it moults to the nymphal stage and feeds again. It now falls to the ground to moult and become a host-seeking adult. Thus, during the course of its life-span, it feeds on two animals: the larva and nymph on one and the adult on another.

As will probably be obvious by now, the larva of a one-host tick seeks a host and remains on this same individual through both moults until eventually dropping off as a fully engorged adult.

All ticks spend considerably more time on the ground than on an animal. The duration of the life-cycle depends on the climate. It may be completed within a single wet season in the tropics but often takes three or more years in temperate or colder regions. The generation time of one- and two-host ticks is generally shorter than that of three-host ticks as the skin provides constant warmth and humidity for those life-cycle stages that develop on the host.

Argasid life-cycle

Soft ticks undergo one larval and several nymphal stages before moulting to become an adult. They take small feeds from many animals, as and when the opportunity arises. They can survive long periods between meals. Mating takes place on the ground. They are more drought-tolerant than hard ticks and are generally found in drier environments, often close to their host's lair, pen or nest. Most species are active mainly at night.

Pathogenesis

The size of the tick lesion depends on the depth of the bite and the array of biologically active substances injected into the host. Some genera, such as *Rhipicephalus*, attach superficially while others, like *Amblyomma*, penetrate deeply into the dermis. Typically, the cement that has been secreted becomes surrounded by a zone of oedema, inflammatory cell infiltration and epithelial hyperplasia.

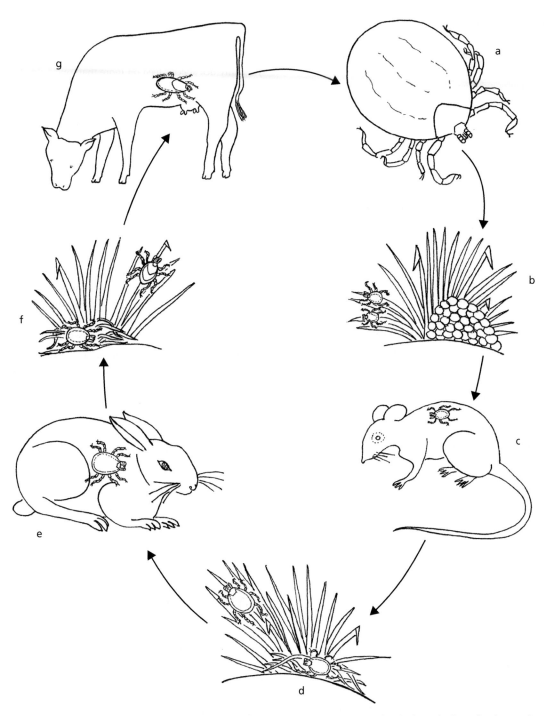

Figure 3.7 Life-cycle of a three-host tick (*Ixodes*): a/b – engorged female lays eggs on ground; c/d – larva feeds on first host and moults on ground; e/f – nymph feeds on second host and moults on ground; g – adult ticks feed on third host (details in text which uses same lettering as shown above).

Extra information box 3.1

Some pharmacological properties of tick saliva

Tick saliva contains a variety of pharmacologically active substances including:
i) histamine blocking agents to minimise the host's inflammatory response;
ii) anticoagulants to ensure a free flow of blood;
iii) cytolysins to enlarge the feeding lesion;
iv) vasoactive mediators and enzymes to increase vascular permeability and facilitate feeding;
v) paralytic toxins; these are produced by some species, although no useful function has yet been established for them. They cause an ascending motor paralysis which can be fatal in smaller animals if respiratory muscles become affected.

The damaging effects caused by ticks can be summarised as:
i)   blood losses (heavy infestations can cause anaemia);
ii) tick worry (discomfort and rubbing, which restrict time for feeding and ruminating);
iii) production losses (reduced weight gain, milk yield and fleece weight/quality); fleece and hide damage (due to puncture wounds and self-inflicted trauma); secondary infection of tick bites by microorganisms, blowfly and screwworm larvae;
iv) tick paralysis (by species producing salivary neurotoxins);
v)   disease transmission (ticks are vectors for a range of protozoal, bacterial, rickettsial and viral agents).

Extra information box 3.2

Immunity to ticks

Ixodid ticks remain attached to their hosts for 5–7 days each time they feed. With some tick species, this level of exposure to salivary antigens enables a partially effective immune response to develop. This acts by interfering with the blood-sucking process. In animals that have been previously exposed, basophilic granulocytes accumulate in the skin around the tick mouthparts. IgE on the cell surface reacts with allergens in the tick saliva causing the basophils to degranulate and produce histamine. This, along with other molecules that are released, disrupts both tick salivation and blood uptake.

Disease transmission

Ticks are very efficient vectors of disease. Reasons for this include:
i)   many tick species feed on more than one animal during their life-cycle (the exception being one-host ticks);
ii) ixodid ticks remain attached to the skin for lengthy periods while feeding, during which time they pump large quantities of saliva, which may contain pathogens, into the wound;
iii) many tick-borne pathogens multiply within the tick;
iv) some organisms invade the tick ovary to become incorporated into developing eggs.

There are two mechanisms involved in the transmission of pathogens by ticks:

a – Trans-stadial: the pathogen is taken up by an immature tick (larva or nymph) and, usually after a series of intermediate steps, invades the salivary gland so it can be transmitted to a new host when a subsequent life-cycle stage (nymph or adult) feeds. This is also known as 'stage-to-stage' transmission.

b – Transovarian transmission: this occurs when pathogens invade the ovary of a female tick and become incorporated into developing eggs, so infection can be subsequently spread by the next generation of ticks. This explains how one-host ticks are able to transmit tick-borne diseases. In some cases, the organisms can be passed down through several tick generations.

Pathogens that congregate or multiply in the tick salivary gland may be released at particular points in the feeding cycle. For example, *Borrelia* (the bacterial agent of Lyme disease) is transmitted from 48 hrs after attachment, whereas *Theileria* (a protozoan parasite) does not appear in tick saliva before the 5th day of feeding.

3.2.2 Hard ticks (Ixodidae)

Whole textbooks have been devoted to ticks and tick-borne diseases. There are numerous tick species, each with its own particular local significance and biological attributes. The scope of this text allows no more than a few examples to illustrate the complexity and significance of this group. Most ixodid ticks of veterinary importance belong to genera listed in Table 3.1. Identification to species level requires expertise, but the features outlined in the table (which are easiest to see in males or unfed females) may give a clue to the probable genus.

Table 3.1 Some important ixodid ticks

	Common names include:	Life-cycle	Identification	Main infections transmitted
Ixodes	Castor bean tick	3-host	Long palps; anal groove curves in front of anus	P: babesiosis; B: Lyme disease, tick pyaemia; R: ehrlichiosis; V: louping ill; paralysis (*I. holocyclus*)
Boophilus[1]	Blue tick	1-host	Mouthparts short; BC-hexagonal	P: babesiosis; R: anaplasmosis
Rhipicephalus	Brown ear tick (cattle); brown dog tick	2- and 3-host species	BC-hexagonal, short palps, festoons	P: theileriosis, babesiosis; R: ehrlichiosis; paralysis (some species)
Amblyomma	Bont ticks; lone star tick	3-host	Long palps, ornate, festoons, banded legs	R: heartwater, Q-fever, Rocky Mountain spotted fever; B: tularaemia
Dermacentor	Rocky Mountain wood tick, American dog tick, Tropical horse tick	3-host (most species)	BC-rectangular, short mouthparts, eyes, ornate,	P: babesiosis; theileriosis; R: Rocky Mountain spotted fever, anaplasmosis, Q-fever; B: tularaemia, Lyme disease; V: equine infectious encephalitis etc.; paralysis (some species)

B = bacterial; BC = basis capituli; P = protozoal; R = rickettsial; V = viral. [1] Now regarded as a subgenus of *Rhipicephalus.*

Minor genera include *Haemaphysalis*, which transmits a nonpathogenic *Babesia* species of cattle, and *Hyalomma*. In veterinary practice, the latter is most often seen on tortoises recently-imported from the wild.

Ixodes

Ixodes species are mostly found in temperate or cooler climates. The most widely distributed member of the genus is *I. ricinus*, which acts as vector for a number of life-threatening protozoal and microbial diseases, including babesiosis and Lyme disease. Other species are more localised such as *I. scapularis* (also known as *I. dammini*) and *I. pacificus* which transmit Lyme disease in eastern and western parts of the USA, respectively. *I. canisuga* has a narrower host range and is associated with dog kennels and foxes in Europe. *I. holocyclus* seems relatively innocuous when feeding on its natural host, the Australian bandicoot, but its saliva is capable of paralysing or even killing a dog, calf or foal.

Ixodes ricinus

I. ricinus will feed on any vertebrate host. The immature stages tend to favour smaller creatures (e.g. rodents) while adults prefer larger animals such as sheep, cattle and dogs. It is a three-host tick with a life-cycle extending over 2–7 years depending on weather conditions and availability of hosts. Host-seeking activity is seasonal, peaking in the spring, but where warmer summer temperatures accelerate off-host development, there may be an additional autumnal rise, particularly in the number of questing nymphs. Well-managed pastures do not provide the microclimate needed for off-host survival and so infestation is generally associated with rough grazing, moorland, hedgerows and woodland.

Lyme disease (borreliosis)

Lyme disease is a trans-stadial tick-borne bacterial condition caused by the spirochaete, *Borrelia burgdorferi*. It induces acute lameness in dogs and is characterised in humans by a fever followed by erythema and arthritis. In eastern USA, immature stages of the vector, *I. scapularis*, feed on small mammals, which are the reservoir for *B. burgdorferi* infection, and adult ticks mainly on deer. Canine and human disease is therefore seen most often in wooded suburbs or where leisure pursuits take people into environments with large deer populations.

Boophilus

This one-host tick is the scourge of cattle production in many hot, humid climates. It is a vector for babesiosis (see Section 4.8.1) and anaplasmosis (a rickettsial infection producing debilitating anaemia, jaundice and abortion). In the wet tropics, these diseases curtail the use of highly productive European breeds, which have to be cross-bred with, or replaced by, tick-resistant *Bos indicus*-type or other indigenous cattle (see Section 8.2.4). The main

Boophilius species are *B. annulatus*, which has a widespread distribution, although mostly eradicated from the USA, and *B. microplus* in Australia, South Africa and Latin America. They spend about three weeks on the host and the generation time can be as little as two months, so large numbers of host-seeking ticks can build up on pastures during the wet season.

Rhipicephalus

Rhipicephalus appendiculatus

Of the several species of *Rhipicephalus* infesting livestock in sub-Saharan Africa, *R. appendiculatus* is particularly devastating. It congregates in the ears of cattle and other animals, where it can do substantial damage (see Figure 3.8), often exacerbated by secondary infection and myiasis. Toxins in its saliva can provoke general malaise ('tick toxicosis'). If that were not enough, *R. appendiculatus* is the principle vector of East Coast Fever (theileriosis – see Section 4.8.2) and several other microbial diseases.

Rhipicephalus sanguineus

This is the brown dog tick. Adults are usually found between the toes or in the ears, while larvae and nymphs are often on the back of the neck. *R. sanguineus* transmits canine babesiosis and ehrlichiosis (a rickettsial infection) and can sometimes cause paralysis. Although primarily a canine parasite, it can also feed on other animals and humans. It has a very widespread distribution but is generally absent from cooler regions (including the UK). It is well adapted for living inside buildings

and, if introduced from an endemic area, can establish in heated quarantine kennels or houses in climates otherwise too cold for its development.

Amblyomma

Amblyomma is perhaps the most attractive of the ticks as the scutum is highly ornate. The long mouthparts, however, penetrate deeply causing a painful wound prone to secondary infection. Most species infest a range of mammals, including cattle, preferring the head, ears and neck. They are of greatest significance in Africa, where they transmit rickettsial diseases such as heartwater and Q fever.

One species, *A. americanum*, is widespread in the USA. It is known as the Lone Star Tick as the female has a large white spot on the scutum (see Figure 3.9). Amongst the diseases it transmits are Rocky Mountain spotted fever and tularaemia. It is a three-host tick with a three year life-cycle. Like *I. ricinus*, its immature stages tend to feed on smaller host species and adults on larger hosts, such as farm livestock, horses and deer.

Dermacentor

Species of *Dermacentor* important in the USA include: the Rocky Mountain wood tick, *D. andersoni*, which parasitizes cattle and other herbivores in the Northwest, the American dog tick, *D. variabilis*, which is mostly found on the eastern side of the country, and *D. nitens*,

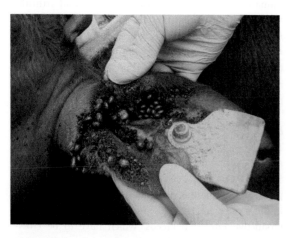

Figure 3.8 *Rhipicephalus* feeding on ear. Reproduced with permission of I. Morrison.

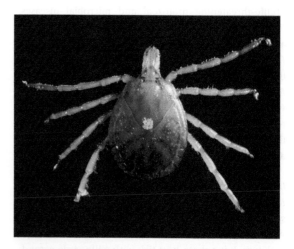

Figure 3.9 *Amblyomma americanum* (unfed adult female): note the white spot on the scutum and the festoons around the posterior margin of the body. Reproduced with permission of R.C. Krecek and L. Wadsworth.

Table 3.2 Some important argasid ticks

	Common names include:	Hosts	Distribution
Otobius	Spinose ear tick	Cattle, horses, dogs etc.	Americas, India, southern Africa
Ornithodorus	Sand tampan	Small and large mammals	Tropics and subtropics
Argas	Fowl tick	Birds	Warmer climates

the tropical horse tick, found in Central America and neighbouring areas. In southern Europe and parts of Africa, *D. reticulatus* plays a similar role in transmitting a long list of protozoal and rickettsial diseases in cattle, horses and dogs. The American species are the principal vectors of Rocky Mountain spotted fever and can sometimes produce paralysis, particularly in calves.

3.2.3 Soft ticks (Argasidae)

There are only three argasid genera commonly affecting domesticated animals: *Argas*, *Ornithodorus* and *Otobius* (see Table 3.2).

Otobius

Otobius megnini is known as the 'spinose ear tick' which gives a clue to both its appearance and life-cycle, the parasitic stages being spent deep in the external ear canal. *O. megnini* is different from other soft ticks as it uses only one individual animal during its life-span. The larva seeks a host and stays on it for several weeks, by which time it has moulted twice to the second nymphal stage. When this is fully engorged, it is up to 1 cm long, blue-grey, covered in spines and ready to leave the animal. All further development takes place off the host and the adults, which do not feed, complete their biological functions hidden in cracks and crevices.

The feeding activities of larvae and nymphs invoke inflammatory responses and a waxy exudate. Secondary bacterial infection and myiasis may follow. The resulting distress can lead to further self-inflicted damage.

Ornithodorus

Ornithodorus species are small argasid ticks, the largest growing to a little over 0.5 cm long (see Figure 3.10). They are generally associated with animal burrows and so only occasionally spill over to livestock to become established in stock pens. One African/Middle Eastern species buries itself in sand in shady places and feeds on the lower legs of cattle. Tethered animals or sleeping

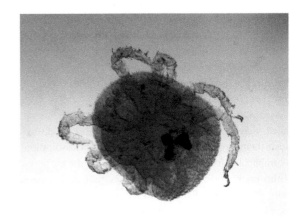

Figure 3.10 Adult *Ornithodorus*.

humans can suffer from multiple bites or tick toxicosis. *Ornithodorus* spp. can carry numerous diseases. It is an important vector of the African swine fever virus and transmits *Borrelia* species causing human relapsing fever.

Argas

The poultry tick, *Argas persicus*, is a common parasite of poultry in warmer climates. They are straw coloured when unfed and spend the day hiding within crevices in poultry houses. They take a blood meal at night, usually selecting a site beneath the wing. Although generally of minor clinical significance, they can reduce productivity. Large numbers cause anaemia and even death, especially in young birds. They transmit spirochaete and rickettsial infections and some species invoke tick paralysis. They are sometimes found on migratory birds visiting temperate regions.

3.3 Mange mites

Like ticks, mites are eight-legged arthropods belonging to the Acarina (see Figure 2.1). Unlike ticks, which are exclusively parasitic, mites occupy countless terrestrial and aquatic niches with only a tiny minority adopting a partial or completely parasitic lifestyle.

Some free-living mites do nevertheless have veterinary significance. For example, some species of forage mite, which are pests of stored food products such as cereals, hay or straw, can induce allergic reactions if they come into contact with animal or human skin. Pasture mites (also called 'oribatid mites') are part of the natural fauna of permanent grasslands and can be very numerous, particularly during summer months. They are relevant to veterinary medicine for a completely different reason – they act as intermediate hosts for anoplocephalid tapeworms (Section 5.3.5), transmitting the infection when they are accidentally swallowed by grazing animals.

As most parasitic mites are associated with a skin disease called 'mange', they are called 'mange mites' to distinguish them from free-living relatives. Their classification is complex but fortunately can be ignored for the purposes of this book. For clinical consideration, mange mites are more conveniently divided into two groups according to their location on the host: subsurface (or burrowing) and surface (or nonburrowing) mites.

3.3.1 Key concepts

Almost all mange mites complete their life-cycle on the host. Transmission is therefore mainly by direct contact between hosts. Mites progress from a six-legged larva through one to three nymphal stages to the adult. Females lay only one large egg at a time (see Figure 3.11) but, as generation times are relatively short, large infestations can build up quickly.

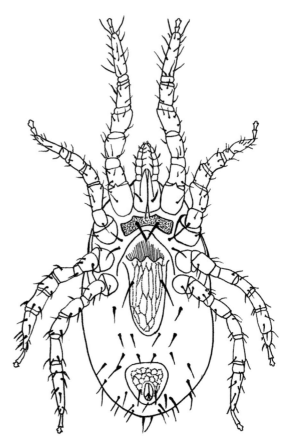

Figure 3.12 A surface mite (the poultry mite, *Dermanyssus*). Redrawn after Hirst, 1922 from Roberts and Janovy Jr., 1996 with permission of McGraw Hill Education.

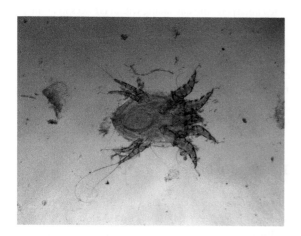

Figure 3.11 Female *Psoroptes* mite with egg.

Anatomically, there are many similarities with ticks (see Figure 3.12). Mites are, however, much smaller. Many are barely visible at less than 0.5 mm long. They have a soft body, although some possess chitinous plates or bars. There is no head but projecting mouthparts comprise sensory palps and chelicerae. The hypostome, which is such a prominent feature of tick mouthparts, is absent from all but a very few parasitic mites. The position of the anus is sometimes useful for identification.

3.3.2 Subsurface mites

Subsurface mites can be recognised as they have short stumpy legs (see Figure 3.13), whereas surface mites have long legs that project much further from the body (e.g. see Figure 3.12).

Help box 3.1

Ticks and mange mites compared

Ticks and mange mites are both eight-legged wingless arthropods. They both belong to the Acarina and so have many similarities but there are also fundamental differences, including:

	Ticks	Mange mites
Size	Large (~0.5 cm)	Small (~0.5 mm)
Time on host	Only to feed; most of life spent on ground	Most spend entire life on host
Eggs laid	In clusters on ground	Singly on host
Duration of life-cycle	Often protracted (months or years)	Short (days or weeks)
Host to host transmission	Questing ticks on vegetation etc.	Direct physical contact
Disease transmission	Vectors of many pathogenic organisms	Vectors for very few pathogens

Two of the three most important subsurface mites belong to the same family and so have much in common. These are *Sarcoptes*, found on mammals, and *Knemidocoptes*

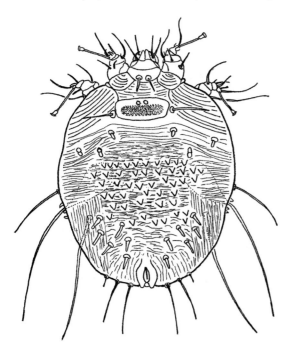

Figure 3.13 A subsurface mite, *Sarcoptes*. Redrawn and modified after Bedford, 1932 from Lapage, 1962 with permission of Wolters Kluwer Health - Lippincott, Williams & Wilkins.

on birds. *Sarcoptes* causes scabies in humans and sarcoptic mange on animals, both highly pruritic and contagious conditions. The third genus, *Demodex*, differs in appearance and lifestyle. It causes demodectic mange (also called demodicosis) which occurs most commonly in dogs and can be very difficult to manage.

Sarcoptes and *Knemidocoptes*

The genus *Sarcoptes* contains only one species, *S. scabiei*, though host-adapted 'strains' are found on all domesticated animals and humans. A strain adapted to one host species can be transmitted to another host and may cause transient clinical signs. However, the mite is unlikely to establish and reproduce on an 'abnormal' host, so infestations usually resolve spontaneously. A closely related genus, *Notoedres*, is occasionally seen on cats.

Help box 3.2

Mange mites and mange: pronunciation

Knemidocoptes the 'K' is silent. It is sometimes spelt *Cnemidocoptes*, but still pronounced 'Nem – ido – cop – teez'.
Cheyletiella the 'Ch' is pronounced as a 'K' ('kay – let – ee – ella').

Sarcoptes

Sarcoptes is a small, round mite with prominent dorsal pegs and spines (see Figure 3.13). Only the anterior two pairs of legs are visible, the others being hidden under the body. The life-cycle is illustrated in Figure 3.14:

a – The fertilised female mite creates a tunnel ('egg-laying pocket') in the upper layers of the epidermis in which she lays eggs while feeding on liquid oozing from damaged tissues (see Figure 3.15).

b – The eggs hatch in under a week releasing 6-legged larvae which crawl to the surface of the skin. They in turn burrow into the epidermis forming 'moulting pockets' where they become 8-legged nymphs. These moult twice before becoming adults.

c – The males look for unfertilised females either on the surface or in a moulting pocket.

The whole life-cycle is completed in about 3 weeks. New hosts are infected by close contact, usually by the transfer of mites on the skin surface. Mites can

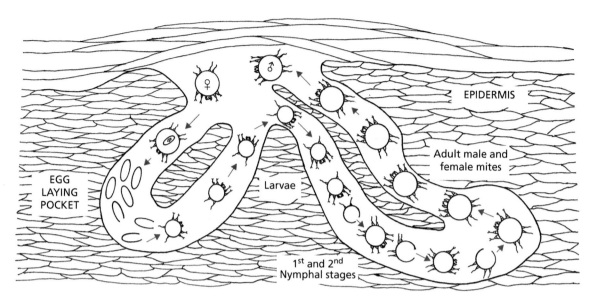

Figure 3.14 Life-cycle of *Sarcoptes* (details in text).

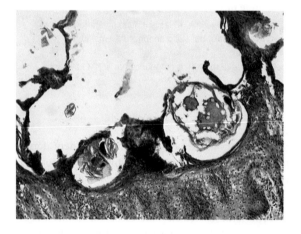

Figure 3.15 Section through *Sarcoptes* mites in superficial skin tunnels.

Help box 3.3

Definition of some dermatology terms

Alopecia   Absence of hair in an area where it is normally present.
Crust   Presence of a dried exudate (serum, blood, pus).
Erythema   Redness of skin (caused by increased blood flow through capillaries).
Papule   Raised solid elevation of the skin < 1 cm diameter (cf. nodule > 1 cm).
Pruritus   A sensory experience (itching) that stimulates a desire to scratch the affected part of the body (or rub, lick, bite, chew, nibble, roll, etc.).
Scale   An accumulation of loose cornified fragments of the stratum corneum.
Urticaria   A skin rash with raised pruritic plaques or bumps.

survive for short periods off the host so, for example, a shared rubbing post might act as a transitory source of infection.

Initially, the burrowing activity of the mites, together with antigenic substances in their saliva and faeces, induce erythema with papule formation and later scale and crust formation with alopecia. Intense pruritus starts about one week postinfection leading to self-inflicted trauma. Epidermal hyperplasia progresses to thickening and wrinkling of the skin.

Antigenic substances in mite saliva and faeces induce hypersensitivity reactions which may present as a pruritic rash within hours of reinfestation. The skin may become thickened, scaly and crusty in chronic infestations and there may be hair loss over affected areas.

Sarcoptic mange is seen most frequently in dogs and pigs, but all animals can be affected. The canine condition (see Section 9.2.3) is a serious welfare issue in neglected and stray dogs in many poorer countries as well as being a common diagnosis in veterinary clinics worldwide. Mild infections in pigs are often overlooked even though the energy expended on scratching and rubbing to relieve pruritus can have a significant effect on food-conversion and growth. The mite is transmitted from sow to piglets during suckling, and from boars to gilts at service.

Sarcoptes is potentially a severe infestation in cattle and sheep but has been brought under control in many regions. It is a notifiable disease in some countries (i.e. its actual or suspected occurrence must be reported to the appropriate national or local veterinary authority). Lesions are seen on the neck and tail of cattle and the face, ears, axillae and groin of sheep. They cause hide damage as well as affecting productivity. The equine condition is now rare in many countries. Lesions spread from head, neck and shoulders to the rest of the body.

Knemidocoptes

Knemidocoptes is the only genus of burrowing mites on birds. It is similar in appearance to *Sarcoptes* except that it lacks dorsal pegs and spines and has a distinct 'U'-shaped chitinous bar behind the mouthparts (see Figure 3.16). Different species cause diseases such as 'scaly leg' and

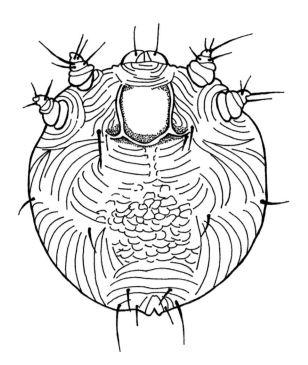

Figure 3.16 *Knemidocoptes*. Redrawn after Urquhart *et al.*, 1987.

'depluming itch' in poultry and 'scaly beak' in cage birds (see Section 8.4.2).

Demodex

This burrowing mite is found on all domesticated animals and humans, but each species is host specific. Some hosts have more than one species. *Demodex* normally lives as a harmless commensal in the skin. Most animals (including humans) carry small numbers without ill-effect. Clinical signs are seen, however, if population numbers are unrestrained by host defence mechanisms. This happens most often in dogs, occasionally in pigs, cattle and goats but rarely in cats or other animals. The condition in cattle is not of clinical concern but distended sebaceous glands, which can contain several thousand mites, reduce the value of the hide for the leather industry, particularly in warmer climates.

Demodex is cigar-shaped, with four pairs of stumpy legs that barely project beyond the body margin (see Figure 3.17). Its structure is well adapted to its lifestyle as it spends its entire existence in hair follicles and sebaceous glands (see Figure 3.18). The life-cycle is completed in 3 weeks. Infestation passes from dam to offspring during suckling.

Immune factors are important in determining the occurrence and severity of demodicosis. These include:

a – Hereditary predisposition: Puppies born to some bitches are genetically more susceptible to infection. This is thought to be associated with a deficiency in the effectiveness of the innate immune system.

b – Parasitic immunosuppression: If present in large numbers, *Demodex* suppresses normal T-cell responses.

c – Induced immunosuppression: Demodicosis can flare up when dogs are given immuno-depressant drugs, such as corticosteroids, for controlling other conditions.

3.3.3 Surface mites

This section deals with a diversity of surface-dwelling mites (see Table 3.3). Most feed on skin scales or suck tissue fluids or exudates. Because their mouthparts are so small, the lesions they produce are shallow and pathogenicity is mostly associated with inflammatory and hypersensitivity reactions to mite antigens. Their life-cycles are similar to that of *Sarcoptes* (see Figure 3.14) except that they do not burrow into the skin.

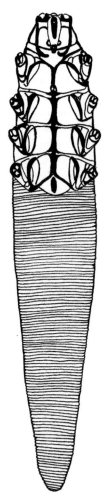

Figure 3.17 *Demodex* (ventral view). Redrawn after James and Hardwood, 1969 from Cheng, 1986 with permission of Elsevier.

Three of the most important surface mites, *Psoroptes*, *Chorioptes* and *Otodectes*, belong to one family while a

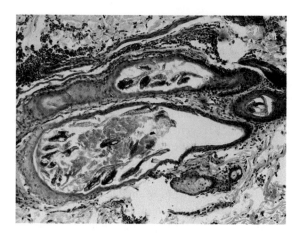

Figure 3.18 *Demodex* mites in hair follicle.

fourth, *Cheyletiella*, is only distantly related. Yet further removed are the poultry mites (*Dermanyssus* and *Ornithonyssus*) and the harvest mite, *Neotrombicula*.

Psoroptes and *Chorioptes*

Psoroptes ovis (see Figure 3.19 and Figure 3.11) is the sheep scab mite. It is highly contagious and can cause great distress to its host. It has pointed mouthparts which it uses to abrade the skin as the first step in generating its liquid diet. The microwounds become contaminated with mite faeces which provoke an intense inflammatory response and a copious serous exudate. The associated pruritus induces rubbing, scratching and self-inflicted damage. There appear to be a number of different strains of *P. ovis* which vary in pathogenicity including one (which may be a different species) that lives in the external ear canal and is relatively nonpathogenic. Other species occur on cattle, horses, rabbits and camelids.

Table 3.3 Some important surface mites

	Most important in:	Off-host life-cycle stages?	Contagious?	Pathogenicity	Zoonosis?	More information in Section:
Psoroptes	Sheep (cattle, rabbits, horses)	No	▼▼▼	▼▼▼	No	8.2.4
Chorioptes	Cattle, horse (sheep)	No	▼	▼	No	8.2.4
Otodectes	Dogs, cats	No	▼▼	▼▼	No	9.2.3
Cheyletiella	Dogs, cats, rabbits	No	▼▼▼	▼▼	Yes	9.3.2
Trombiculids	Dogs (and other animals)	Yes	No	▼	Yes	
Dermanyssus/ *Ornithonyssus*	Poultry (can bite other animals)	*D*: Yes *O*: No	*D*: No *O*: Yes	▼▼	Yes	8.4.2

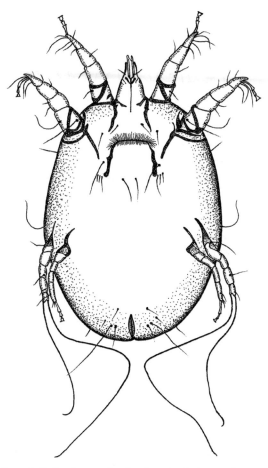

Figure 3.19 The sheep scab mite, *Psoroptes*. Redrawn after Mönnig from Lapage, 1962 with permission of Wolters Kluwer Health - Lippincott, Williams & Wilkins.

Extra information box 3.3

History of sheep scab in Great Britain

Sheep scab was eradicated from England, Scotland and Wales in 1952, but reappeared in 1973 and has since been endemic. Sheep scab is a serious animal welfare issue so why has it proved impossible to control the disease a second time?

Legislation introduced in 1928 to control sheep scab involved:

i) compulsory dipping of all sheep at specified times of year (under supervision within infected areas);
ii) regular inspection of sheep flocks with all suspect cases to be reported to the authorities;
iii) restricted movement of sheep within, and out of, infected areas.

Control measures introduced after reintroduction of the disease failed because:

i) modern acaricides are less robust than the sheep dips previously employed (now withdrawn because of adverse environmental effects), so reliable results are obtained only if they are used strictly according to label recommendations;
ii) regular inspections and supervision are no longer economically feasible and so universal compliance with regulations and treatment recommendations cannot be guaranteed.

Sheep scab remains a notifiable disease in Australia and New Zealand where the disease has been eradicated and strict regulations have prevented its reintroduction.

Chorioptes bovis is more benign than *P. ovis* as it has rounded mouthparts designed for chewing skin debris. It is only half the size of *Psoroptes* and is found mostly on cattle and horses. *Psoroptes* and *Chorioptes* can be differentiated most reliably by microscopic examination of the ends of their legs (see Figure 3.20): *Psoroptes* has a funnel-shaped sucker mounted on a segmented stalk; while *Chorioptes* has a cup-shaped sucker mounted on a shorter unsegmented stalk.

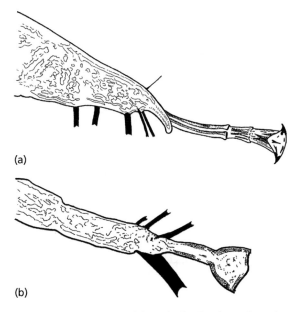

(a)

(b)

Figure 3.20 Close up view of the pedicel and sucker at the end of the leg of (a) *Psoroptes* and (b) *Chorioptes*. (The black bars are long hairs which have been cut short for the diagram.) Adapted from MAFF 1986 with permission. © Crown copyright 1986.

Otodectes

Otodectes cynotis is the commonest mange mite of cats and dogs worldwide. It also affects foxes and ferrets. It inhabits the external ear, mostly deep down near the eardrum and is easily recognised as whitish moving specks. For confirmation, it is long-legged and the females have suckers only on the front two pairs of legs. Also, chitinous bars behind the front legs on either side of the underside of the body meet to form a characteristic 'V' shape (see Figure 3.21). The mites feed on superficial debris and the life-cycle is completed in 3 weeks. They are able to live off the host for a short time.

Although a majority of cats harbour *Otodectes*, only a few show clinical signs. Infestation is probably acquired by kittens from the queen during suckling. In contrast, *Otodectes* is a common cause of 'otitis externa' in dogs although the severity of the condition varies considerably between individuals (see Section 9.2.3).

Cheyletiella

Different *Cheyletiella* species occur on dogs (*C. yasguri*) and cats (*C. blakei*). A third species can be found on pet rabbits. They are highly contagious but clinical signs in animals are usually mild and easily overlooked, being restricted to the presence of an excessive amount of scurf ('dandruff') and slight itchiness.

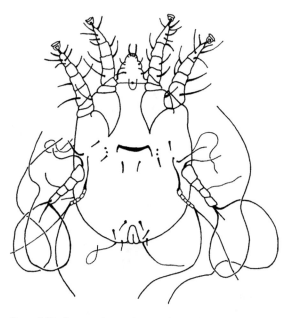

Figure 3.21 The ear-mite *Otodectes*. Redrawn after Urquhart *et al.*, 1987.

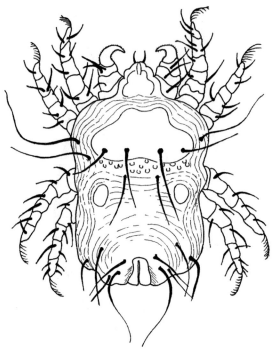

Figure 3.22 *Cheyletiella*. Diagram partly based on Urquhart *et al.*, 1987 and 1996 with permission of John Wiley & Sons Ltd.

Cheyletiella lives in the fur and is highly motile. At about 0.4 mm in length it is just visible to the naked eye and has earned the nickname 'walking dandruff'. Under the microscope, it can be seen to have a slightly elongated body with a definite 'waist' (see Figure 3.22). There are prominent clawed palps on either side of blade-like mouthparts. There are also comb-like structures at the end of each leg.

Extra information box 3.4

The itch mite, *Psorergates*

Psorergates ovis provokes wool loss and matted fleece in Australasia, southern Africa and the Americas. It occurs mostly in Merino sheep. Although technically a surface mite, it spends much of its life-cycle within the superficial layers of the skin, which become thickened and pruritic. Because of this lifestyle, it is not very contagious but spreads through a flock slowly, transfer taking place when sheep are tightly penned, especially after shearing. Skin scrapings are needed to demonstrate its presence. It is very small (0.2 mm) and round with legs stretched out as though it has just done a star-jump.

The mites feed by superficially piercing the skin and sucking fluid. They stick their eggs to hairs with silky threads a little above skin level. The egg is relatively large enabling the larval stage to be completed before hatching takes place. Consequently, only nymphs and adults are found in the fur. The life-cycle is completed in 2 weeks.

Other surface mites

This section embraces a miscellany of troublesome parasites that have more in common with sap-feeding plant parasitic mites than with other animal parasitic genera. They show gradations in parasitic adaptation: *Neotrombicula* is parasitic only in the larval stage; *Dermanyssus* is mostly free-living but nymphs and adults seek a host at night to take a blood meal; while all life-cycle stages of *Ornithonyssus* spend much of their time on the host.

Trombiculids

There are some 50 trombiculid mites that attack livestock and pets. Most have a very wide potential host range and have various local names including 'harvest mites' (Europe), 'chigger mites' (America) and 'scrub itch mites' (Australia). The nymphs and adults are predators, hunting and eating other arthropods. Eggs are laid in damp soil. The larvae climb vegetation to transfer onto an animal. They are therefore most often found on the lower limbs and around the face.

The six-legged parasitic form is small (0.2 mm) with a round, orange body covered in stout hairs (see Figure 3.23). It inserts its chelicerae into the skin, injects cytolytic enzymes and feeds on partly digested tissue. This causes irritation and, with successive attacks, the development of a hypersensitivity reaction. Mite numbers are greatest in late summer in temperate areas, though present throughout the year in tropical regions.

Dermanyssus

This genus includes the 'red mite' of poultry, *D. gallinae*, which is also found on pigeons, wild birds and occasionally mammals, including humans. The adult is about 1 mm long and spider-like in appearance with long legs and pointed mouthparts (see Figure 3.12). In the unfed state it is greyish-white, becoming red when it takes a blood meal. Anaemia will result if sufficient numbers of mites are present.

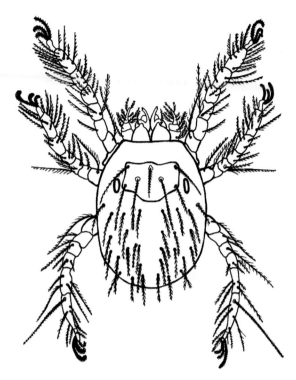

Figure 3.23 Larva of the European harvest mite, *Neotrombicula*. Redrawn after Wall and Shearer, 1997.

Dermanyssus is nocturnal, leaving its favoured habitats (e.g. crevices in wooden poultry houses) only to feed. Eggs are laid off the host and the life-cycle can be completed in as little as one week, so large populations can build up quickly. Numbers are highest in winter. The larvae do not feed, but the two nymphal stages and the adult do. Adults can survive several months without feeding, so empty poultry houses, aviaries and nests can act as a reservoir of infestation for future occupants or farm workers.

A related genus, *Ornithonyssus* (which includes the northern and tropical fowl mites), is very similar to *Dermanyssus* in many ways but has more hairs on its body. It has ensured itself a constant food-source by adapting to near-permanent residency on its host. The nasal mite, *Pneumonyssus*, has gone one step further by adopting a specialised habitat providing greater warmth and humidity. Infestation with the canine species is mostly subclinical but rhinitis and other problems may occur.

Help box 3.4

Summary of mite infestation – which infests what

	Cattle	Sheep	Pig	Horse	Dog	Cat	Rabbit	Birds	Humans	Notes
Subsurface mites										
Sarcoptes	▼	▼	▼	▼	▼	(1)	▼		▼(2)	Different strains
Knemidocoptes								▼		
Demodex	▼	▼	▼	▼	▼	▼	▼		▼	Different species
Surface mites										
Psoroptes	▼	▼		▼			▼			(3)
Chorioptes	▼	▼		▼						Same species
Otodectes					▼	▼				Same species
Cheyletiella					▼	▼	▼		(4)	Different species
Other mites										
Trombiculids	▼	▼	▼	▼	▼	▼	▼	▼	▼	Wide host range
Dermanyssus								▼	(4)	

(1) Cats have *Notoedres*, but *Sarcoptes* can occur; (2) both human strain and zoonotic infestations occur; (3) cattle/sheep same species; others different; (4) zoonotic infestation.

Extra information box 3.5

Varroa in bee-hives

Parasitism by mites is not confined to warm-blooded animals. Many use invertebrates. A relevant example is *Varroa destructor* which lives in bee-hives. It lays its eggs in the central brood-rearing area and feeds on bee larvae and adults by sucking haemolymph. This weakens the bees and makes them prone to other diseases and debilitating factors. European bees are very susceptible and, since its introduction in the 1970s, *Varroa* has slowly swept across the continent causing considerable damage to bee colonies. The mite is now almost global in distribution.

3.4 Other arthropods

The great majority of parasitic arthropods are insects, ticks or mites, but some crustaceans also impact veterinary medicine. The Crustacea differ from other arthropods in that each of their legs has a segmented branch. The group contains shrimps, lobsters, barnacles, etc. Also included are copepods and crabs that act as intermediate hosts for parasites with aquatic phases in their life-cycle, such as the pseudophyllidean tapeworms (see Section 5.4.1), some zoonotic trematodes and the anisakid roundworms (see Section 9.3.1).

The tongue worm, *Linguatula*, is worthy of brief consideration as a curiosity occasionally brought to animal clinics for identification. This strange creature belongs to a group of uncertain taxonomy. They are usually assigned to the Crustacea but some experts consider them to be a separate Phylum. The adult, which can grow to more than 10 cm in length, lives in the nasal passages of vertebrates. Their elongated bodies are transversely striated with four small claws at the broader anterior end (see Figure 3.24). Eggs are expelled with nasal discharges or swallowed and passed in the faeces. If ingested by a grazing animal, the hatched larva migrates to a mesenteric lymph node where it develops to become an infective nymph inside a small cyst (< 1 mm). The final host become infected if it eats raw or under-cooked viscera. The nymph crawls into the nasal passages via the soft palate. Tongue worms survive about a year and can provoke sneezing, coughing and a wet nose. The veterinarian is usually consulted when an adult *Linguatula* is forcibly ejected from the nose of a sneezing dog in view of the owner.

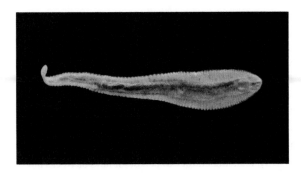

Figure 3.24 *Linguatula* sneezed out by a greyhound.

Extra information box 3.7

Sea lice

Sea lice are of major economic importance to the fish farming industry in both Northern Europe and North America. Although called 'lice', they are crustacean and in no way related to the Phthiraptera. Sea lice are red-brown in colour and often described as looking like tiny horseshoe crabs. The females grow to 1 cm long and trail long egg sacs behind them. They have five pairs of legs, three for swimming and two pairs that assist eating.

The life-cycle is complex but can be briefly summarised as follows: eggs are released from egg sacs into the environment; they hatch to produce, in succession, two nonparasitic larval stages and seven parasitic larval stages before reaching the adult stage. This takes 3 weeks to 4 months, depending on water temperatures.

Migrating wild salmonids often carry low numbers of sea lice. They bring infestation to coastal waters, where large parasitic populations can build up on farmed fish in sea cages. Sea lice browse on the epidermis using a mouth tube with a toothed ridge. Heavy infestations cause abrasions and haemorrhage, and are also immunosuppressive. This lowers productivity and creates a welfare problem.

3.5 Ectoparasiticides

Ectoparasiticides are chemicals used for the control of parasites on, or in, the skin or hair coat. The term 'veterinary ectoparasiticide' encompasses both veterinary insecticides (active against insects) and veterinary acaricides (active against ticks and mites), as the same compounds are often, but not always, effective against both types of arthropod. A further term 'endectocide' is sometimes used to describe the macrocyclic lactones, reflecting their spectrum of activity which embraces a wide selection of endoparasites as well as some ectoparasites (see Section 7.3.2).

A distinction is made between ectoparasiticides which kill the target organism by interacting with vital body functions and insect growth regulators (IGRs) which function by disrupting developmental processes in juvenile life-cycle stages.

3.5.1 Key concepts

Ectoparasiticides are often applied directly onto the skin or coat by means of sprays, dips, shampoos, powders etc. Alternatively, some are given by mouth or injection so the active ingredient is carried to the skin via the blood-stream.

A convenient and popular method of administration is the 'pour-on' (for farm animals) or 'spot-on' (for pets). These involve relatively small volume liquid formulations that are applied along the dorsal midline at sites that cannot be reached by licking. Two mechanisms enable the active compound to spread from the point of application to the whole body surface (see Figure 3.25):

a – surface diffusion: the active compound spreads out from the point of application by migrating along the lipid layer of the skin;

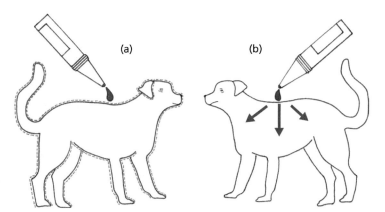

Figure 3.25 How spot-on formulations reach all parts of the skin: a – by surface diffusion; b – distributed via the blood (details in text).

b – transcutaneous: the compound is absorbed locally and distributed via the blood circulation.

Products are also available for household application directly onto carpets, furniture etc. (e.g. to control off-host life-cycle stages of the flea). Large scale environmental use (e.g. for the control of farm animal pests) is, however, generally uneconomic and ecologically unacceptable.

Modes of action

Arthropods are covered by a protective exoskeleton and so ectoparasiticides have to overcome this barrier to exert their toxic effect. There are two main mechanisms for doing this:

a – contact poisons: which are absorbed across the intersegmental membranes that allow component parts of the exoskeleton to move independently;

b – stomach poisons: which have to be ingested before they can be absorbed.

Many ectoparasiticides act on the parasite nervous system at synaptic or neuromuscular junctions. Selective toxicity is achieved in most cases because the arthropod receptor has a greater affinity for the compound ('toxicant') than the mammalian or avian equivalent.

IGRs do not kill adult arthropods directly but interrupt the life-cycle by preventing egg-formation or hatching, and/or larval development, feeding or metamorphosis. These effects can be achieved in two ways:

a – Insect juvenile hormone analogues: these interfere with the hormonal control of sequential development. Examples include methoprene and pyriproxyfen.

b – Chitin inhibitors (also called Insect Development Inhibitors or IDIs): interference with chitin synthesis disrupts the development of vital structures such as larval mouthparts. Examples include cyromazine, dicyclanil and lufenuron.

Both IGR modes of action are specific to insect physiology, hence mammalian toxicity is low.

Special properties

Although all ectoparasiticides used for animal treatment should achieve their therapeutic purpose if used appropriately, there are subtle differences in the way this effect is achieved. An understanding of these properties optimises the choice of product for individual clinical situations.

a – Knock-down: in the broader field of applied entomology, this term describes the ability of a toxicant to bring down a flying insect (without necessarily killing it). In veterinary usage, however, it is employed to describe the immediate effect that a compound has on those ectoparasites present on the animal at the time of treatment. Thus, 'knock-down' is a short-term curative effect providing immediate relief from the deleterious effects of the parasite.

b – Persistent efficacy: some products have residual activity, enabling efficacy to persist for days or weeks after treatment, thereby providing a period of protection from reinfestation. This may result from the toxicant binding to wool, hair or skin, or being released slowly from a body reservoir (for example, sebaceous glands or body fat) or from a device such as a collar, ear-tag or tail-band.

c – Speed of kill: some products have a faster lethal effect than others. This may reflect the inherent biological properties of the compound but can also be influenced by formulation. In the case of flea control, for example, speed of kill for different products ranges from a few minutes to 48 hrs.

d – Repellency: some compounds discourage flies and other arthropods from landing or taking residence on a treated animal. There are two types of repellency:

    i)   vapour phase – the arthropod is affected by the 'smell' of the product. Examples include citrus oils such as Oil of Citronella;

   ii)   contact – the arthropod has to touch the treated surface before it retreats (e.g. synthetic pyrethroids).

e – Antifeeding effects: repellency, a quick knock-down and behavioural changes induced by the compound may, separately or in combination, substantially reduce opportunities for arthropods to bite and feed.

f – Spectrum of activity: narrow spectrum products are active against a restricted range of parasites or life-cycle stages. Broad spectrum products control a wider variety, sometimes including species from widely differing taxonomic groups (e.g. the endectocides).

g – Ovicidal activity: some IGRs (e.g. lufenuron, methoprene, pyriproxyfen) do not kill adult arthropods on the host but prevent them from laying fertile eggs.

h – Larvicidal activity: compounds that target larvae rather than adults can be useful for animal treatments (e.g. to control blowfly strike) or for environmental application (e.g. to control off-host life-cycle stages of fleas).

3.5.2 Some important ectoparasiticides

Historically, a broad spectrum of activity and long persistency were considered essential for ectoparasite control on farm animals. Some sheep dips, for example, gave more than 14 weeks protection against ticks, scab mites and blowfly strike. Such performance came at a cost, however, and substances such as the organochlorines (e.g. DDT and dieldrin) were found to damage ecological systems. Environmental pollution with these compounds led to the accumulation of persistent tissue-residues in wild-life food-chains. The modern approach, therefore, is to use safer and less persistent compounds sparingly in a more sophisticated and targeted manner.

Synthetic pyrethroids

Synthetic pyrethroids (SPs) can often be recognised by their chemical names as these usually end in -methrin (e.g. permethrin). They are surface-acting compounds with a rapid knock-down effect. They are used mainly against nuisance flies, biting flies and lice. Some also have a powerful contact repellent action. This effect is exploited, for example, in impregnated dog collars used to discourage the bites of phlebotomine sandflies (the vectors of leishmaniosis).

When arthropods are exposed to an SP, the permeability of neuronal membranes for Na^+ ions is increased, leading to hyperexcitability and death (see Figure 3.26). This effect is dramatically displayed when an SP spray is used in the home and flies are seen spinning round on the windowsill. Domestic fly sprays may contain piperonyl butoxide as a synergist, which enhances the activity of the SP by inhibiting detoxification enzymes.

Licensed products containing SPs generally have a wide safety margin if used as directed in the product literature. Cats, however, are more sensitive to SPs than other animals and consequently high concentration formulations, such as those used for flea control on dogs, must not be used on this species. Fish and aquatic invertebrates are also very susceptible to SP toxicity and care must be taken to prevent water pollution.

Organophosphates and carbamates

The organophosphates (OPs) and carbamates have been in use for several decades. Most have good on-animal persistency and a broad spectrum of activity against insects, ticks and surface mites. Some have been discontinued because of safety concerns, especially possible neurological effects in humans resulting from repeated low-level exposure (e.g. farmers dipping sheep without

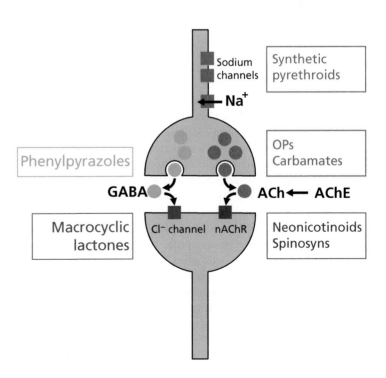

Figure 3.26 Diagrammatic representation of an insect nerve synapse showing the site of action of each major group of insecticides. Adapted from I. Denholm with permission.

adequate protective clothing). Others, e.g. diazinon, continue to meet modern regulatory requirements if used with appropriate precautions. Examples of carbamates currently in use include carbaryl and propoxur.

Both these groups act as anticholinesterases (see Figure 3.26). By inhibiting the enzyme cholinesterase, they prevent the breakdown of acetylcholine (ACh) at neuromuscular junctions following neural discharge. Accumulation of ACh leads to paralysis and death.

Neonicotinoids and spinosyns

These are both relatively new chemical groups already widely used in crop protection. At the time of writing, only a few such compounds, including imidacloprid, nitenpyram and spinosad, have been developed for veterinary use, mainly for flea control.

The neonicotinoids are synthetic compounds while the spinosyns are metabolites formed during a fermentation process employing a soil-dwelling actinomycete. The two groups act on different sets of postsynaptic nicotinic acetylcholine receptor binding sites (nAChRs). This disrupts the nervous system (see Figure 3.26). Selective toxicity is thought to be due to a dissimilarity of insect and mammalian nAChRs.

Macrocyclic lactones

The macrocyclic lactones (MLs) are based on fermentation products from different species of the mould *Streptomyces*. They are used mostly for worm control (i.e. as anthelmintics) and are discussed in greater detail in Section 7.3.2. Some MLs, such as ivermectin, doramectin and moxidectin, are anthelmintics which also have useful insecticidal and/or acaricidal properties. Selamectin was developed specifically as a flea-control product but it also has useful activity against a range of other ectoparasites and nematodes in pet animals. MLs are systemic drugs with greatest potency against tissue-dwelling and blood-sucking arthropods.

MLs act by opening glutamate-gated chloride channels in postsynaptic membranes, producing hyperpolarisation and inhibiting neurotransmission (see Figure 3.26). Some individual dogs, most often rough-coated collies, lack an efflux transporter protein that removes ML from the CNS (central nervous system), allowing toxic, and sometimes fatal, concentrations to accumulate. MLs licensed for use in dogs, such as selamectin (for flea control) or ivermectin (for heart-worm control), were selected for this purpose as they carry only a low risk of CNS toxicity at the dose-rate recommended for that particular usage.

Phenylpyrazoles

Compounds in this group, including fipronil and pyriprole, are used mostly for flea and tick control on pet animals. They block transmission of signals by the arthropod inhibitory neurotransmitter GABA and inhibit the flux of Cl⁻ into nerve cells (see Figure 3.26). They are contact poisons. Fipronil attains its persistency by accumulating in sebaceous cells and being released slowly onto the skin.

Other ectoparasiticides

Amitraz

Amitraz acts on receptor sites of the invertebrate neurotransmitter, octopamine, thereby increasing nervous activity. It has been employed for many years in cattle dips and sprays, particularly in regions where tick resistance to other acaricides is a problem. It is now used mostly in small animal medicine for the treatment of demodicosis, a condition that does not always respond satisfactorily to other therapies. It is also useful in tick control on dogs as even sublethal doses disrupt attachment behaviour and have an anti-feeding effect. It also causes rapid detachment of ticks that are already established. These effects can be used to reduce the risk of Lyme disease and other conditions which are transmitted by ticks at a late stage of the feeding process.

Metaflumizone and indoxacarb

These, at the time of writing, are the most recently introduced compounds for flea control, belonging to the semicarbazone and oxadiazine chemical groupings, respectively. Both block Na⁺ channels in nerve axon membranes, thereby preventing the passage of nerve impulses and causing paralysis and death. Indoxacarb is a pro-drug that requires bioactivation by enzymes in the insect's mid-gut. Metaflumizone is active against ticks as well as fleas.

Inert inorganic insecticides

Fine-flowing powders have been prepared from inert substances such as sodium polyborate, which can be used in homes infested with fleas or other arthropod pests (e.g. dust mites). The powder is blown under pressure into cracks in floors and walls, the pile of carpets, furniture etc. They appear to act by desiccating the organism or by clogging its respiratory spiracles.

3.5.3 Insect growth regulators

By interrupting arthropod life-cycles at the egg or larval stages (see Section 3.5.1), IGRs can be useful adjuncts to conventional ectoparasiticides. They can be used in a number of ways:

a – To prevent cutaneous myiasis: the presence of IGR residues in the fleece of summer grazing sheep, for example, will ensure that larvae hatching from clusters of eggs deposited by blowflies will fail to develop to a stage that can cause significant damage. Cyromazine and dicyclanil are used in this way.

b – To prevent contamination of domestic environment: in flea control, treating animals with an IGR, such as lufenuron, will ensure that, should infestation of a pet animal occur, any eggs dropping to the ground will be sterile and therefore unable to contribute to the environmental reservoir of developing off-host life-cycle stages (see Section 9.2.3).

c – To aid control of off-host life-cycle stages: in a flea-infested household, larval habitats can be targeted:

   i)   directly, by spraying IGRs onto 'hotspots' (see Section 2.2.2);

   ii) indirectly, by appropriate animal treatments with some IGRs (e.g. pyriproxyfen), which result in trace amounts being subsequently transferred from the animal's coat to its close environment (e.g. its blanket) in amounts sufficient to eliminate any larvae that may be developing there.

d – To prevent development of resistant strains: IGRs (e.g. methoprene) are sometimes administered in combination with an ectoparasiticide so that any treatment survivors will produce only infertile eggs. This prevents any selection for resistance genes that might otherwise occur.

3.5.4 Problems with ectoparasiticides

Some ectoparasiticides can be hazardous if used carelessly. The risk is particularly high when they are being used in large volumes in sprays or baths. These often have to be prepared by diluting potentially dangerous concentrates. Appropriate safety precautions, such as wearing protective clothing (see Figure 3.27), must be adopted in these circumstances. Environmental protection measures may

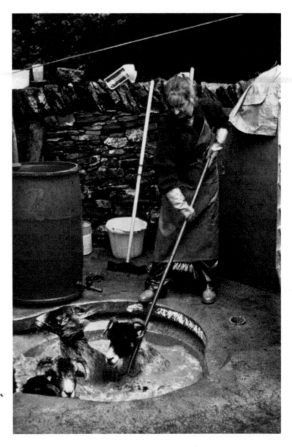

Figure 3.27 Dipping sheep: note the protective clothing in use. The facemask on the wall is used when handling concentrated solutions for preparing or replenishing the dipwash. Reproduced with permission of C. Lewis © 2014 Eli Lilly and Company or affiliates.

also be needed. In some countries, such as the UK, only trained and certificated operators are allowed to perform certain procedures.

Particular hazards associated with ectoparasiticides include:

a – Acute toxicity: to the animal being treated, to people preparing or administering the medication and to those who handle treated animals.

b – Chronic toxicity: animal handlers may suffer as a result of repeated low level exposure to some toxicants if appropriate precautions are not taken. This may come about by aerosol inhalation as well as by splashing onto the skin.

c – Residues: good compliance with product withdrawal periods safeguards against residues in meat and milk, but the wool industry has to cleanse fleeces before further processing to ensure that there are no undesirable residues in textiles and carpets.

d – Environmental contamination: to protect waterways and groundwater reservoirs, high volume sprays or dips must not be used where run-off from treated animals, or the disposal of surplus materials, might cause pollution.

e – Resistance: the development of parasite populations resistant to chemicals that were previously effective is a problem that seriously impacts livestock management systems in many regions (e.g. tick and blowfly control in Australia; sheep scab in South America, etc.). An overview of the nature of resistance and strategies for its control was provided in Chapter 1 (see Section 1.6.3).

CHAPTER 4

Protozoa (single-celled parasites)

4.1 Introduction

Although protozoa are single-celled organisms, they are not necessarily primitive. They have much greater complexity than other unicellular life-forms, such as bacteria. Like multicellular animals and plants, their DNA is mostly packaged into chromosomes within a nucleus. They have many subcellular structures similar to those in metazoan cells but, in addition, each protozoan species possesses specialised organelles that enable it to live and function as an independent organism within its own ecological niche. Most protozoa are free-living although many coexist with animal hosts. This chapter focuses on those that are potentially pathogenic. Many others are benign ('commensals') or even beneficial to their host, e.g. the symbionts that digest cellulose in the rumen or caecum of herbivores.

Principles of Veterinary Parasitology, First Edition. By Dennis Jacobs, Mark Fox, Lynda Gibbons and Carlos Hermosilla.
© 2016 John Wiley & Sons, Ltd. Published 2016 by John Wiley & Sons, Ltd.
Companion website: www.wiley.com/go/jacobs/principles-veterinary-parasitology

Practical tip box 4.1

Diagnosis of protozoal disease

Care! Finding protozoa in faeces or other diagnostic materials does not necessarily identify the cause of the disease under investigation. Many protozoa are harmless inhabitants of the alimentary tract, especially in herbivores. Even some potentially pathogenic protozoal infections can be asymptomatic unless the host is stressed or otherwise compromised.

4.2 Key concepts

4.2.1 Classification

There is a great diversity of pathogenic protozoa. Those of greatest economic, welfare or zoonotic significance are covered below, but many others are encountered less frequently or are yet to be recognised as pathogens. A simplified classification chart (see Figure 4.1) makes a useful framework for understanding veterinary protozoology as it reflects differences in structure, behaviour and life-cycle, which, in turn, often determine disease processes.

4.2.2 Locomotion

One of the most obvious features separating the major protozoan groups is the way they move, as summarised in Table 4.1.

Ciliates (see Figure 4.2) can be recognised by the thousands of tiny hairs ('cilia') covering the body surface. To propel the organism along, these bend in coordinated ripples (like Mexican waves round a sports stadium).

Amoebae are amorphous jelly-like blobs (see Figure 4.3) that progress by pushing out a finger-like protrusion ('pseudopodium') which enlarges as cytoplasm flows

Table 4.1 Some important characteristics of major protozoan groups

	Locomotion by:	Intracellular stages?
Ciliates	Cilia	No
Amoebae	Pseudopodia	No
Flagellates	Flagellae	Some spp.
Apicomplexa	Gliding	Yes

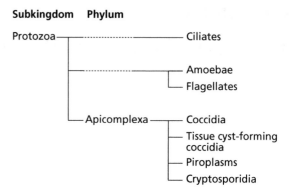

Figure 4.1 The major groups of protozoan parasites of veterinary importance.

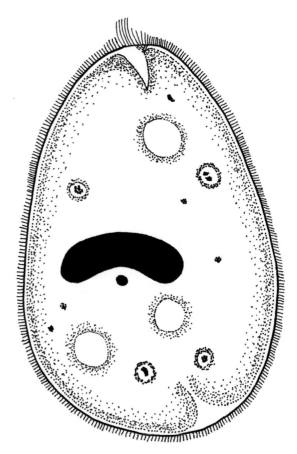

Figure 4.2 *Balantidium* trophozoite. Redrawn after Cheng, 1986 with permission of Elsevier.

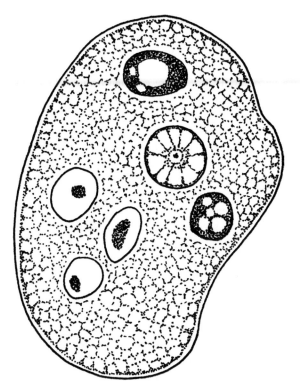

Figure 4.3 *Entamoeba* trophozoite. Redrawn after Jeanne Robertson from Roberts and Janovy Jr, 1996 with permission of McGraw-Hill Education.

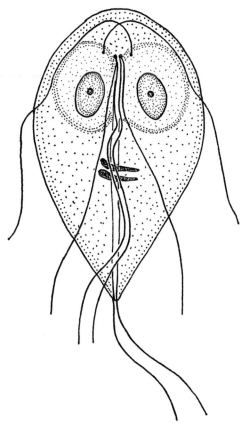

Figure 4.4 *Giardia* trophozoite. Redrawn after William Ober from Roberts and Janovy Jr., 1996 with permission of McGraw-Hill Education.

into it. Amoebae need a suitable substrate for active movement.

The flagellates, in contrast, are strong swimmers employing one or more long contractile fibres ('flagellae' – see Figure 4.4) that flex in a whiplike fashion. They are well suited for life in blood or other body fluids.

The intracellular life-cycle forms of apicomplexans are immobile but the forms that leave one host cell to find another, such as the *Toxoplasma* merozoites illustrated in Figure 4.5, have sleek, crescent-shaped bodies that appear to glide along a spiral trajectory. This effect is achieved by intracellular contractile microfilaments that induce subtle alterations along the body surface. These propel the organism along an excreted slime trail in a manner analogous to the progress of a snail. Once a suitable host cell is located, penetration is achieved by means of a specialised structure, the 'apical complex'.

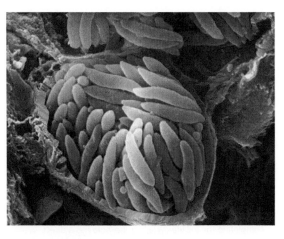

Figure 4.5 Schizont: SEM (with artificial colouring) showing merozoites (pink) within host cells (blue). Reproduced with permission of D.J. Ferguson.

4.2.3 Nutrition

Protozoa feed mainly on particulate material. The cell membrane indents and folds slowly over, thereby entrapping a small quantity of food and drawing it into the cell. This process is known as pinocytosis or phagocytosis, depending on the size of the particle (in ascending order). In ciliates, food particles are directed by the action of cilia towards the base of a funnel-like structure (the 'cytostome'). When sufficient food has accumulated in this, a vacuole forms which is engulfed into the cytoplasm. Many parasitic protozoa are also able to absorb liquid nutrients and in some cases this may be their main source of nourishment.

The feeding stage in a protozoan's life-cycle is called a 'trophozoite'. For many species this is the only form that exists, but others have a succession of stages with different functions, appearances and, of course, names.

4.2.4 Transmission

Trophozoites adapted to a parasitic existence are often vulnerable to unfavourable conditions in the external environment. Those of many species, therefore, secrete a protective wall around themselves to form a resistant 'cyst' prior to leaving their host.

Passage from host to host can take place in many ways, ranging from passive transfer of trophozoites or cysts (by faecal-oral transfer, for example) to transmission of various life-cycle stages by arthropod vectors or the ingestion by carnivores of organisms within intermediate hosts.

Extra information box 4.1

Explanation of life-cycle jargon

Protozoan life-cycles can be direct (i.e. completed without an intermediate host) or indirect (with an essential intermediate host) and, for simplicity, this is the terminology used in this book. Other terms may be found elsewhere:

Homoxenous (or monoxenous) The parasite uses a single host species during its life-cycle, e.g. *Eimeria* (see Section 4.6.2);
Heteroxenous More than one host is needed for the parasite to pass through all its different life-cycle stages, e.g. *Babesia* has to alternate between a mammalian host and a tick vector (see Section 4.8.1);
Facultatively heteroxenous The parasite needs more than one host if it is to pass through all its different life-cycle stages, but it can nevertheless sustain the species without completing the full life-cycle, e.g. *Isospora* has a direct life-cycle maintained by faecal-oral transmission, but some species can, in addition, utilise an optional intermediate host (see Table 4.4).

4.2.5 Reproduction

All protozoa reproduce asexually (i.e. by mitosis), although many are able to exchange genetic material within the species. Ciliates, for example, have both a macro- and a micronucleus (see Figure 4.2) and occasionally come together ('conjugate') to switch micronuclei.

The apicomplexans have complex life-cycles, which, in addition to asexual divisions, also include a sexual phase during which male and female gametes are formed by meiotic division. In some genera, the fertilised cell generates a protective wall to become an 'oocyst' (see Figure 4.6).

Asexual reproduction can occur in different ways depending on species and life-cycle phase:

a – Binary fission: the nucleus divides and the cytoplasm parts to form two similar daughter organisms.

b – Budding: the cytoplasm divides unequally so that small offspring bud off from a parent cell.

c – Multiple fission: this is a prolific type of asexual multiplication seen particularly in the Apicomplexa. It is also known as schizogony or merogony. The nucleus replicates repeatedly but the cytoplasm does not divide until shortly before the cell (now termed a 'schizont' or 'meront') bursts to release numerous daughter organisms ('merozoites').

d – Sporogony: this term is used to describe the cell divisions that occur within an apicomplexan oocyst (see Figure 4.6). As a result of this process, mature ('sporulated') oocysts contain two or more infective organisms ('sporozoites'), often arranged in bundles within separate enclosing walls ('sporocysts'). The number of sporocysts and sporozoites within an oocyst is a useful characteristic for diagnostic purposes.

4.3 Ciliates

The ciliates are generally harmless commensals. They are easily recognised by the hairs (cilia) covering the body, the funnel-shaped depression leading to the mouth (cytostome) and the kidney-shaped macronucleus (see Figure 4.2). The small micronucleus is less obvious.

Balantidium and similar genera occur in the lumen of the large intestine of pigs, cattle, primates and some other animals. The trophozoites are about 80 µm long and may become invasive if the intestinal mucosa is damaged by another pathological process (see Figure 4.7). This

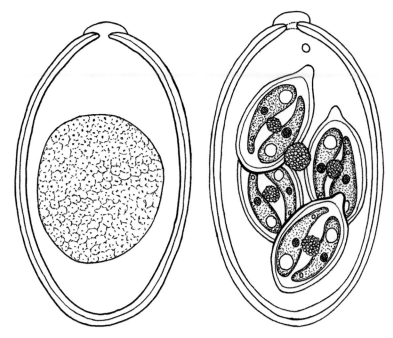

Figure 4.6 *Eimeria* oocysts: unsporulated (left); sporulated (right). Based on Roberts and Janovy Jr, 1996. Reproduced with permission of McGraw-Hill Education.

process can lead to ulceration and dysentery in pigs and primates (including humans).

Infections spread by excretion of cysts in host faeces. The cysts are slightly smaller than the corresponding trophozoite. They are thick-walled, but this does not obscure the macronucleus which provides a useful diagnostic feature (see Figure 4.8). Human and canine infections are usually derived from pigs.

4.4 Amoebae

Amoebic infections are often caused by opportunistic free-living aquatic species that take advantage of chance encounters with susceptible hosts (such as humans in a contaminated swimming pool).

One species, *Entamoeba histolytica*, is a true parasite transmitted by the faecal-oral route. It provokes a

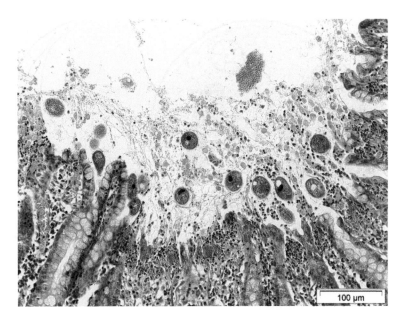

Figure 4.7 *Balantidium* trophozoites on eroded surface of large intestine.

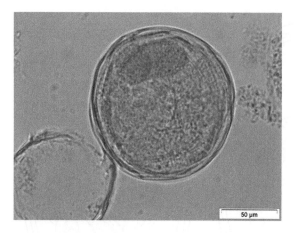

Figure 4.8 *Balantidium* cyst: note macronucleus in upper part of cyst.

disease called amoebic dysentery in primates and can pass from humans to dogs and cats. It occurs more commonly in warmer climates.

Faecal smears from infected patients may contain motile amoebae (see Figure 4.3) or small (10 μm) cysts containing four nuclei (see Figure 4.9). Autopsy will reveal deep ulcers in the large intestine and abscesses in the liver.

4.5 Flagellates

The flagellates are those protozoa propelled by one or more whiplike contractile fibres. Most are commensals

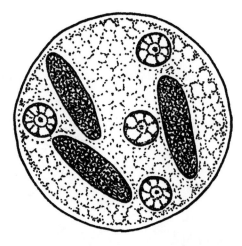

Figure 4.9 *Entamoeba* cyst. Redrawn after Jeanne Robertson from Roberts and Janovy Jr, 1996 with permission of McGraw-Hill Education.

or symbionts although some are dangerous pathogens. It is convenient to divide the latter into the haemo-flagellates (see Section 4.5.1) that live within body tissues, particularly blood and lymph, and those that do not penetrate into the tissues but remain within the lumen of the alimentary tract, uterus or prepuce (see Section 4.5.2).

4.5.1 Haemoflagellates

The haemoflagellates include two major genera: *Trypanosoma* and *Leishmania*, both of which are of greatest importance in tropical and subtropical climates.

Both genera have indirect life-histories that include a succession of morphologically different life-cycle stages. There is little purpose in describing those that occur in the insect vector as they currently have little diagnostic application, but the two forms found in the mammalian host are:

a – Trypomastigote: this is found in blood plasma and is typical of all *Trypanosoma* species (see Figure 4.10). It is elongated, motile and has a long flagellum which is partly bound to the body and partly free.

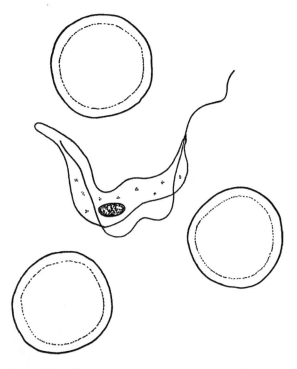

Figure 4.10 A *Trypanosoma* trypomastigote surrounded by red blood cells.

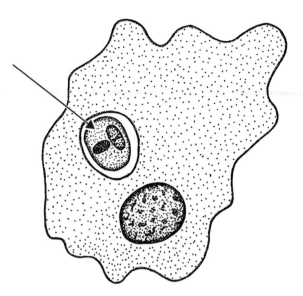

Figure 4.11 A *Leishmania* amastigote (arrowed) in the cytoplasm of a host cell. Redrawn after IPZ, S. Ehrat from Deplazes *et al.*, 2013 with permission of Enke Verlag.

b – Amastigote: this is the intracellular form (see Figure 4.11). It is rounded with a rudimentary flagellum. Not all haemoflagellates have an amastigote stage, but it is a feature of *Trypanosoma cruzi* and *Leishmania* infections.

Trypanosoma

Trypanosomes are responsible for serious disease in humans (sleeping sickness in Africa and Chagas disease in parts of Latin America). They also impose severe constraints on agricultural production throughout large areas of sub-Saharan Africa, inflicting death and chronic disease on both food-providing ruminants and the draught animals needed to cultivate crops and to carry produce to market.

Trypomastigotes of *Trypanosoma* are mostly around 20 µm in length, although some species are longer and some shorter. A single flagellum originates near the hind end of the organism from a dark-staining basal body ('kinetosome'). It meanders initially along the length of the body and is held in place by the 'undulating membrane' which gives the trypanosomes their characteristic appearance (see Figure 4.10). The remainder of the flagellum lies free and protrudes anteriorly. Trypanosomes swim with a corkscrew movement.

Life-cycle

Most trypanosomes have indirect life-cycles using insect vectors which become infected while taking a blood meal from a mammalian host. After an initial period of multiplication in the insect gut, the life-cycle proceeds in one of two ways, depending on species:

a – Salivarian transmission: trypanosome species using tsetse-flies as vector pass forward from the insect gut to the salivary glands where they multiply. The next time the fly feeds, infective organisms in its saliva are inoculated into a new host animal.

b – Stercorarian transmission: trypanosome species that use reduviid bugs or keds as vector multiply in the rectum of the insect and are transmitted when it defecates onto the skin of the next host it feeds upon. The excreted trypanosomes have to be rubbed into the bite wound, other abrasion or onto a mucous membrane (such as the conjunctiva) for the life-cycle to proceed.

There are, however, two trypanosome species of veterinary importance that do not multiply within a vector. The first of these, *T. evansi*, relies on mechanical transfer of infected blood from host to host by tabanid flies, stable flies or vampire bats. If any of these are disturbed while feeding, they will seek a new animal to satisfy their appetite. Trypanosomes transported in this way will die if not quickly transferred to a new host.

Another species, *T. equiperdum*, does not use a vector at all but is transmitted directly from host to host during coitus. It is therefore a venereal parasitosis.

After entering a new host, trypanosomes multiply in the skin, causing a transitory inflammatory swelling before entering the blood-stream. In most *Trypanosoma* species, the trypomastigotes stay in the blood to replicate by binary fission. Those of *T. cruzi*, however, do not divide but instead enter various tissues of the body and proliferate as intracellular amastigotes before reentering the circulation as a new generation of trypomastigotes.

Epidemiology

The distribution of the various trypanosome-associated diseases is largely dependent on the presence and abundance of potential vectors. Different species of tsetse fly, for example, have different feeding preferences and are restricted to either riverine, savannah or forest habitats in sub-Saharan Africa. The reduviid bugs that carry *T. cruzi* are found in parts of Latin America living inside buildings. They emerge from their hiding places at night to take blood meals.

Help box 4.1

> ### Reminder: incidence and prevalence
>
> Incidence: the number of new cases of infection per unit time
> Prevalence: proportion of host population infected at a point in time

Host factors can also influence the incidence and severity of disease. Some indigenous breeds of African cattle, for example, are less vulnerable to the effects of infection than imported European cattle. Trypanotolerant wild animals can remain parasitaemic for prolonged periods without showing signs of disease, thereby acting as reservoirs of infection. *T. brucei* infects antelope as well as cattle, horses and donkeys in Africa, while *T. cruzi* infects armadillos and possums as well as humans in South America.

Susceptible animals that survive the acute phase of infection are able to mount an effective immune defence but this gives only temporary protection. African trypanosomes are able to evade host immune responses by varying the surface antigens on their glycoprotein coat (by a number of processes including trans-splicing RNA). This they can do repeatedly, thereby outmanoeuvring each successive immune attack. The result of this see-saw battle between host and parasite is a relapsing parasitaemia (see Figure 4.12).

Pathogenesis

The pathogenicity of trypanosomosis varies with host species and breed, and with parasite species and strain.

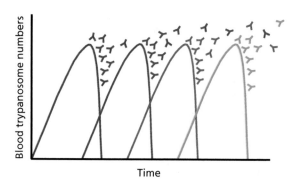

Figure 4.12 Diagrammatic representation of the relapsing parasitaemia associated with trypanosomosis. Each coloured curve depicts the number of trypanosomes expressing a particular surface antigen. Host antibodies generated in response to each antigen are represented by 'Y'-shaped symbols in the corresponding colour.

Infections are usually chronic with fever and malaise marking each parasitaemic episode. Lymph nodes and spleen are swollen due to plasma cell hyperplasia, which in turn leads to high nonspecific IgM blood levels and eventually to lymphoid exhaustion. Immunity to other pathogens is thereby compromised. Animals also develop a haemolytic anaemia and there is progressive weight-loss. Fertility and work capacity are reduced.

T. cruzi infections are generally asymptomatic but considerable tissue damage can accrue in humans as a result of intracellular parasite replication in heart, oesophageal and intestinal muscles.

Table 4.2 Some important *Trypanosoma* species

	Host	Zoonotic?	Vector	Transmission	Distribution	More information
T. congolense	Wide host range	▼	Tsetse fly	Salivarian	Sub-Saharan Africa	
T. brucei	Wide host range, varies with subspecies	▼▼▼ (some subspecies cause sleeping sickness)	Tsetse fly	Salivarian	Sub-Saharan Africa	2.2.5 8.2.3
T. vivax	Wide host range		Tsetse fly	Salivarian	Africa, South America	
T. evansi	Wide host range	▼	Biting flies, vampire bats	Mechanical	North Africa, Asia, Latin America	
T. equiperdum	Horse		None	Venereal	Mediterranean area, South Africa, South America	9.1.4
T. cruzi	Armadillo, possum, human	▼▼▼ (Chagas disease)	Reduviid bug	Stercorarian	Latin America	2.2.4 9.3.2

Important trypanosomes

Tsetse-transmitted species

T. congolense, T. brucei and *T. vivax* are all major pathogens of cattle in sub-Saharan Africa, although they affect other domesticated animals and wild reservoir hosts as well (see Table 4.2). *T. congolense* and *T. vivax* are responsible for both acute and longer-term disease while *T. brucei* tends to be more chronic. There are several subspecies of *T. brucei*, some of which are more important as human pathogens while others are primarily of veterinary significance. The clinical picture associated with *T. brucei* infection is complicated by the fact that it can invade extravascular tissues such as myocardium and CNS.

Trypanosoma evansi

T. evansi is spread mechanically in North Africa and Asia by biting flies and, in Latin America, also by vampire bats. The associated disease is called 'surra' and occurs mainly in cattle, buffalo, pigs, horses and camels, but *T. evansi* can infect many other animals as well.

Trypanosoma equiperdum

The venereally transmitted *T. equiperdum* replicates in subcutaneous and other tissues provoking transitory urticarial plaques and oedema of the genitalia and adjacent tissues. Progressive loss of condition and neurological complications may lead to a fatal outcome. Donkeys are often asymptomatic. This condition is known as 'dourine' and occurs widely but has been eradicated in North America, most European and some other countries.

Leishmania

Leishmania species are closely related to the trypanosomes. Only one morphological form, the amastigote, occurs in mammalian hosts. This is found inside phagocytic cells such as macrophages, monocytes and polymorphonuclear neutrophils. The amastigote is oval with a rudimentary flagellum that does not protrude beyond the body (see Figure 4.11). *Leishmania* is responsible for serious disease in humans, dogs and wild animals (see Figure 4.13). About 30 morphologically indistinguishable species have been recorded,

mainly in the Mediterranean region and parts of Asia, South America and Africa. The European species is *L. infantum*, but this comprises several distinct strains ('zymodemes').

Life-cycle

Each species of *Leishmania* uses a specific phlebotomine sandfly vector. Infected host cells are ingested when the fly takes a blood meal. The organism multiplies in the insect gut and migrates to the proboscis where it waits to be inoculated into a new host. Transmission can also take place if the fly is crushed onto abraded skin. Successive cycles of replication follow in the mammalian host as amastigotes multiply within and then destroy their host cells before seeking others to parasitize.

Epidemiology

Disease risk is largely determined by the distribution of the sand-fly vectors: *Phlebotomus* spp. in the Old World and *Lutzomyia* spp. in the Americas. In Europe, canine leishmaniosis is particularly prevalent along the Mediterranean coast, with some inland foci of transmission. Many infected dogs are asymptomatic. These provide an unsuspected source for onward transmission to other dogs or humans. There are also reservoirs of infection in some wild animals, especially rodents.

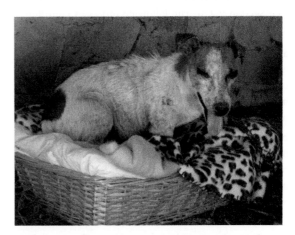

Figure 4.13 Cutaneous leishmaniosis: an advanced case showing ulceration on the nose and general alopecia. Reproduced with permission of L.H. Kramer.

Leishmaniosis is not endemic in northern Europe, although isolated cases do occur. This happens as local dogs have no opportunity to develop immunity and are therefore highly susceptible to infection if taken south on vacation. Such animals are a potential danger to their owners and in-contact pets at home as mechanical transmission can take place in the absence of sand-flies if infected material is rubbed into a skin abrasion (see Section 9.3.2).

A well-documented outbreak of leishmaniosis, caused by a particular strain of *L. infantum,* occurred recently in hunt kennels in New York State. Infected fox-hounds plus a few dogs of other breeds have since been found in other parts of the USA. Circumstantial evidence suggests that, with no sandflies in the region, direct transmission by close contact may have been responsible in this instance. Infection can also be passed from dog to dog by blood transfusion.

Dogs are the main reservoir for human infection in the Mediterranean basin and parts of South America. Wild animals play a significant role in many rural environments, although human-to-human transmission via sandfly bites predominates in some regions.

Pathogenesis

Leishmaniosis is a slowly progressing and relapsing disease. Young dogs are most vulnerable. The first clinical signs may not become evident until months or years after infection. The events taking place during this long incubation period are complex and lead to two main clinical presentations in dogs: cutaneous and visceral (see Section 9.2.3). The following processes contribute to these outcomes:

a – Macrophage destruction: The continuing infection and disruption of large numbers of macrophages provokes the formation of granulomatous lesions in many tissues, including the skin. These give rise to loss of hair, ulceration and other dermatological signs.

b – Reticulo-endothelial involvement: Amastigotes become disseminated throughout the reticulo-endothelial system and infect cells of the monocyte-macrophage line causing generalised swelling of lymph nodes (lymphadenopathy) and enlargement of the spleen.

c – Immune-complex formation: The parasites induce an exaggerated antibody response. As a result, immune-complexes are deposited in a number of locations producing polyarthritis, inflammation of and protein-loss from renal tubules (glomerulonephritis), ocular lesions and other deleterious effects.

4.5.2 Other flagellates

Although the flagellates covered in this section do not invade host tissues, they are nevertheless very damaging in their different ways. *Giardia* is a common cause of diarrhoea, with an estimated two million human cases occurring annually in the USA, for example. This parasite is also found in wild and domesticated mammals. The trichomonads are a group of parasites responsible for diseases ranging from infertility in cattle and digestive upsets in cats to feeding problems in birds. *Spironucleus* is a common cause of mortality in game bird poults, while *Histomonas* is responsible for 'blackhead' in turkeys. All reproduce by binary fission and have simple, direct life-cycles. *Giardia* and *Spironucleus* encyst to enhance their chances of survival outside the host, but the trichomonads are transmitted as naked trophozoites. *Histomonas* is unique in that it uses a nematode worm to transport itself from host to host.

Giardia

Giardia may be found in the upper small intestine of a wide range of mammalian hosts (see Figure 4.14). Although it can provoke acute, intermittent or chronic diarrhoea of varying severity, many infections are asymptomatic. There are several species but that of greatest importance in veterinary and human medicine is *G. duodenalis* (also known as *G. intestinalis* or *G. lamblia*). Accumulating evidence suggests that *G. duodenalis* is not a single species but a series of morphologically identical forms with differing biological attributes that can only be differentiated at a molecular level.

Giardia trophozoites are 15–20 μm long and pear-shaped with four pairs of flagellae (see Figure 4.4). They are bilaterally symmetrical with a separate nucleus on either side of the body (see Figure 4.15). They also have a large anterior disc used for attachment to the intestinal wall (see Figure 4.16).

Because the epithelial cells lining intestinal villi are continually being shed (as part of a normal physiological

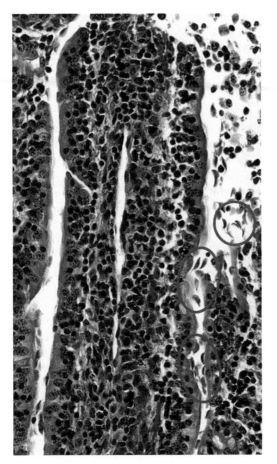

Figure 4.14 *Giardia* in small intestine: trophozoites (circled) can be seen between villi, some adhering to the epithelium. Reproduced with permission of AHVLA, Carmarthen © Crown copyright 2013.

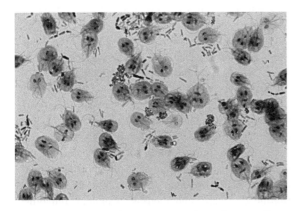

Figure 4.15 *Giardia* trophozoites growing in a culture medium.

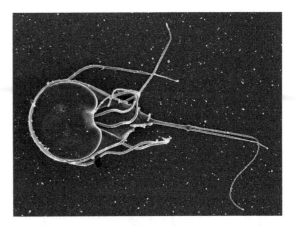

Figure 4.16 SEM of *Giardia* trophozoite showing attachment disc and flagellae. Reproduced with permission of R.C.A. Thompson.

process), *Giardia* trophozoites have to relocate at frequent intervals. Heavy infections may be associated with a flattening of the intestinal mucosa (villous and crypt atrophy), leading to decreased production of digestive enzymes, malabsorption of nutrients, enhanced gut motility and consequently weight loss.

Trophozoites finding themselves in the lower small intestine form resistant cysts (see Figure 4.17). These are ovoid, measure 10 µm in diameter and have four nuclei. They are passed in the faeces of infected animals at irregular intervals, commencing a few days after infection. They are immediately infective and can be transmitted to a new host by faecal-oral transfer or via faecal contamination of drinking water.

After the cyst is swallowed, the released organism immediately splits into four individuals, thereby enhancing its chances of establishing in its new host. Serious disease can be initiated by ingestion of just a few cysts, which is why polluted water supplies can be a potent source of infection.

Epidemiology

Giardia infections may be abbreviated by host immune responses or they can persist for many months. Prevalence rates up to 15% have been recorded in European and North American dogs and cats, with the highest figures coming from urban areas and in younger animals. Such statistics, however, tell only part of the story, as the percentage of the host population carrying the

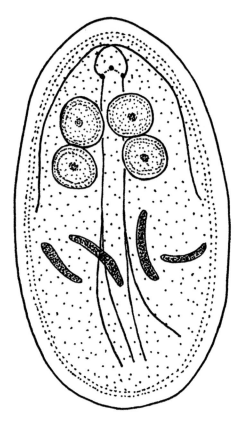

Figure 4.17 *Giardia* cyst. Redrawn after William Ober from Roberts and Janovy Jr., 1996 with permission of McGraw-Hill Education.

various *G. duodenalis* genotypes (called 'assemblages') varies considerably from place to place. This is of veterinary public health significance as not all genotypes occurring in pet animals are potentially zoonotic (see Table 4.3).

Table 4.3 Major *Giardia duodenalis* genotypes

Assemblage	Species name*	Host specificity	Hosts
A, B	A – *G. duodenalis*	Broad	Human, dogs, cats, livestock and wildlife
	B – *G. enterica*		
C, D	*G. canis*	Narrow	Dogs
E	*G. bovis*	Narrow	Livestock
F	*G. cati*	Narrow	Cats
G	*G. simondi*	Narrow	Rats

* These are proposed species names not yet in common usage at the time of writing.

Two assemblages, A and B, have a very broad host range and these are the ones that pose a zoonotic hazard. There are well-documented cases of human epidemics being caused by the contamination of rivers or reservoirs with *Giardia* cysts originating from wildlife (e.g. beavers) or grazing livestock. There is also the possibility of direct faecal-oral transmission from pets to humans, or vice versa. Other assemblages are host specific and so household dogs infected with C or D, or cats with F, are unlikely to expose their owner to any risk. The part played by pets in the epidemiology of human giardiosis and the reverse role of humans in initiating canine/feline disease is still ill-defined and is the subject of on-going investigation.

Trichomonads

Many trichomonad species are commensals in the large intestine but some are pathogenic. Genus names within the group often reflect the number of forward-pointing flagellae. A feline example has five such flagellae and is therefore called *Pentatrichomonas*. An exception is *Trichomonas gallinae* which has four anterior flagellae. *T. gallinae* causes a serious and often fatal disease in pigeons and wild birds (e.g. finches) characterised by necrotic nodules in the oesophagus and crop.

The most important trichomonad in veterinary practice is *Tritrichomonas foetus*, which causes reproductive problems in cattle and digestive disorders (typhlocolitis) in cats.

Bovine trichomonosis

T. foetus is a venereally transmitted trichomonad that lives in the uterus of cows and the preputial cavity of bulls. It occurs worldwide, although it has become rare or absent in countries where artificial insemination is widely employed.

This pear-shaped protozoan is 10–25 μm long. It has three anterior flagellae and another projecting backwards which is bound by an undulating membrane for most of its length (see Figure 4.18). When seen in vaginal or preputial washings, the organisms swim with jerky movements. The body is supported by an obvious longitudinal rod ('axostyle').

Chronically infected bulls show no clinical signs. In cows, infection may induce early abortion or may manifest as an irregular oestrous cycle or infertility. Uterine discharge, endometritis, pyometra and other reproductive dysfunctions may also occur.

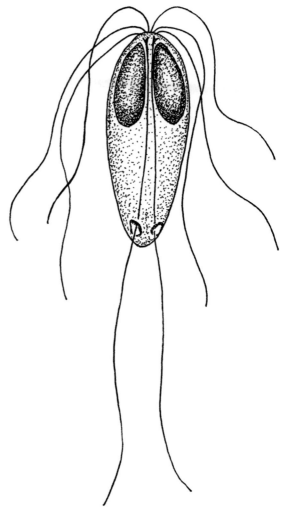

Figure 4.19 *Spironucleus.* Redrawn from Perdue *et al.,* 2008 with permission of the American Association for Laboratory Animal Science.

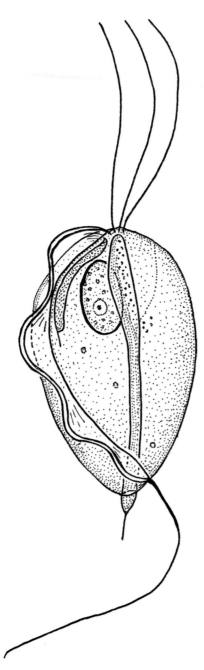

Figure 4.18 *Tritrichomonas foetus.* Redrawn from William Ober from Wenrich and Emmerson, 1933 in Roberts and Janovy Jr, 1996 with permission of McGraw-Hill Education.

intestine of turkeys and game birds. It causes infectious catarrhal enteritis in poults but older birds are often symptomless carriers. *Spironucleus* is small (less than 10 μm) and when seen in mucosa scrapings moves characteristically fast and straight. It is bilaterally symmetrical with a nucleus and three flagellae on each side of a narrow body. A further two flagellae trail behind (see Figure 4.19).

Histomonas

Histomonas infects turkeys, game birds and free-range chickens. The associated disease, infectious

Spironucleus

This flagellate was until recently called *Hexamita*. It resides in the lumen and crypts of the upper small

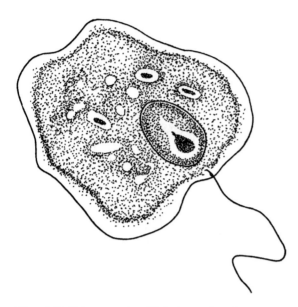

Figure 4.20 *Histomonas meleagridis.* Redrawn after Cheng, 1986 with permission of Elsevier.

entero-hepatitis, is known colloquially as 'blackhead' as the head and wattle sometimes become cyanotic (blue, due to deficient blood supply). It is seen mostly in young turkeys and there can be a high mortality rate.

Histomonas is irregularly round or oval, measuring between 6 and 20 μm (see Figure 4.20). A single flagellum is present on histomonads in the caeca, but not on those in the liver.

Infection can take place by simple faecal-oral transfer within a contaminated area. Wider transmission, however, is an intricate process which starts when an intestinal histomonad invades the tissues of another parasite co-inhabiting the caeca of the avian host. This is the nematode worm, *Heterakis* (see Section 7.1.3). The protozoan travels to the ovary of the worm and is incorporated into an egg which eventually passes into the environment with the bird's droppings. The worm eggs are tough and long-living. If an egg is subsequently ingested by an earthworm, the nematode larva contained within hatches and remains inside its newly adopted transport host. Thus, the histomonad is now inside a nematode larva which, in turn, is inside an earthworm (see Figure 4.21). If and when the earthworm is caught and eaten by another bird, two parasitic transmission cycles (*Heterakis* and *Histomonas*) are completed.

On arrival in a new host, histomonads invade the caecal wall and multiply, producing ulcers. They travel by way of the hepatic portal system to the liver where they continue to reproduce, forming necrotic lesions throughout the parenchyma. In histological section, the parasites do not stain readily and appear as pale, amorphous 'ghosts' (see Figure 4.22). It is not known if these histomonads return to the intestine or if their presence in the liver is accidental and a biological dead-end.

4.6 Coccidia

4.6.1 General characteristics

The coccidia are a very large group containing many parasites of considerable importance to veterinary and human medicine. They may be divided into those genera that produce tissue cysts in intermediate hosts (discussed in Section 4.7) and those that do not. Some, such

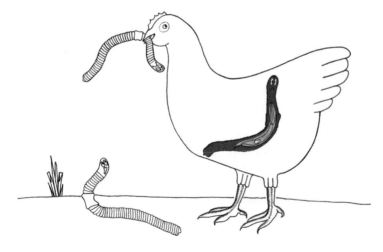

Figure 4.21 Transmission of *Histomonas*: the histomonad (yellow) is inside the nematode larva (blue), which is inside the earthworm (red), which has been swallowed by the bird.

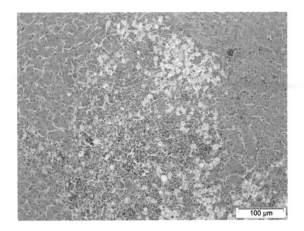

Figure 4.22 Histomonads in the liver: the parasites appear as pale pink 'ghosts'.

as *Isospora*, do not fall conveniently into either category but seem to be intermediary as they do not form tissue cysts seen by light microscopy, yet molecular evidence suggests genetic affinity with those that do.

Coccidian life-cycles form a chain of increasing complexity ranging from the 'simple' pattern displayed by *Eimeria*, which undergoes sexual and asexual development in the same host, via *Sarcocystis*, which alternates between final and intermediate hosts, to *Toxoplasma* and *Neospora*, which can cycle indefinitely in intermediate host populations but retain the genetic advantages of sexual replication when opportunity arises (see Table 4.4).

The dominant genus amongst the 'simple' coccidia (i.e. those that do not form tissue cysts) is *Eimeria*. This is of greatest significance in the poultry industry but it also causes disease in ruminants and some other animals. *Isospora* is of relatively minor importance but can be detrimental to the health of piglets, dogs and cats.

Another genus, *Cryptosporidium*, which until recently was considered an atypical 'simple' coccidian, is now known to be a very distant relative. As it differs fundamentally in some aspects of its biology, it will be considered separately (in Section 4.9).

4.6.2 *Eimeria*

The genus *Eimeria* is widespread in nature with multiple species occurring in virtually every vertebrate host. With a few exceptions, all *Eimeria* species are host specific. Most inhabit the epithelial lining or deeper tissues of the alimentary tract, although a few are found in other locations such as bile ducts or renal tubules. Many are relatively harmless but others are serious pathogens.

Life-cycle

In broad outline, the *Eimeria* life-cycle involves three stages of replication (see Figure 4.23):

a – Schizogony: This initial phase of abundant asexual reproduction takes place in the host.

b – Gametogony: Prolific sexual replication follows, the products of which are egg-like 'oocysts'.

c – Sporogony: A more modest phase of asexual division occurs within the oocyst after it has been shed into the environment.

During sporogony, the fertilised cell divides into four pairs of daughter organisms (sporozoites). Each pair of sporozoites is held within an enclosing wall (the 'sporocyst'). Thus, an *Eimeria* oocyst contains four sporocysts each containing two sporozoites (see Figure 4.6). The oocyst is now capable of infecting a new host and is said to be 'sporulated'.

Table 4.4 Examples of coccidian life-cycles

Genus:	Tissue cyst forming?	Life-cycle[1]	Transmission
Eimeria	No	One host only	Horizontal
Isospora	No	Some species: FH →FH only Other species: FH→FH ↔ (IH optional)	Horizontal
Sarcocystis/ Besnoitia[2]	Yes	Alternating FH ↔ IH	Horizontal
Neospora/ Toxoplasma	Yes	IH ↔ IH (↔ FH optional)	Horizontal and vertical

[1] FH = final host; IH = intermediate host; [2] the life-cycle of *Besnoitia* is still poorly understood.

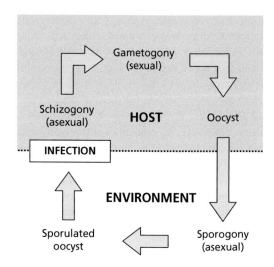

Figure 4.23 Overview of *Eimeria* life-cycle (details in text).

cycle stage of each *Eimeria* species has its own particular predilection site along the alimentary tract.

b – The parasite grows within the host cell and divides by multiple fission ('schizogony') to form a bunch of banana-shaped daughter organisms ('merozoites') called a 'schizont' (see Figure 4.5).

c – The host cell bursts and merozoites disperse to invade further epithelial cells. Each *Eimeria* species has a fixed number of schizogony cycles (usually two to four). Depending on species and stage of infection, therefore, the merozoite either develops into another schizont or progresses to the next phase of the life-cycle (gametogony).

d – A merozoite entering gametogony develops either into a single female macrogametocyte, which grows to occupy most of the volume of its host cell, or into a male microgametocyte, which divides to become a mass of small motile male gametes. On their release, these seek out and fertilise macrogametocytes.

e – A protective wall forms around the zygote forming the oocyst. This is released into the intestinal contents (or into the bile ducts or renal tubules in the case of hepatic or renal species).

f – The oocyst is not infective until it has sporulated. This happens only after the oocyst has exited the host. Sporogony is temperature dependent and will occur only if there is sufficient humidity and oxygen. Transmission is by direct faecal-oral transfer.

More detail has to be added to the above overview of the *Eimeria* life-cycle to provide an adequate foundation for understanding the epidemiology, pathogenesis, diagnosis and control of coccidiosis (see Figure 4.24):

a – When a sporulated oocyst is swallowed by a suitable host, the sporozoites contained within are released and each invades an epithelial cell. Every life-

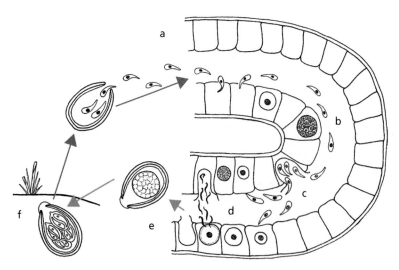

Figure 4.24 Life-cycle of a typical *Eimeria* species: a – sporozoites from swallowed oocyst invade intestinal cell; b – schizogony; c – merozoites released; d – gametogony; e – oocyst formation and release; f – sporulation (details in text which uses same lettering as shown above). Based on Soulsby, 1982 with permission of Wolters Kluwer Health - Lippincott, Williams & Wilkins.

Help box 4.2

Summary of names used in *Eimeria* life-cycle

Life-cycle phase	Life-cycle stages*
Schizogony (1st asexual phase – in host)	Schizont[1] $\Rightarrow$ Merozoites
Gametogony (sexual phase – in host)	Microgametocyte[2] $\Rightarrow$ Male gametes (microgametes)
	Macrogametocyte[3] $\Rightarrow$ Female gamete (macrogamete) $\Rightarrow$ Oocyst
Sporogony (2nd asexual phase – inside oocyst)	Sporocysts $\Rightarrow$ Sporozoites

* Some textbooks use an alternative terminology: [1]meront; [2]microgamont; [3]macrogamont.

Epidemiology

Eimeria oocysts are ubiquitous, robust and able to survive months or years in the environment. They are blown about as dust particles and strict biosecurity is required to minimise the introduction of infectious material into buildings. Chicks become infected by pecking the ground when placed into a poultry house. Organisms derived from a single infection go through the succession of parasitic developmental stages synchronously and leave the body almost simultaneously as oocysts. The coccidian life-cycle is therefore self-limiting in the absence of reinfection, although in reality most hosts are continually exposed to reinfection.

Help box 4.3

Definition: prepatent period

Strictly speaking, the prepatent period is the time that elapses between infection of a host and the ability of a clinician to demonstrate the presence of the aetiological agent by any means (observation, serology etc.). In parasitology, the term is usually confined to the interval between infection and the appearance of life-cycle stages in faeces, blood or other sampled fluid or tissue. In the case of coccidia, the onset of patency is indicated by the occurrence of the first oocysts in avian droppings or mammalian faeces.

A 'patent' infection is one where, for example, oocysts, eggs or larvae are being shed into the environment, or infective forms (such as trypanosomes) are circulating in the blood.

The phases of asexual and sexual multiplication taking place during the coccidian life-cycle ensure that for every oocyst ingested by a host, the potential exists for many thousands to be subsequently passed. The prepatent period varies with species but is usually about a week, so the generation time is short. Sporulation of oocysts can happen in as little as 2–3 days if environmental conditions are optimal. The biotic potential of the parasite is therefore enormous and massive infections can build up very rapidly. A protective immunity develops but only slowly. So, in agricultural systems with high stocking densities, the situation can become explosive if precautionary measures are not taken. There is no cross immunity between species, so hosts surviving infection with one species remain vulnerable to others.

Practical tip box 4.2

Diagnosis of coccidial infections by faecal or litter examination

Coccidian oocysts are usually round or ovoid and can vary from 10 to 50 μm in length depending on species. Care is needed when examining samples as other similarly sized objects, such as pollen grains can easily be mistaken for oocysts (see Figure 4. 25).

Unsporulated oocysts in fresh samples are useful for indicating the presence of a coccidial infection but more information can be gleaned by incubating the material to promote sporulation. This enables *Eimeria* oocysts, which each have four sporocysts containing two sporozoites, to be differentiated from those of *Isospora*, which have two sporocysts each containing four sporozoites.

Species recognition, however, is a job for the expert and is dependent upon observing or measuring the following: size (length and width); shape (oval, round, etc.); thickness and appearance of oocyst wall; colour (colourless, yellow-brown, etc.); and the presence or absence of a micropyle (a 'cap' at one end of the oocyst as can be seen in Figure 4.6). Some species have to be cultured in the laboratory to the sporulated oocyst stage before identification can be made.

Reference is then made to an appropriate identification key. Mixed infections are the rule rather than the exception and so it may be necessary to calculate the proportion of each species in the sample in order to judge clinical significance. Not all species are equally pathogenic and so a high oocyst count is not necessarily indicative of a disease process. To complicate matters still further, oocysts can be absent from host faeces if clinical signs occur during the prepatent period of a highly virulent infection or are due, as in the case of some mammalian infections, to damage persisting beyond the period of patency.

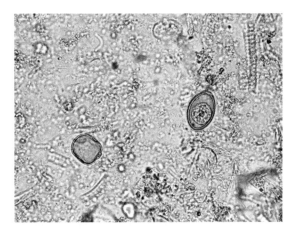

Figure 4.25 An *Eimeria* oocyst (right) and a pollen grain (left).

Pathogenicity

Eimeria species vary considerably in their pathogenicity. The damage they cause depends on the size and position of each life-cycle stage. On this basis, the coccidia are divided into two major clinical categories:

a – The malabsorption group. This includes species in which all life-cycle stages are found in relatively superficial locations along the alimentary tract. Infection induces villous atrophy and mucoid enteritis, but little haemorrhage. The resulting digestive and absorptive abnormalities lead to impaired food utilisation and reduced weight-gain, with diarrhoea in severe cases.

b – The haemorrhagic group. This embraces species which have a particularly large life-cycle stage (often the second generation schizont) situated in a subepithelial position at the base of an intestinal crypt. When parasitized host cells rupture by cytolysis to release the merozoites within, deep erosions are formed and crypt stem cells are destroyed. Thus, in addition to the villous atrophy mentioned above, there is marked haemorrhage into the gut leading to blood stained faeces. The outcome is often severe disease or death.

Histopathology

In histological sections, the mature life-cycle stages (schizogony and gametogony) each have a characteristic appearance although developmental forms can be less easy to recognise. This is not normally a problem as field cases mostly display numerous parasites at various stages of maturation. Thus, a diagnosis of 'coccidiosis' is relatively easy to confirm. To deduce which *Eimeria* species is responsible, however, involves consideration of the location of the lesion along the digestive tract, the size of the parasitized cells and their precise position (e.g. in villous/crypt epithelium or in the lamina propria).

Trophozoites appear in histological section as small, rounded, basophilic objects with a single nucleus. Close inspection reveals that each lies within a parasitic vacuole in the host cell cytoplasm. A mature schizont is a spherical cluster of merozoites. If these are fortuitously cut lengthways, their banana shape is obvious, but more often they are seen in tangential or transverse section as numerous small basophilic oval or circular objects within the cell (see Figure 4.26).

Gametogony (see Figure 4.27) is marked by the presence of macrogametocytes and microgametocytes. The female parasite has a single large nucleus and eosinophilic granules which later become clear wall-forming bodies. These coalesce after fertilisation to form the layers of the oocyst wall. The male organism is multinucleate. As microgametes differentiate, they congregate around the periphery of the cell. Microgametocytes can easily be confused with immature schizonts, but in the former the densely basophilic microgametes often present a characteristic 'swirling' appearance.

4.6.3 Coccidiosis

Avian coccidiosis

Intensive poultry production is dependent upon effective control of coccidiosis (see Section 8.4.1). Five

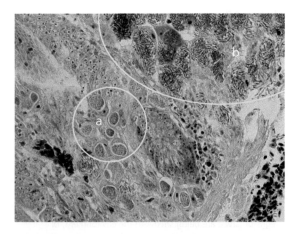

Figure 4.26 An *Eimeria* infection – section of caecal wall showing schizogony: a – immature schizonts; b – mature schizonts.

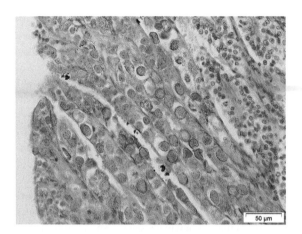

Figure 4.27 An *Eimeria* infection – section of intestinal wall showing gametogony with numerous macro- and microgametocyes. A few oocysts (with dark staining walls) can also be seen.

of the seven *Eimeria* species in chickens are of major economic importance. Turkeys have a different set of seven species. Buildings and management systems must be designed, maintained and fine-tuned to minimise opportunity for oocysts to accumulate and sporulate. The judicious use of chemoprophylactic medication or vaccination is often an integral component of control programmes, but should augment, not replace, good husbandry practices.

Mammalian coccidiosis

While coccidia are of greatest importance in poultry, they can also cause disease in mammals. Sheep and cattle have numerous *Eimeria* species (see Section 8.2.1); horses just one (see Section 9.1.1); while pigs can have both *Eimeria* and *Isospora* (see Section 8.3.1). The only 'simple' coccidian genus in dogs and cats is *Isospora* (see Section 9.2.1), although oocysts of several tissue-cyst forming genera may also be passed with their faeces.

Many coccidian species in mammals are of little pathogenic importance and high faecal oocyst counts may be found in healthy animals. Pathogenicity is related to the size, position (whether superficial or deep) and location of the life-cycle stages. For instance, some pathogenic species in ruminants grow into large macroschizonts (over 300 µm in diameter and containing hundreds of thousands of merozoites) within endothelial cells lining the lymphatic vessels in intestinal villi (lacteals). Coccidia developing in the small intestine may cause

digestive disturbances, while those in the large intestine interfere with water absorption. If tissue destruction is confined to a small area, the disease process is ameliorated by physiological compensation in unaffected parts. Extensive mucosal damage, however, requires a prolonged recovery period after removal of the parasites.

As exposure leads to protective immunity, disease (usually watery diarrhoea or dysentery along with weight loss) is usually seen in young animals and is often associated with overcrowded or unhygienic conditions. Adult animals often have low-level subclinical infections and thereby act as a source of contamination for the environment into which their offspring are born.

4.7 Tissue cyst-forming coccidia

The tissue cyst-forming coccidia include *Toxoplasma*, which is a major zoonotic hazard responsible for widespread disease, including abortion and stillbirths in sheep and humans; *Neospora* and *Besnoitia*, whose detrimental effects include significant losses to the cattle industry; and others that are mostly of lesser or uncertain clinical significance, such as *Sarcocystis* and the minor genera *Hammondia* and *Frankelia*.

Despite ongoing research, large gaps in scientific knowledge and understanding of the tissue cyst-forming coccidia still exist. For example, the life-cycles of *Besnoitia besnoiti* and *Sarcocystis neurona* have yet to be fully elucidated. Another major pathogen, *Neospora caninum*, remained unrecognised until the 1980s and important information on its biology continues to emerge. It is likely that the occurrence or clinical significance of others in the group await discovery.

The life-cycles of the tissue cyst-forming coccidia vary in complexity and detail but all involve a final host and an intermediate host (see Figure 4.28). The sequence of events in the final host is generally similar to that occurring in the 'simple' coccidia (see Figure 4.23), i.e. infection leads to schizogony followed by sexual reproduction and the production of oocysts, which subsequently sporulate to attain infectivity. In this case, however, the sporulated oocysts have two sporocysts each containing four sporozoites.

Further stages of prolific intracellular asexual multiplication take place in an intermediate host. Initially, waves of rapid replication are associated with the widespread dissemination of organisms (called 'zoites' or

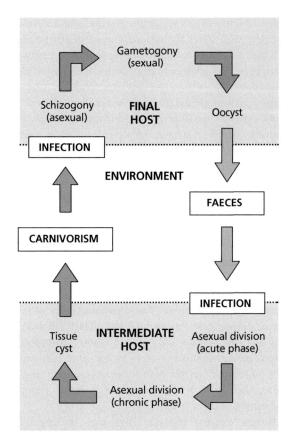

Figure 4.28 Overview of the general life-cycle of tissue cyst-forming coccidia (details in text).

'tachyzoites') throughout the body. Eventually, this acute phase of infection is superseded by slowly-dividing intracellular organisms that produce parasitic tissue cysts. The size, structure and locality of the cysts vary between genera and species. By the time the cyst is fully formed, it is packed with numerous banana-shaped organisms ('bradyzoites' or 'cystozoites') which are now infective and waiting for their host to be eaten by another animal suitable for the continuation of the life-cycle.

4.7.1 *Sarcocystis*

There are many different species of *Sarcocystis*. The intestinal life-cycle stages in the final host are non-pathogenic. The tissue cysts ('sarcocysts') in the intermediate host are also innocuous in most cases. The most serious pathogenicity associated with this genus occurs during the intervening acute phase of infection in the intermediate host and is characterised by transitory, but sometimes serious, pyrexia. The true incidence of this condition is unknown but is probably more common than generally realised. *S. neurona*, is particularly troublesome as it causes equine protozoal myeloencephalitis (EPM), the most commonly diagnosed neurological condition of horses in the USA. Other species, such as *S. cruzi* and *S. suicanis*, have been associated with chronic wasting disease in cattle and pigs, respectively.

Each species of *Sarcocystis* is host specific, generally alternating between one final and one intermediate host. The names of newly discovered species reflect this strict rotation. Thus, *S. suicanis* has the pig as intermediate host and the dog as final host. Unfortunately, the rules of international zoological nomenclature do not allow this practice to be applied retrospectively and long-standing species such as *S. cruzi* have to keep the name they were originally given.

Although there are some variations that affect pathogenicity and diagnosis, the life-cycle of *Sarcocystis* (see Figure 4.29) is otherwise very similar to the general outline given for the tissue cyst-forming coccidia (see Figure 4.28):

a – The final host is infected by swallowing tissues containing a sarcocyst.

b – Organisms (bradyzoites) invade the small intestine and penetrate deeply into subepithelial tissues. There is no schizogony phase and so the bradyzoites develop directly into gametocytes. The oocysts that eventually form take a long time to work their way passively from the lamina propria back to the lumen of the intestine. Consequently, they are released gradually over a prolonged period (weeks or months), by which time they have already sporulated.

c – The oocysts have a very delicate wall (see Figure 4.30) which soon disintegrates so 'naked' sporocysts are passed out with the faeces. The life-cycle continues if and when these are swallowed by an intermediate host.

d – Initially, rapid asexual multiplication takes place within vascular endothelial cells. Other cell types may be used in later stages, depending on species.

e – The tissue cysts (sarcocysts) develop slowly within striated muscle cells (see Figure 4.31). Eventually they become surrounded by a thick outer wall with

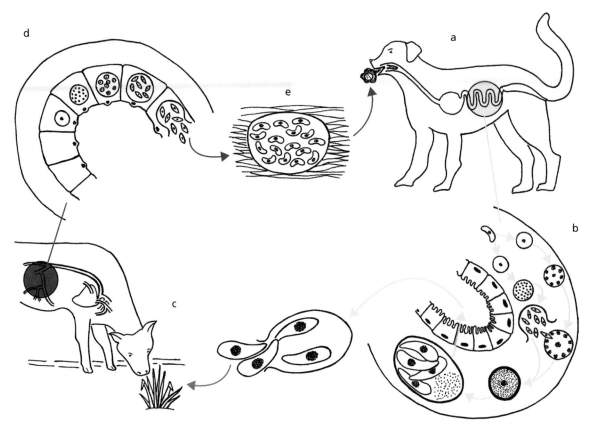

Figure 4.29 Life-cycle of a typical *Sarcocystis* species: a – tissue cyst swallowed by final host; b – gametogony in intestinal lamina propria; oocysts form and sporulate; c – sporocysts released and swallowed by intermediate host; d – rapid asexual reproduction in cells lining blood vessels; e – tissue cysts form in muscles and fill with infective bradyzoites (details in text). Redrawn from Dubey, 1976 with permission of the American Veterinary Medical Association; sporocyst redrawn after Roberts and Janovy Jr, 1996 with permission of McGraw-Hill Education.

internal partitions forming compartments that fill with bradyzoites.

Dogs and cats act as final hosts for a number of *Sarcocystis* species. Together, these infect a wide range of intermediate hosts including cattle, sheep and pigs. Dogs are also responsible for some of the sarcocysts found in horses. Humans can be a source of contamination for cattle and pigs.

Sarcocysts vary in size from microscopic to several centimetres in length according to species and stage of development (see Figure 4.32). Larger ones may result in infected carcases being condemned on aesthetic grounds at meat inspection.

Practical tip box 4.3

Detection of *Sarcocystis*

There is rarely any cause for diagnosticians to look for *Sarcocystis* in faecal samples but naked sporocysts may occasionally be found fortuitously during routine faecal examination (see Figure 4.30). They are small (up to 15 μm) and usually very few in number.

Sarcocysts in meat appear as ivory-white streaks or nodules. In pigs, care is needed to distinguish them from *Trichinella* cysts (see Section 7.1.6) and histology may be required to confirm diagnosis.

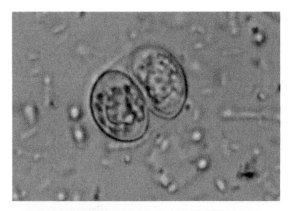

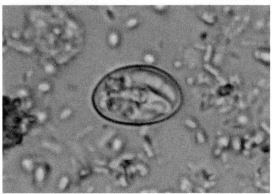

Figure 4.30 *Sarcocystis*: sporulated oocyst (above) and naked sporocyst (below) – not to same scale. Reproduced with permission of J.W. McGarry.

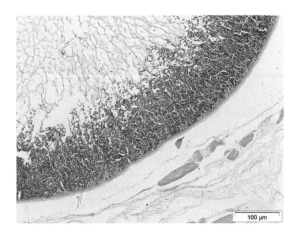

Figure 4.31 Section through part of a sarcocyst showing numerous banana-shaped bradyzoites clustered inside the periphery of the cyst.

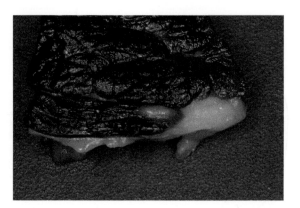

Figure 4.32 A sarcocyst in beef. Reproduced with permission of AHLVA, RVC Surveillance Centre © Crown copyright 2013.

Sarcocystis neurona

Sarcocystis neurona is the causal agent of equine protozoal myeloencephalitis, an emerging disease in the Americas (see Section 9.1.4). It has certain species of American opossum as final host. The natural intermediate host is unknown but sarcocysts develop in experimentally infected racoons and some other animals.

S. neurona is unusual and dangerous because it attempts to establish in some animals that are not true intermediate hosts. These aberrant hosts, which include the horse, are physiologically incapable of supporting the whole life-cycle. Consequently, the parasite undergoes the early stages of asexual multiplication in the CNS but fails to form infective sarcocysts.

Disease similar to that seen in horses also occurs in some wild animals, e.g. Californian sea-otters, causing welfare and conservation issues. Equine cases have occasionally been diagnosed in parts of the world where there are no opossums, suggesting the existence of other *Sarcocystis* species or related genera which can produce similar effects. A *Sarcocystis* species is known to cause meningoencephalitis in European and North American pigeons.

4.7.2 Besnoitia

Bovine besnoitiosis is widely distributed in Africa and Asia. It also occurs in southwest Central Europe where the endemic zone has been steadily extending in recent years.

Besnoitia is similar to *Sarcocystis* in that it has an alternating carnivore-herbivore two-host life-cycle. Unlike *Sarcocystis*, the intestinal phase in the final host includes

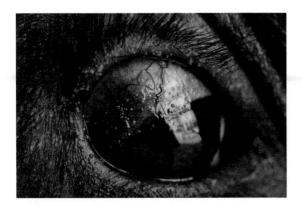

Figure 4.33 *Besnoitia* cysts on the conjunctiva of a cow. Reproduced with permission of A. Gentile.

both schizogony and gametogony and thus conforms more closely to the general life-cycle illustrated in Figure 4.28. The oocysts are released soon after they are formed and sporulate in the external environment. They are similar in appearance to those of *Toxoplasma* (see Figure 4.36).

In the intermediate host, asexual division occurs first in endothelial cells and then in a variety of tissues. Ultimately, bradyzoites form and accumulate within fibroblasts and epithelial cells which swell to produce firm nodules 0.5 – 1 mm in diameter (see Figure 4.33). Parasitized cells are surrounded by a thick hyaline capsule (see Figure 4.34). Cysts are particularly numerous in subcutaneous tissues, muscle fascia and blood vessel walls, but can be found in the supporting connective tissue of any organ, including the eye and testes.

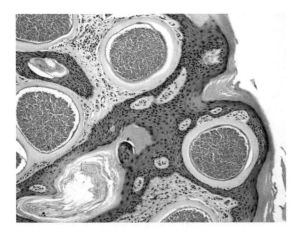

Figure 4.34 *Besnoitia* cysts containing bradyzoites in bovine skin. Reproduced with permission of G. Militerno.

The final host for *B. besnoiti*, the causal agent of bovine besnoitiosis, is unknown but wild felids are suspected. Tissue cysts have been found in some wild ungulates although disease has not been reported in these. The epidemiology is poorly understood but there is a suggestion that biting flies, such as tabanids and stable flies, can act as mechanical vectors, allowing horizontal transmission to take place between cattle.

The disease in cattle varies greatly in severity between individuals with the worst cases progressing from an acute febrile phase to a chronic form characterised by thickened skin, alopecia and loss of condition, sometimes with cysts visible on the conjunctivae.

4.7.3 *Toxoplasma*

There is only one known species in this genus, *Toxoplasma gondii*, but it is nevertheless one of the most widely distributed of all parasites as it can utilise almost any warm-blooded animal as intermediate host. Only felids, however, can act as final host.

T. gondii is responsible for serious disease in intermediate hosts, especially humans and sheep. Most infections are, however, relatively innocuous because:

a – not all *T. gondii* genotypes are virulent; and

b – host immunity generally develops quickly after exposure.

The biology of this parasite is complicated but a detailed understanding is required for the provision of effective veterinary, medical and public health advice and control measures.

Life-cycle

In broad outline, the basic life-cycle of *T. gondii* is similar to that of other tissue cyst-forming coccidia (see Figure 4.28) except that there are a greater number of potential routes of transmission between hosts (see Figure 4.35). These are:

a – The feline final host can become infected in **two** ways:

  i)   by eating tissues from an intermediate host harbouring tissue cysts (e.g. natural predator – prey relationships);

  ii) by ingesting sporulated oocysts from the environment (i.e. faecal – oral transmission).

Of these, the first route is the more efficient as almost all susceptible cats infected this way start to shed oocysts within 3–10 days. In contrast, infections take

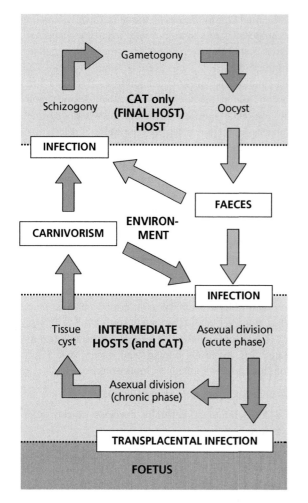

Figure 4.35 Overview of *Toxoplasma* life-cycle (details in text).

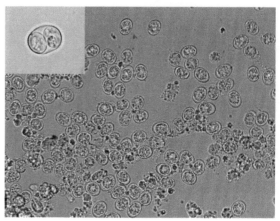

Figure 4.36 Unsporulated *Toxoplasma* oocysts from cat faeces. Inset (at higher magnification): a sporulated *Toxoplasma* oocyst. Reproduced with permission of D. Buxton.

longer to become patent and establish in fewer than 50% of cats swallowing sporulated oocysts.

b – Intermediate hosts can acquire infection in **three** main ways:

i) by ingesting sporulated oocysts from the environment (faecal – oral transmission);

ii) by eating infected tissues from another intermediate host (carnivorism, omnivorism, cannibalism);

iii) vertical transmission (known as transplacental, congenital or prenatal infection). This occurs most frequently in humans, sheep and rodents.

In the special case of farmers, veterinarians or students handling foetal membranes while assisting ewes at lambing time, there is a risk of rubbing infective

material into skin abrasions or transferring organisms to the mouth if appropriate precautions are not taken.

T. gondii infections have also been transmitted as an unintended consequence of transplant surgery.

When a cat becomes infected for the first time, incoming sporozoites or bradyzoites invade enterocytes lining the small intestine and initiate multiple cycles of schizogony. This leads to gametogony with the production and excretion of millions of unsporulated oocysts (see Figure 4.36) over a period of 1–2 weeks. The cat will not shed oocysts again during its lifetime unless immunity wanes or is compromised. *T. gondii* oocysts are very small (~10 μm) and sporulate in 2–3 days in favourable conditions.

Some bradyzoites from ingested tissue cysts penetrate more deeply into the intestinal mucosa and induce a somatic infection culminating in the production of tissue cysts in feline tissues. Thus, the cat acts simultaneously as a final and an intermediate host.

When an intermediate host becomes infected for the first time, the acute phase of infection (see Figure 4.37) continues until the onset of an effective immune response (up to two weeks). At this turning point, any tachyzoites that happen to be travelling around the body will be killed, but those protected inside host cells become slow-dividing, cyst-forming organisms. When mature, the tissue cysts measure 60–100 μm and are spherical or ovoid (see Figure 4.38). They have a thin (< 0.5 μm), elastic outer wall which encloses tens or hundreds of banana-shaped bradyzoites. *T. gondii* cysts

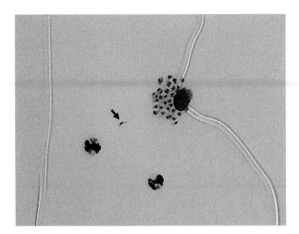

Figure 4.37 Acute *Toxoplasma* infection (brain imprint smear) showing tachyzoites in a host cell and one free tachyzoite (arrowed).

are particularly numerous in muscle and nervous tissues, including the eye, but they can be found in other sites. They retain their viability and infectivity for the lifetime of their host.

If host immunity is compromised at a later date, bradyzoites can escape from their parasitic cysts and revert to replicating rapidly, thereby initiating new generations of tachyzoites. These disperse widely through the body and provoke a recrudescence of clinical signs. This phenomenon, known as postnatal toxoplasmosis, is particularly dangerous in human HIV-AIDS patients. It is also a common complication in dogs suffering with immunosuppressive viruses such as canine distemper.

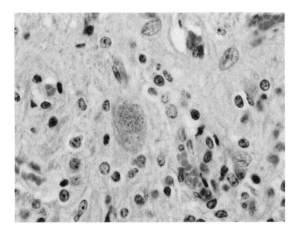

Figure 4.38 *Toxoplasma* tissue cyst in brain of an unborn lamb. Reproduced with permission of D. Buxton.

Extra information box 4.2

Immune effector mechanisms against protozoa

T helper-cells can, through their associated cytokines like IFN-γ, induce the synthesis of active N- and O-metabolites which can kill or damage intracellular infections (e.g. the amastigote stage of *Leishmania* in macrophages). In a separate mechanism, cytotoxic T-cells recognise and destroy infected cells marked by MHC-I. This cannot, however, influence parasites such as *Babesia* and *Theileria* in mammalian erythrocytes, as nonnucleated cells lack MHC-I molecules.

In toxoplasmosis, it is the production of *T. gondii*-specific Th1-cells that forces intracellular tachyzoites to convert into bradyzoites. The Th1-cells secrete the cytokine INF-γ which leads to increased macrophage activation and NO-synthesis. This binds covalently to iron thereby inhibiting the mitochondrial Fe-dependent enzymes that the aerobic tachyzoites need to survive. In contrast, bradyzoites have an anaerobic metabolism and can therefore survive this NO-mediated effector mechanism. This constraint is removed in immunocompromising infections such as HIV which deplete the numbers of functional T helper (CD4$^+$) cells.

Pathogenicity

Intestinal infection in the cat affects only superficial cells at the tips of the villi. Damage is therefore highly localised and damaged cells are quickly replaced. The consequences are, therefore, clinically insignificant.

The initial phase of infection in intermediate hosts can cause acute febrile disease. In humans, this takes the form of a 'flulike' episode, often with swollen lymph nodes. The disease can progress to more serious complications such as pneumonia and encephalitis. Once the acute phase of infection has passed, the tissue-cysts normally cause few problems, unless they are situated in a particularly sensitive tissue such as the retina of the eye. There is a suggestion that *T. gondii* infection could be a risk factor contributing to the onset of specific types of mental illness but this link is as yet unproven.

Transplacental infection happens when a susceptible nonimmune host is exposed to *T. gondii* during pregnancy. During the acute phase of infection, tachyzoites can invade the placenta of some host species (particularly sheep and humans) thereby gaining access to the foetus.

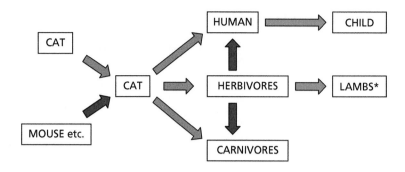

Key:
Red arrow horizontal transmission (carnivorism)
Brown arrow horizontal transmission (faecal-oral)
Pink arrow vertical transmission (transplacental)
*Vertical transmission herbivores – sheep only

Figure 4.39 Overview of the general epidemiology of *Toxoplasma* infections.

Epidemiology

Three factors described in previous paragraphs contribute to the complicated web of transmission pathways utilised by *Toxoplasma* in nature (see Figure 4.39):

i)   Almost any warm-blooded animal can act as intermediate host.

ii) Infection can be transmitted either by ingestion of oocysts from felids or tissues cysts from any intermediate host.

iii) Vertical (transplacental) transmission occurs in some hosts.

Thus, meat-producing animals are generally infected by ingesting oocysts, although lambs can acquire the parasite *in utero* (see Section 8.2.5). Humans can be infected from cat faeces, by eating undercooked meat or congenitally (see Section 9.3.2). In addition, there are many wild-life cycles in which infections are perpetuated by predation, cannibalism or scavenging.

4.7.4 Neospora

Neospora is morphologically identical to *Toxoplasma*, but is biologically and immunologically distinct. The life-history of the main species, *N. caninum*, has only recently been elucidated. Dogs and other canids (e.g. wolves) act as final host, but otherwise the life-cycle has many similarities with that of *T. gondii* (see Figure 4.35). There is, however, one important feature not seen in the *Toxoplasma* life-cycle: tissue cysts persisting in the final host often become reactivated during pregnancy. This results in the production of tachyzoites, which invade the placenta and infect the foetuses. Thus, congenital infection occurs in the canine final host as well as in some intermediate hosts, especially cattle.

N. caninum uses a relatively limited range of intermediate hosts. This includes some bovidae, sheep and wild ungulates. The tissue cysts, measuring 30–100 μm, occur mainly in the central nervous system (see Figure 4.40). They resemble those of *T. gondii* (see Figure 4.38), except that the cyst walls are usually thicker (up to 4 μm).

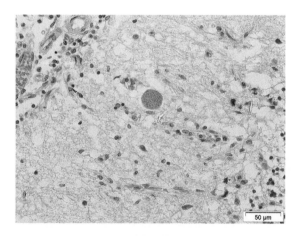

Figure 4.40 *Neospora* cyst in brain section showing bradyzoites within thick (pink-staining) cyst wall.

The daily output of *N. caninum* oocysts from infected dogs is often very small and lasts for two to three weeks. Reinfection sometimes leads to a resumption of oocyst production. The oocysts are similar in size and appearance to those of *Toxoplasma* (see Figure 4.36).

Neosporosis is a serious condition in cattle and dogs (see Sections 8.2.5 and 9.2.4). Vertical transmission is a regular feature in both these species and can happen in successive pregnancies. *N. caninum* is an occasional cause of abortion in sheep, but the extent to which this happens is currently unclear. Another species, *N. hughesi* occurs in horses and is associated with equine myeloencephalitis in the USA and possibly elsewhere, but little is known of its biology.

Bovine neosporosis

Vertical transmission is the most important route of infection for *N. caninum* in cattle and neosporosis is one of the commonest causes of bovine abortion worldwide. Disease is provoked when actively proliferating tachyzoites invade the placenta. Many full-term calves born to infected dams are, however, healthy. Nevertheless, they are likely to be harbouring tissue cysts that will persist into later life. These, in turn, may be reactivated by pregnancy to repeat the process. Vertical transmission within a breeding herd makes control programmes difficult to design and expensive to execute.

The tachyzoites that invade the placenta to induce abortion or effect transmission to the next generation can originate in two ways (see Figure 4.41):

a – Exogenous: due to the recent ingestion of sporulated oocysts (i.e. horizontal transmission from dogs via the faecal-oral route).

b – Endogenous: due to the reactivation of congenitally-acquired tissue cysts (i.e. a long-standing infection derived by vertical transmission).

There is great variability between herds both in the proportion of cows that are seropositive and the rate at which uninfected animals seroconvert (an indication of exposure to sporulated oocysts). As a general rule, dam to calf transmission seems more common than postnatal infection.

Canine neosporosis

Canine infection via horizontal transmission (see Figure 4.41) can occur as a result of eating infected raw meat, foetal membranes or other tissues and can result in neurological disease in dogs of any age, although many infections are asymptomatic. Infected bitches give birth to apparently healthy litters, but a proportion of the pups will nevertheless have acquired infection *in utero*. Some of these are likely to develop myositis and encephalomyelitis with a risk of becoming paralysed during the first months of life.

4.8 Blood-borne apicomplexans

Blood-borne apicomplexans encompass two zoological groups, the haemosporidia and piroplasms, whose life-histories share some broad similarities. Both utilise

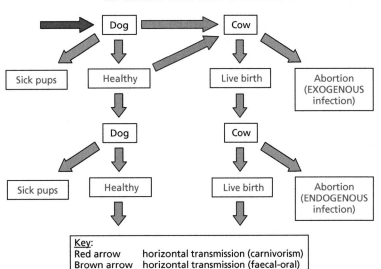

Figure 4.41 Overview of the epidemiology of *Neospora* infections.

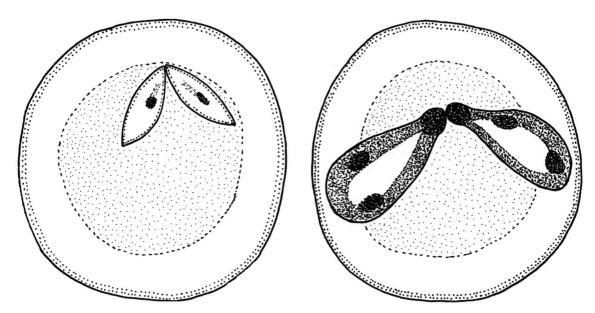

Figure 4.42 Red blood cells containing a small *Babesia* species (left) and a large *Babesia* species (right). (Left: redrawn from Cheng, 1986 with permission of Elsevier; right: drawn from a photomicrograph by © M. Sloboda 2008.)

vertebrate blood cells for part of their life-cycle and both are transmitted by haematophagous arthropods. Sexual reproduction takes places in the invertebrate host giving rise to sporozoites which accumulate in the salivary gland to await onward transmission.

The haemosporidia are primarily of importance in human medicine with several species of the mosquito-borne genus *Plasmodium* being responsible for different forms of human malaria. Another species, *Plasmodium gallinaceum*, causes avian malaria, which is particularly prevalent in SE Asia and the Indian subcontinent but can also occur elsewhere. Haemolytic anaemia is sometimes accompanied by paralysis when parasitized cells clog brain capillaries. Related genera, such as *Leucocytozoon*, are also associated with avian disease.

The piroplasms are of greater veterinary interest. They are tick-borne pathogens. Two genera are of particular importance in tropical animal production: *Babesia*, associated mainly with red blood cells and *Theileria*, which parasitizes leukocytes as well.

4.8.1 *Babesia*

Babesiosis is a potentially fatal disease characterised by fever and anaemia. It tends to be sporadic in occurrence but it can exert a heavy toll on animals newly introduced to an endemic area. The susceptibility of European cattle breeds to this disease is a major factor limiting their use in tropical regions. Alternative and regional names for bovine babesiosis include 'piroplasmosis', 'redwater' and 'Texas fever'.

Babesia species are described as 'small' or 'large' depending on their relative size when fully formed within the erythrocyte (see Figure 4.42). Their morphology varies with the stage of development, but the form seen most frequently in blood smears is the pear-shaped trophozoite.

Life-cycle

Each *Babesia* species is restricted to one or a few mammalian hosts and a similarly narrow range of ticks. For simplicity, the life-cycle diagram shown in Figure 4.43 illustrates a hypothetical *Babesia* species that uses a one-host tick as vector (see Section 3.2.1):

a – Each time an organism divides within a mammalian red blood cell (RBC), the two daughter merozoites escape by lysing the host cell and enter new erythrocytes. Here, the trophozoite grows and passes through a transitory ring (annular) form before dividing into two further merozoites. This on-going cycle can continue for the life-span of the animal, although it is usually dampened down or, less often, eliminated by host immunity.

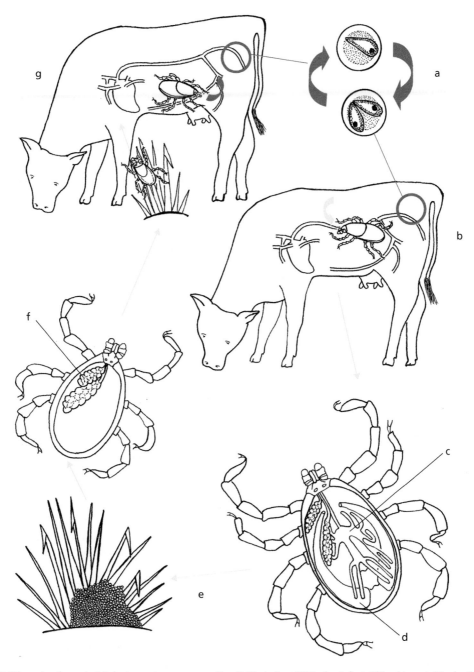

Figure 4.43 Life-cycle of a typical *Babesia* species: a – merozoites divide in host RBCs; b – infected blood ingested by feeding tick; c – sexual replication occurs in tick mid-gut and organisms disperse through body; d – organisms multiplying in tick ovary incorporated into eggs; e – infected tick eggs deposited on ground; f – sporozoites form in salivary gland of new generation of ticks; g – infective sporozoites injected into new host when tick feeds (details in text). Adult tick redrawn from Edwards, Goddard and Varela-Stokes, 2009 with permission of Midsouth Entomological Society.

b – Some merozoites on entering an RBC transform into a nondividing stage, which is infective when ingested by a suitable tick.

c – Sexual reproduction takes place in the tick gut. After fertilisation, further multiplication produces large numbers of organisms ('kinetes') that are distributed via the tick's haemolymph system to a variety of tissues and organs, including the salivary glands and ovaries, where several cycles of asexual multiplication take place.

d – Organisms multiplying in the ovaries become incorporated into eggs. The parasite is thereby passed on to the next generation of ticks ('transovarian transmission').

e – Typically, only a small percentage of the cluster of eggs laid by the tick will be infected with *Babesia*.

f – When the hatched tick finds a new host and starts to feed, kinetes in the salivary glands divide to form infective sporozoites.

g – Transmission takes place when the tick, as part of its feeding process, pumps saliva containing sporozoites into the mammalian host.

The life-cycles of *Babesia* species utilising two- or three-host ticks are more complicated, but follow the same general pattern. In some cases, a tick that has acquired infection by feeding on an infected host while in the larval stage is capable of transmitting the parasite after moulting to the nymphal or adult stages ('transstadial transmission'). In other species, transovarian transmission is the more usual route. Either way, the adult tick seems more efficient at transmitting *Babesia* to cattle than immature stages.

A feature of *Babesia* infections is the persistence of a low level parasitaemia despite a strong immune response. The mechanisms for this are incompletely understood for most species, but when *B. bovis* enters an erythrocyte it is able to remodel the surface of the host cell forming ridges. These greatly enhance the tendency of infected RBCs to stick to capillary endothelium, thereby reducing their chances of being caught and phagocytosed by spleen macrophages.

Pathogenicity

When merozoites lyse their erythrocytes, parasite antigen is released into the blood plasma. This becomes adsorbed onto other RBCs, which are then removed by the host reticulo-endothelial system. The haemolytic anaemia associated with babesiosis can therefore be much greater than would be expected from the degree of parasitaemia.

Haemolysis is accompanied by haemoglobinuria, fever and sometimes diarrhoea. Some species, e.g. *B. bovis*, stimulate the production of vasoactive substances resulting in dilation and increased permeability of capillaries, which in turn leads to hypotension. *B. bovis* also promotes clumping of erythrocytes in capillaries, especially in the brain and kidneys, which can produce tissue hypoxia and neurological signs. Death ensues within a few days if the acute crisis is not abbreviated soon enough by the onset of host immunity.

Epidemiology

An unusual factor in the epidemiology of bovine babesiosis is the fact that calves up to 6 months of age are relatively refractory to the disease. The explanation for this seems to be associated with a more rapid production of IL-12 and IFN-γ (see Help box 1.4) in the spleen of calves as compared with older cattle. Additionally, innate NK cells, which are an important source of IFN-γ in cattle, are more abundant in young calves than in adults. The practical consequence is that calves exposed to infection will respond more effectively to the parasite, thereby limiting clinical impact.

Older cattle surviving initial infection quickly develop a good protective immunity. This is sometimes called 'premunity' as in many cases small numbers of organisms persist. The term 'carrier state' is also used as such animals can still infect the tick population thus perpetuating the risk of babesiosis occurring on the farm. Stress can trigger a resurgence of clinical signs and immunity wanes after about two years in the absence of reinfection.

Where calf-hood exposure is common, disease will be sporadic and confined to animals that are stressed or, for one reason or another, have not had an opportunity to acquire immunity.

Disease risk is determined by the balance maintained between herd immunity and the numbers of infected ticks (especially adults) seeking a blood-meal (tick pressure). Counter-intuitively, risk decreases as the numbers of infected ticks increases, as will become apparent by comparing these two scenarios:

a – Enzootic stability: This epidemiological state is associated with a *high* rate of transmission-

many infected ticks, therefore:

calf-hood infection common;

immunity boosted throughout life;

high level of herd immunity maintained;

consequently, a low (sporadic) incidence of overt disease.

b – Enzootic instability: This is associated with a *low* rate of transmission-

few infected ticks, therefore:

infrequent exposure during calf-hood and later life;

immunity wanes or is absent in many individuals;

low level of herd immunity (i.e. a high proportion of susceptible animals);

consequently, a higher incidence of overt disease.

The geographical occurrence of babesiosis at regional and local levels is determined by the distribution of the tick vectors. Thus, in the UK, the disease is associated with rough grazing or pastures adjacent to rocky outcrops, hedgerows etc. in the wetter parts of the country, as these factors provide the microclimate needed to support the vector, *Ixodes ricinus*.

Babesiosis/piroplasmosis

There are a number of *Babesia* species that differ in their host specificity, pathogenicity and geographical distribution (Table 4.5). Two names are in common usage for the associated disease, babesiosis and piroplasmosis. The former is preferable but the second, older term persists in some contexts.

Babesiosis in ruminants

Although a confusing variety of species names can be found in the literature, taxonomic studies have shown that there are only four valid *Babesia* species in cattle. Two of these, *B. bovis* and *B. bigemina*, are major pathogens in warmer regions of the world, while a third, *B. divergens*, is a sporadic problem in parts of the UK and other European countries. The fourth species, the only 'large' *Babesia* in cattle, is considered to be relatively harmless.

Small ruminants have at least two *Babesia* species, but they are generally of minor clinical significance.

Babesiosis in small animals

The epidemiology of canine babesiosis is complicated and still being unravelled. This is partly because modern molecular techniques indicate that there are more species involved than was previously realised, and partly because some species are extending their endemic range as a result of climate change and pet travel.

Traditionally, infections with 'large' forms of *Babesia* (see Figure 4.44) were all ascribed to the species *B. canis*. This has now been split into three well-defined entities that are called 'species' by some authors or 'subspecies' by others. The one known as *B. canis canis* is largely confined to southern European countries but is spreading. *B. canis vogeli* is found in warmer regions of the Americas, Europe, Asia, Australia and Africa, while *B. canis rossi* is confined to the African continent. A fourth large form has recently been discovered in immunocompromised dogs in eastern USA.

The main 'small' species, *B. gibsoni* (see Figure 4.45), is endemic in SE Asia but foci of infection have become established in parts of the USA, Europe and elsewhere. This species can be transmitted directly from dog to dog via bite wounds. A virulent form of '*B. gibsoni*' occurring in California is now known to be a genetically distinct

Table 4.5 Some important *Babesia* species

Host	Species	Morphology	Region	Tick vector	Pathogenicity	More information
Cattle	*B. bovis*	Small	Tropics and warmer regions	*Boophilus microplus*	▼▼▼	8.2.3
	B. bigemina	Small	Tropics and warmer regions	*Boophilus* and *Rhipicephalus*	▼▼	
	B. divergens	Small	Northwest Europe	*Ixodes ricinus*	▼▼	8.2.3
	B. major	Large	Temperate regions	*Haemaphysalis*		
Dogs	'*B. canis*'[1]	Large	See text	See text	▼▼	9.2.2
	B. gibsoni	Small	Asia, USA, Europe	*Haemaphysalis*	▼▼▼	9.2.2
Horses	*B. caballi*	Large	Widespread	Several genera	▼▼	9.1.2
	'*B. equi*'[2]	Large	Widespread	Several genera	▼▼▼	9.1.2

[1] Three subspecies; [2] more correctly called *Theileria equi* (see text).

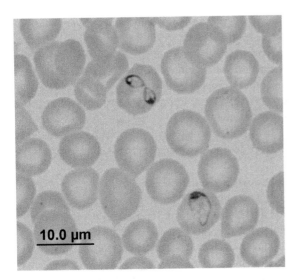

10.0 μm

Figure 4.44 Blood smear from a dog infected with a 'large' *Babesia* species (*B. vogeli*): note the annular form of the parasite in one RBC (below) and an organism dividing into two merozoites in another (above). Reproduced with permission of P.J. Irwin.

entity, while a 'small' *Babesia* causing disease in Spain and Croatia seems to have greater affinity with a common rodent species.

At the time of writing, no canine *Babesia* species are endemic in the UK. Consequently, British dogs have no immunity to babesiosis and are highly vulnerable when taken out of the country.

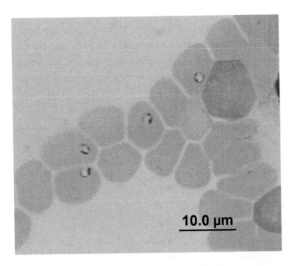

10.0 μm

Figure 4.45 Blood smear from a dog infected with a 'small' *Babesia* species (*B. gibsoni*). Reproduced with permission of P.J. Irwin.

A cat species occurs in South Africa, but otherwise feline infections are rarely reported.

Extra information box 4.3

Rangelia vitelli

Dogs exposed to ixodid ticks in Brazil sometimes fall victim to a disease similar to canine babesiosis but with persistent bleeding from the nose, mouth and pinnae as prominent clinical signs. Molecular studies have confirmed that the aetiological agent, *R. vitellii*, is a piroplasm but it differs from *Babesia* as life-cycle stages have been observed in white blood cells and capillary endothelial cells as well as in erythrocytes.

Equine piroplasmosis

Equine piroplasmosis occurs in southern Europe, South and Central America, the Caribbean and Asia. Strict regulations are enforced to prevent its entry into nonendemic zones such as the USA and Canada, Australasia, Japan and some European countries (including the UK). Of the two species causing this condition (see Table 4.5), *B. equi* is the more pathogenic. This species is unusual in that four merozoites often form in the RBC, giving a 'Maltese cross' appearance. There is also a pre-erythrocytic life-cycle stage which suggests that it is fundamentally different from other *Babesia* species and may have a closer affinity with the genus *Theileria*. The alternative name *Theileria equi* is therefore gaining acceptance. *B. equi* also differs from *B. caballi* as there is no transovarian transmission in ticks, but there can be transmission *in utero* from mare to foal.

4.8.2 *Theileria*

There are a number of *Theileria* species of varying pathogenicity that parasitize livestock in different parts of the world, including *T. annulata* which affects cattle in the Mediterranean region and Asia. In Africa, East Coast Fever, caused by *T. parva*, is a debilitating and often fatal disease which has a major impact on cattle production. An equine species, *T. equi*, was discussed in Section 4.8.1 under the heading '*Equine piroplasmosis*'.

T. parva is transmitted by the brown ear tick, *Rhipicephalus appendiculatus* (a three-host ixodid tick). Infection is usually acquired by the nymphal stage and passed on by the adult. There is no transovarian transmission.

After gametogony has taken place in the tick gut, kinetes invade the salivary gland. Here they replicate and differentiate into infective sporozoites which are subsequently passed to the mammalian host when the tick feeds.

The sporozoites invade lymphocytes and induce them to divide continuously as lymphoblasts ('clonal expansion'). Each host cell division is synchronised with parasite replication and, as a result, infected cells become widely distributed through the host's lymphoid system. After 2–3 weeks, attacking cytotoxic T-cells initiate a massive destruction of parasitized lymphoblasts. Meanwhile, parasitic organisms start to invade erythrocytes and differentiate into the life-cycle stage infective to ticks.

Constant tick challenge establishes a state of endemic stability which minimises losses in indigenous cattle, but any factor upsetting this delicate balance can precipitate an epidemic.

Extra information box 4.4

Hepatozoon

Hepatozoon is a cause of lethargy, fever and weight-loss in dogs in some warmer regions of the world. Although it is only distantly related to *Theileria*, there are similarities as gametogony takes place in the tick vector and parasitized white blood cells occur in the mammalian host. In this case, however, the sporozoites remain within the tick. Transmission occurs when the dog swallows the feeding tick while grooming. *Hepatozoon* multiplies in the liver, spleen and lymph-nodes. The stage infective for the tick circulates primarily in neutrophils where they can be detected in stained blood smears.

4.9 Cryptosporidia

Cryptosporidium is an apicomplexan genus of minute size that nestles into the microvillous brush border of epithelial cells lining the alimentary and respiratory tracts. It diverged from other apicomplexan lineages in ancient evolutionary history and has since developed many unique features. It is an enigma as it is an intracellular parasite that lives in an extracytoplasmic location. It accomplishes this feat by sitting on top of the host cell, covered only by a host-derived membrane, and using an intricate feeder organelle to connect with the cytoplasm below.

Cryptosporidium is a highly sophisticated parasite that draws many more biosynthetic molecules directly from the host than any other parasitic protozoon. This reduces the number of active biochemical pathways that can act as a target for chemotherapy and explains why so few drugs have any effect on this parasite.

Cryptosporidium species can only be differentiated by molecular techniques and studies to elucidate their host range, epidemiology and zoonotic potential are ongoing. Disease in domesticated animals and man was previously attributed mostly to *C. parvum* but it is now known that cattle, for example, harbour at least five different species or genotypes; sheep at least eight; while humans have at least seven, of which the most common are *C. parvum* and *C. hominis*.

4.9.1 *Cryptosporidium parvum*

Cryptosporidiosis caused by *C. parvum* is an important water-borne zoonosis and is a serious potential complication in human HIV-AIDS patients. Livestock are thought to be the main source of contamination for water supplies, but rabbits have also been incriminated. Children may be at risk via the faecal-oral route when visiting farms with young calves or lambs.

In histological sections, cryptosporidia are seen as tiny round objects sitting on the luminal surface of intestinal or respiratory cells (see Figure 4.46).

Life-cycle

Apart from size and location, the *Cryptosporidium* life-cycle (see Figure 4.47) is superficially similar to that of

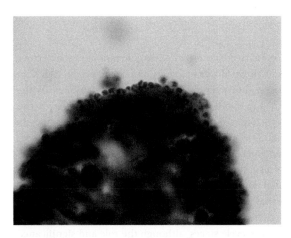

Figure 4.46 Numerous cryptosporidia sitting on epithelial cells at the tip of an intestinal villus.

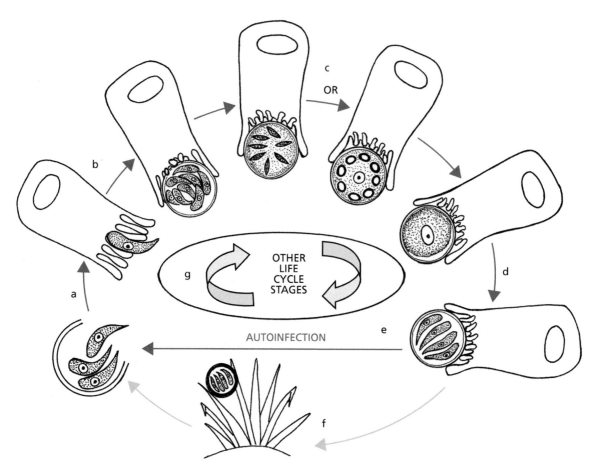

Figure 4.47 Life-cycle of *Cryptosporidium parvum:* a – sporozoites released from oocyst settle in microvilli of epithelial cells; b – schizogony; c – gametogony; d – oocysts form and sporulate; e – thin-walled oocysts release sporozoites within host; f – thick-walled oocysts exit host in faeces; g – other extra-cellular life-cycle stages may exist. Parasites redrawn after Gardiner *et al.,* 1988 with permission of USDA.

Eimeria (see Figure 4.24). Two generations of schizogony are followed by gametogony and oocyst production. The oocyst, however, contains just four sporozoites (without any sporocysts). A fundamental difference is the occurrence of two types of oocyst: thin-walled oocysts that autoinfect the host in which they were produced; and thick-walled oocysts which are excreted in faeces to disseminate infection. The latter are already sporulated when passed and so are immediately infective. The prepatent period is less than a week.

There is also evidence of additional extracellular parasitic life-cycle stages, although the role and significance of these is as yet poorly understood.

Pathogenicity

Cryptosporidiosis is most frequently seen in neonatal animals. A mild to moderate diarrhoea is associated with intestinal villous atrophy. Many infections are asymptomatic but large numbers of oocysts are excreted over a few days. Uncomplicated cases resolve within a few days as protective immunity builds up, but small numbers of oocysts can continue to be shed intermittently in later life, especially after calving.

4.9.2 Avian cryptosporidiosis

The most widespread avian *Cryptosporidium* species is *C. bayleyi* which affects a number of birds, including poultry.

The parasites are most numerous in the bursa of Fabricius and cloaca, but clinical signs are provoked by those replicating in the air passages, from the nasopharynges to the bronchi. Mucosal hyperplasia leads to a mucous discharge, sneezing and difficulty in breathing.

4.10 Antiprotozoal drugs

Antiprotozoal drugs encompass a great diversity of chemistry and modes of action. To review all of these would be beyond the scope of this book and so discussion is restricted to some general considerations and a brief overview of the chemical control of avian coccidiosis.

4.10.1 Key concepts

The life-cycles of 'microparasites', such as protozoa and bacteria, are fundamentally different from 'macroparasites' such as arthropods or helminths. Microparasites multiply within their host and consequently each organism entering the body is capable of initiating a massive infection if not checked by natural host defences or chemotherapy (see Figure 1.2). The primary objective for antiprotozoal therapy is therefore to disrupt parasite replication, thereby ensuring that the parasite population does not grow to a level that will overwhelm host immunity. In the case of African bovine trypanosomosis, for example, the most commonly used drugs disrupt nucleic acid synthesis by intercalating into parasite DNA.

4.10.2 Anticoccidial drugs

Coccidiosis control is critical for the poultry industry (see Section 8.4.1). Anticoccidial drugs belong to a variety of chemical classes but can be divided into two general categories on the basis of their effect on the parasite:

a – Coccidiocides: kill intracellular stages of *Eimeria* spp. and are particularly useful for the treatment of clinical disease; they are usually administered in drinking water (rather than the usual medicated feed) as sick birds have a reduced appetite.

b – Coccidiostats: inhibit growth and replication of the parasite without necessarily killing it; these are employed prophylactically as feed additives.

The distinction between these categories is often blurred as the effect on the parasite can depend on dose-rate and duration of exposure. The spectrum of activity of the various anticoccidial drugs differs, especially with regard to the life-cycle stages targeted. Counter-intuitively, the most efficacious anticoccidials do not always provide optimum field performance. This is because they have two inherent disadvantages:

a – Delayed immunity: if a highly effective treatment stops parasitic development at a very early stage in the life-cycle, opportunities for antigen presentation to the immune system are limited and birds will remain susceptible to reinfection;

b – Enhanced risk of drug resistance: selection pressure is high with highly effective treatments as the few organisms that survive treatment undergo prolific asexual multiplication within the host before producing gametes. Thus, there is potential for enormous numbers of oocysts carrying resistance genes to be shed into the environment. Resistance can build up quickly if subsequent parasite generations are also exposed to the same drug (see Section 1.6.3).

Historically, many anticoccidial compounds have become obsolete as resistance problems progressively eroded their usefulness. As a result, few compounds are currently available for treating clinical outbreaks of coccidiosis and these should be reserved for emergency use.

Fortunately, a greater number of compounds are available for prophylactic use. They should be used strategically as part of a planned management programme (see Section 8.4.1). Their mode of use differs for broiler production and for replacement breeding and egg-laying stock. In the former case the aim is to optimise health and productivity for the duration of their short life-span (although there must be no chemical residue in the meat at slaughter). Replacement stock, on the other hand, has to be given opportunity to develop immunity.

Ionophores

The ionophores are the most widely used chemical group for controlling coccidiosis in chickens. They are fermentation products prepared from *Streptomyces* moulds. Examples include monensin, salinomycin and narasin. They act on extracellular life-cycle stages in the intestine (sporozoites, merozoites and microgametocytes) by allowing an influx of Na^+ ions. This produces osmotic imbalance and structural damage. The Na^+

pump has to work overtime to rectify the situation and this exhausts the parasite's energy reserves. The parasite eventually succumbs to these combined effects.

Ionophores substantially reduce, but do not completely eliminate, oocyst production in treated birds. As a result, they suppress clinical and subclinical coccidiosis, reduce the build-up of oocysts in the litter and allow immunity to develop. As they exert relatively little selection pressure on the parasite population, resistance has been very slow to develop to this chemical class.

Caution is needed when disposing of unused medicated chicken feed, or when treating other animals, as some members of the ionophore group are toxic to horses, turkeys and game birds.

Sulphonamides

The sulphonamides and a number of other older remedies are antagonists of para-amino benzoic acid (PABA) which is a precursor of folic acid. Coccidia have to manufacture folic acid in large amounts during schizogony as it is needed for DNA synthesis. Selective toxicity is achieved as mammals and birds obtain their folic acid from dietary sources (it is a B-complex vitamin) and therefore have no need for PABA. Although resistance has curtailed their widespread use, sulphonamides still have niche applications, especially if combined with other folate antagonists, such as pyrimethamine, which provide a synergistic effect. Another older product, amprolium, exerts its effect by antagonising thiamine (vitamin B_1), also needed in quantity by rapidly dividing coccidia.

CHAPTER 5
Platyhelminthes ('flatworms')

5.1 Introduction

Platyhelminths typically have a flattened body with suckers, or similar structures, for attachment to their host. Most are hermaphrodite (i.e. each individual has male and female sex organs). The body surface ('tegument') is metabolically active and therefore structurally and functionally distinct from the arthropod exoskeleton, the cuticle of nematodes or mammalian skin.

The term platyhelminth (meaning 'flatworm') encompasses two major parasitic groups: the Cestoda (tapeworms) and the Trematoda (flukes). Adult cestodes are segmented and ribbon-like, reminiscent of a tape-measure – hence the traditional name 'tapeworm' (see Figure 5.1). They have no alimentary tract and absorb nutrients through the tegument. In contrast, trematodes do have a mouth and internal digestive system. They are leaf-shaped and unsegmented (see Figure 5.2).

Principles of Veterinary Parasitology, First Edition. By Dennis Jacobs, Mark Fox, Lynda Gibbons and Carlos Hermosilla.
© 2016 John Wiley & Sons, Ltd. Published 2016 by John Wiley & Sons, Ltd.
Companion website: www.wiley.com/go/jacobs/principles-veterinary-parasitology

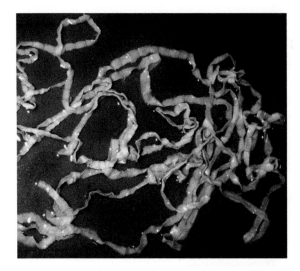

Figure 5.1 A typical tapeworm (*Taenia saginata*). Reproduced with permission of P. Stevenson.

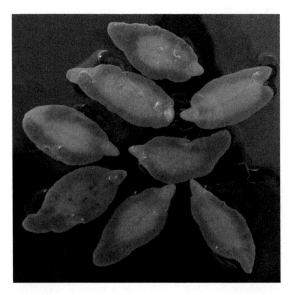

Figure 5.2 A typical trematode (*Fasciola hepatica*). Reproduced with permission of T. de Waal.

5.2 Cestodes

Adult tapeworms generally cause only minor harm despite their impressive size (some grow to several metres in length). Concern lies more with their larval stage which, in some instances, is of greater significance in veterinary practice or public health.

5.2.1 Key concepts

Adult tapeworms are usually found in the small intestine of their host. Their most obvious feature is a chain (strobila) of independently maturing reproductive segments (proglottids). Less apparent at the anterior end of the chain is an attachment organ called the 'scolex' (see Figure 5.3). This is superficially embedded in the intestinal mucosa and maintains the tapeworm's position with the help of suckers or grooves and sometimes hooks. New proglottids are produced at regular intervals from the neck at the base of the scolex. As each one is produced, earlier proglottids are pushed further back along the line. A mature segment can cross-fertilise with its neighbours along the chain or with those of another individual of the same species. This possibly explains why tapeworms are often found in a tangle at autopsy.

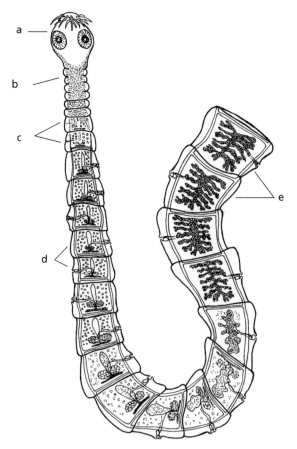

Figure 5.3 A typical cyclophyllidean tapeworm (*Taenia*): a – scolex with hooks and suckers; b – neck; c – immature segments; d – mature segments; e – gravid segments.

Two major cestode groups are of veterinary interest: the Cyclophyllidea and the Pseudophyllidea. These have fundamentally different life-cycles. Microscopic differentiation of the two types of adult tapeworm is straightforward as the cyclophyllidian scolex has four circular suckers and often hooks (see Figure 5.4), while its pseudophyllidean equivalent has two elongated grooves (bothria) instead (see Figure 5.5). Cyclophyl-

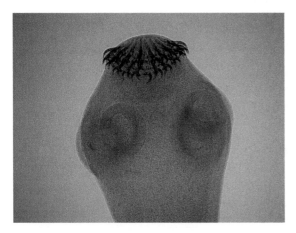

Figure 5.4 Scolex and neck of a cyclophyllidean tapeworm showing hooks and four suckers.

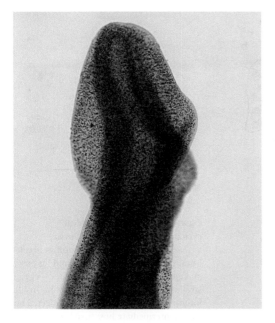

Figure 5.5 A pseudophyllidean scolex: note the presence of longitudinal grooves (and the absence of hooks and suckers).

lidean proglottids have obvious openings (genital pores) on one or both lateral margins while reproductive activity is confined to the centre of the pseudophyllidean segment.

5.3 Cyclophyllidean tapeworms

Four cyclophyllidean families are of particular interest (see Figure 5.6). Of these, the family Taeniidae is the most significant because it encompasses two important genera: *Taenia* and *Echinococcus*. Two common tapeworms *Anoplocephala* and *Moniezia* belong to the second family (the Anoplocephalidae) and have similar life-cycles even though they occur in different hosts and are quite different in appearance. A third family contains *Dipylidium*, frequently encountered in dogs and cats, and a number of minor genera found in birds. The only highly pathogenic poultry cestode, *Davainea*, belongs to a fourth family.

5.3.1 Cyclophyllidean life-cycle

The cyclophyllidean life-cycle alternates between a larval form (metacestode) in the intermediate host and the adult tapeworm in the final host (see Figure 5.7):

a – By the time a segment reaches the posterior end of the adult tapeworm, it is full of eggs and is known as a gravid proglottid.

b – The gravid proglottid separates from the chain and is swept through the host's digestive system to emerge into the outside world. The segments are muscular and can crawl through the anus, which is why they are sometimes seen adhering to the host animal's skin or coat. More often they drop to the ground where they squirm around releasing their eggs, which can number hundreds of thousands. In some other species, eggs are not discharged until the proglottid disintegrates.

c – The egg is immediately infective. It hatches when swallowed by an appropriate intermediate host releasing an embryo (the oncosphere) which migrates to its preferred predilection site. Here it transforms into a larval tapeworm (metacestode).

d – The metacestode develops and waits to be ingested by its final host.

Class	Order	Family	Genus

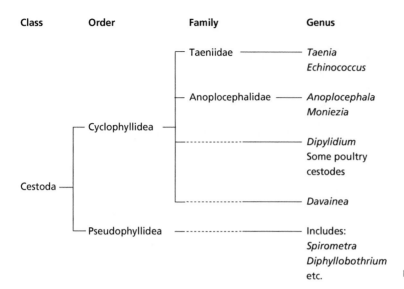

Taeniidae ———— *Taenia*
Echinococcus

Anoplocephalidae ——— *Anoplocephala*
Moniezia

Dipylidium
Some poultry
cestodes

Davainea

Includes:
Spirometra
Diphyllobothrium
etc.

Cyclophyllidea

Cestoda

Pseudophyllidea

Figure 5.6 The major groups of cestodes.

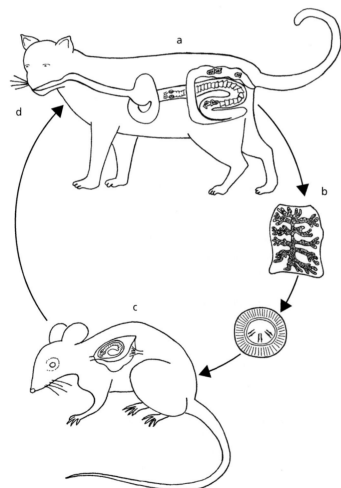

Figure 5.7 Life-cycle of a typical cyclophyllidean tapeworm (*Taenia taeniaeformis*): a – adult tapeworm in small intestine of final host; b – proglottid is passed and ejects eggs into environment; c – egg swallowed and metacestode develops inside intermediate host; d – final host infected by eating intermediate host tissues containing metacestode (details in text which uses same lettering as shown above).

Depending on species, infection of the final host can entail one of the following biological associations:

a – A predator-prey relationship: e.g. a cat eating a mouse infected with *T. taeniaeformis* (as depicted in Figure 5.7);

b – Meat-eating: e.g. a human eating an undercooked steak containing a *Taenia saginata* metacestode;

c – Incidental ingestion: which can come about in at least two ways:

i)   while grazing (e.g. a horse swallowing pasture mites infected with *Anoplocephala*);

ii) while self-grooming (e.g. a cat infested by fleas carrying *Dipylidium*).

Practical tip box 5.1

Diagnosis of cyclophyllidean infections

Faecal examination by microscopy (coproscopy) is unreliable for the diagnosis of cyclophyllidean infections as eggs are often not released until *after* the tapeworm segment has exited the host. The detection of antigen or DNA in faeces is a better approach if a test is available for the tapeworm in question.

5.3.2 Metacestodes

Basically, a metacestode is a thin-walled, fluid filled cyst, although surrounding host tissue responses may make the wall appear thicker. Growing from the inner surface of the cyst wall are one or more tiny tapeworm 'heads' (protoscolices). These are often 'inverted'.

An 'inverted protoscolex' is a tapeworm head that is 'inside out'. This may seem improbable, but a good way to envisage the concept is to think of the finger of an inflated rubber glove (see Figure 5.8). Imagine that you have drawn hooks and suckers on the end with a marker pen. Now push the tip of the finger downwards so it goes inside itself. The hooks and suckers are now

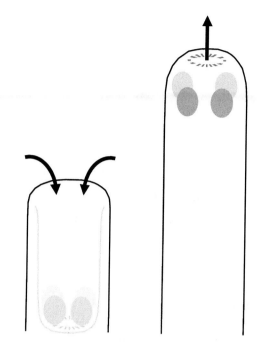

Figure 5.8 Metacestode heads: inverted (left); everted (right). (Details in text.)

on the 'inner' surface. This mimics the arrangement of the inverted protoscolex.

When subject to digestive juices in the small intestine of a final host, the 'finger tip' pops out ('everts'), so hooks and suckers are now externally situated and ready to attach onto the mucosa. The protoscolex is now ready to develop into an adult tapeworm.

In some species, the cyst wall gives rise to multiple tapeworm heads. This is a form of asexual replication and, in these cases, swallowing one metacestode results in the establishment of several or many adult tapeworms.

Six types of metacestode are found in domesticated animals. These are summarised in Table 5.1 and described in greater detail at appropriate points in the chapter:

Table 5.1 The six types of cyclophyllidean metacestode

Metacestode	Number of tapeworm 'heads'	Special features	Illustrated in
Cysticercus	One	Fluid-filled cyst, head attached to cyst wall	Figures 5.10a, 5.12, 5.13
Coenurus	Dozens	Fluid-filled cyst, heads attached to cyst wall	Figures 5.10b, 5.14
Strobilocercus	One	Head separated from cyst by chain of segments	Figures 5.10c, 5.15
Cysticercoid	One	Head within very small cyst; occurs only in invertebrates	Figure 5.23
Hydatid cyst	Up to thousands	Fluid-filled cyst, heads detach from wall into cyst fluid	Figures 5.19, 5.20, 5.22
Alveolar cyst	Up to thousands	As hydatid cyst but new cysts also bud off externally	Figure 5.21

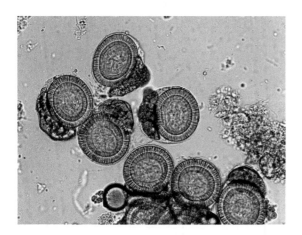

Figure 5.9 Taeniid eggs (taken from a gravid *Taenia* segment).

5.3.3 *Taenia*

Taenia spp. can be easily differentiated from other tapeworm genera by taking into account:

i)   their length (0.5–15 m depending on species);
ii) the shape of their gravid segments, which are roughly rectangular and longer than they are broad (see Figure 5.3);
iii) the presence of just one genital pore on each segment, situated on the lateral margin.

The eggs, however, cannot be distinguished from those of *Echinococcus*. Both taeniid genera produce small (40 μm), round eggs which are surrounded by a radially striated shell-like structure (see Figure 5.9).

Careful microscopic examination reveals that the embryo (oncosphere) inside the egg has six small hooks. A gravid *Taenia* segment contains up to 250 000 such eggs. When within the segment, these have an outer coating covering the striated layer but this is soon lost and not usually seen on eggs recovered from faeces.

There are a number of *Taenia* species of veterinary interest and their most important biological features are summarised in Table 5.2. In most cases, telling the different *Taenia* species apart is a job for the specialist (who will look firstly at the shape of the hooks that are arranged in a double row around the anterior end of the scolex).

Metacestodes

There are three types of metacestode associated with the various *Taenia* species (see Figure 5.10):

a – Cysticercus: a fluid filled cavity lined by a delicate parasitic membrane that has just one easily visible solid protrusion (a single inverted tapeworm head);

b – Coenurus: a coenurus is like a cysticercus but there are multiple (typically dozens) of inverted tapeworm heads that appear as whitish spots on the parasitic membrane;

c – Strobilocercus: this consists of a single tapeworm head which is separated from its parasitic bladder by a chain of segments. The whole is folded up to form a pea-sized sphere. This type of metacestode occurs only with the cat tapeworm *T. taeniaeformis*.

Table 5.2 *Taenia* species and their hosts (adapted from Dunn, 1978)

Taenia species	Final host	Intermediate host	Metacestode	Obsolete name for metacestode[1]
T. saginata	Human	Cattle	Cysticercus in muscle	*C. bovis*
T. solium	Human	Pig		*C. cellulosae*
T. ovis	Dog	Sheep		*C. ovis*
T. hydatigena	Dog	Sheep etc.	Cysticercus in peritoneum	*C. tenuicollis*
T. pisiformis	Dog	Rabbit		*C. pisiformis*
T. multiceps[2]	Dog	Sheep etc.	Coenurus (various sites)[3]	*C. cerebralis*
T. serialis	Dog	Rabbit		*C. serialis*
T. taeniaeformis	Cat	Mouse etc.	Strobilocercus in liver	*C. fasciolaris*

[1]*C* = *Cysticercus*; [2]also known as *Multiceps multiceps*; [3]*T. multiceps* inside skull; *T. serialis* in intermuscular connective tissue.

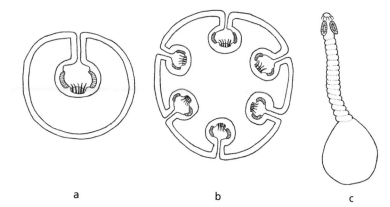

Figure 5.10 The three types of metacestode associated with different *Taenia* species: a – cysticercus; b – coenurus; c – strobilocerus.

a   b   c

Help box 5.1

Nomenclature of metacestodes

Early zoologists did not recognise the connection between adult tapeworms and their metacestodes as they look so different. So, thinking they were different organisms, they were given different names. Unfortunately, some of these obsolete names persist, particularly in meat inspection. For example, you may hear the term '*Cysticercus bovis*' used for what we would now call the 'metacestode of *Taenia saginata*'.

Taenia species of humans

Humans act as final host to at least two *Taenia* species (see Table 5.2). These are the beef tapeworm (*T. saginata*) and the pork tapeworm (*T. solium*). The colloquial names aptly define the intermediate host of each parasite and the method of transmission. *T. saginata* is a relatively minor pathogen but occurs in all beef-eating communities. Its prevalence in any country is determined by the adequacy of human sanitation, meat inspection and food preparation. *T. solium* has been eradicated from many localities but is still a serious zoonotic hazard in parts of Latin America, Africa and Asia.

The beef tapeworm

The life-cycle of *T. saginata* is typically cyclophyllidean, alternating between the human final host and the bovine intermediate host. Humans are infected by eating undercooked beef. The resulting adult tapeworm can reach 15 m in length. Unlike other cyclophyllideans, the scolex of both the adult tapeworm and the metacestode (which is a cysticercus) has no hooks and is said to be 'unarmed'. Cattle are infected by ingesting eggs

on pasture or from utensils contaminated with human faecal material (e.g. calves drinking from a soiled milk-bucket). Transmission to grassland can be:

a – direct: with eggs reaching pasture by direct deposition of human faeces;

b – indirect: by application of inadequately treated sewage sludge as fertiliser;

c – by birds: whole *T. saginata* proglottids can be picked up by sea-gulls, crows etc. feeding at sewage outlets and carried onto pasture-land. If the segment is swallowed, undamaged *T. saginata* eggs can pass through the bird to be voided in its droppings.

The cysticerci of *T. saginata* can settle in any bovine muscle (see Figure 5.11) but the greatest densities (i.e. nos. per kg tissue) tend to be in the heart,

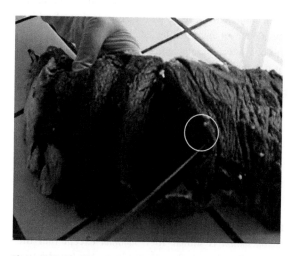

Figure 5.11 *T. saginata* cysticercus (circled) in a joint of beef. Reproduced with permission of R.C. Krecek.

masseters and triceps. They grow to a final size of about
1 × 0.5 cm and are infective after about 3–4 months. If
acquired during calf-hood, they are likely to survive for
the lifetime of the animal; if acquired later in life they
will eventually be killed by host immune responses. In
the latter case, they are gradually replaced by caseous
(cheeselike) material which later calcifies. The size and
condition of cysticerci in a carcase can be used to provide a rough estimate of when the animal was exposed
to infection (which may be helpful in pinpointing the
source of contamination). The presence of *T. saginata*
metacestodes in cattle is known as 'cysticercosis'. The
condition is asymptomatic and therefore only diagnosed
after slaughter.

The epidemiology of bovine cysticercosis differs from
place to place. In the UK, for example, a very low prevalence in the human population coupled with a generally
high standard of sanitation results in a low transmission
rate to cattle. Consequently, bovine prevalence is also
very low (< 5 per 10^3) and there is little or no opportunity for herd immunity to develop. The national herd
therefore remains vulnerable and any group of cattle
that becomes exposed to *T. saginata* eggs will acquire
multiple cysticerci leading to abattoir condemnations.
Such sporadic occurrences are known as 'cysticercosis
storms'.

In contrast, in East Africa for example, a relatively
high prevalence plus a lack of sanitation in some rural
populations results in a high rate of transmission to cattle. Thus, many calves are infected and, although calf-
hood infection persists, these animals are immune to
reinfection. Thus, the general picture is that of a high
prevalence of lightly infected cattle. Meat inspection
will not detect all infected carcases and so the potential
for new human infection is always present.

Extra information box 5.1

Taenia saginata asiatica

This is a recently discovered subspecies of *T. saginata*
that occurs in Asia. It has the pig as its intermediate host
but can be differentiated from *T. solium* as its scolex is
unarmed (i.e. without hooks).

The pork tapeworm

Taenia solium is similar to *T. saginata* except that the
intermediate host is the pig and its scolex has the two
rows of hooks typical of the genus. Although the adult

tapeworm itself is relatively innocuous, *T. solium* is nevertheless a very dangerous human parasite as its cysticerci, normally found in porcine muscle, are also capable of developing in human tissues, particularly in the
brain and musculature. Human cysticercosis can originate in two ways:

a – by swallowing eggs, e.g. if *T. solium* eggs are transferred to the mouth on dirty fingers or on salad crops
grown on soil contaminated or fertilised with human
excrement;

b – retroperistalsis, i.e. abnormal intestinal contractions which move gut contents forwards instead of
backwards. If *T. solium* eggs in a person harbouring a
pork tapeworm are brought forward to the duodenum,
they are stimulated to hatch, releasing oncospheres
which invade the body.

T. solium infections are particularly prevalent in communities where pigs are allowed to scavenge freely
around human habitation.

Taenia species of dogs

At least five *Taenia* species are commonly found in dogs
around the world. Some can also establish in foxes. The
adult tapeworms vary in length from 0.5 to 5 m but they
cause little harm, except that exiting proglottids can sometimes provoke anal pruritus. The life-cycle is typically
cyclophyllidean (see Figure 5.7). Different species use different intermediate hosts (see Table 5.2). Consequently,
the prevalence of each in dog populations is determined
by diet – i.e. whether or not there is opportunity to scavenge carcasses, to eat inadequately cooked meat and offal,
or to catch rabbits. The prepatent period also varies with
species but is generally between 6 and 8 weeks.

Taenia ovis

As can be seen from Table 5.2, the biology of *T. ovis* is
similar to that of *T. saginata* but with the dog as final host
and sheep as intermediate host. The cysticerci are not
infective for humans but nevertheless their presence
in meat leads to condemnation of the carcase at meat
inspection in many countries. It therefore causes significant economic losses in some sheep exporting regions,
for example Australasia.

Taenia hydatigena

T. hydatigena is the commonest *Taenia* species of dogs in
Britain and many other countries. Sheep are the usual

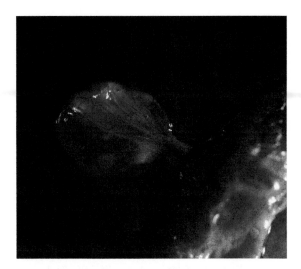

Figure 5.12 Metacestode of *Taenia hydatigena* (cysticercus) on surface of liver.

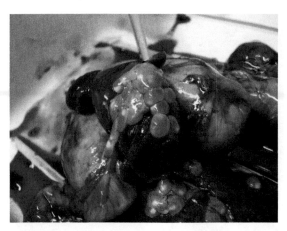

Figure 5.13 Metacestodes of *Taenia pisiformis* (cysticerci) in peritoneal cavity of a hare. Reproduced with permission of L.H. Kramer.

intermediate host, but the cysticerci can also establish in other livestock species.

The cysticerci grow up to 8 cm in the peritoneal cavity and are often found adhering to the omentum (see Figure 5.12). To reach its predilection site, the oncosphere hatches out of the egg in the small intestine and enters the hepatic portal system to be swept to the liver. Here it transforms into a cysticercus and grows rapidly while migrating through the liver parenchyma. After about a month, it breaks through the liver capsule leaving behind necrotic tracks which become fibrotic. The presence of a single metacestode is unlikely to compromise health but if a sheep swallows a whole proglottid, the simultaneous passage of many thousands of cysticerci will cause massive liver damage and sudden death. This condition, known as 'cysticercosis hepatica', is superficially similar to acute fasciolosis (see Section 5.6.2) but is a rare event usually affecting only a single animal in a flock.

Help box 5.2

Avoid common mistakes!

- Don't confuse *Taenia hydatigena* with the hydatid cyst. They are not connected.
- The metacestode of *T. hydatigena* is a cysticercus.
- The hydatid cyst is the metacestode of *Echinococcus granulosus*.

Taenia pisiformis

T. pisiformis is similar to *T. hydatigena* except that the cysticerci are pea-sized and are found in the peritoneal cavity of rabbits and hares (see Figure 5.13).

Taenia multiceps

T. multiceps is also known as *Multiceps multiceps*. It is of widespread distribution, although not reported from the USA or New Zealand. It is the dog *Taenia* that most commonly produces disease in sheep. After the egg is swallowed, the hatched oncosphere enters the circulation and travels to the central nervous system, usually the brain. Here it migrates across the tissues to settle in the cranial cavity as a slow-growing coenurus. This has multiple scolices arranged in small clusters. It attains a final size of some 5 cm (see Figure 5.14). In so doing, it acts as a space occupying lesion inducing atrophy of adjacent brain and skull tissues. The clinical outcome depends on the site affected. It is often asymptomatic but, if near the cerebellum, can induce walking in circles, a staggering gait, an abnormal head position, blindness and other neurological disturbances. The coenurus may be found in other livestock species and humans on rare occasions.

Taenia serialis

The coenurus of *T. serialis* forms in intermuscular connective tissues of rabbits. Cases in pet rabbits are often presented as a soft subdermal swelling and probably originate from eggs shed by urban foxes.

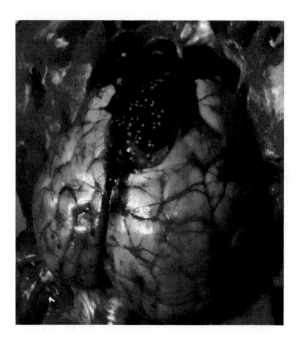

Figure 5.14 *Taenia multiceps* metacestode (coenurus) on brain of sheep (upper right). Clusters of tapeworm heads appear as white dots on the cyst wall. Reproduced with permission of A. Longstaffe.

Taenia species of cats

T. taeniaeformis is the only *Taenia* species commonly found in cats. Although growing to 70 cm, it causes little if any distress. The intermediate hosts are mice and other rodents (see Figure 5.7). The metacestode is a strobilocercus occurring as a pea-sized nodule in the liver (see Figure 5.15).

Practical tip box 5.2

Diagnosis of tapeworm infections in dogs and cats

Accurate diagnosis to genus level of adult tapeworms in dogs and cats is necessary for two reasons. Firstly, this knowledge is essential for advising pet owners how to prevent reinfection. Secondly, not all cestocidal drugs are equally effective against all tapeworm genera (see Table 9.7).

Often the only available evidence of tapeworm infection is a poorly preserved proglottid passed by the pet and collected by the client. In this case, soak the segment in a drop of water on a microscope slide and break it open to reveal the eggs inside. If *Taenia*, they will be typically taeniid in appearance (see Figure 5.9) and separate, i.e. not in packets like those of *Dipylidium* (see Figure 5.30).

If *Taenia* is identified in a dog, then reinfection can be avoided by denying access to raw or undercooked meat and offal. Cats are more difficult – a good hunter will inevitably become reinfected.

5.3.4 *Echinococcus*

The two major *Echinococcus* species, *E. granulosus* and *E. multilocularis*, rarely cause clinical problems in domesticated animals but they are nevertheless of considerable importance in veterinary public health.

Echinococcus differs from the closely related genus, *Taenia*, in a number of important respects. At only about 0.5 cm long, the adult worm is very much smaller (see Figure 5.16). It comprises a scolex and just three or four proglottids (see Figure 5.17). The anterior part of the worm snuggles deeply into the mucosal villi covering the wall of the small intestine (see Figure 5.18).

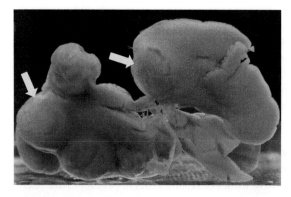

Figure 5.15 Museum specimen: mouse liver with several *Taenia taeniaeformis* strobilocerci (appearing as nodular lesions, arrowed).

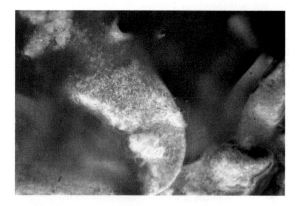

Figure 5.16 *Echinococcus* adults attached to wall of small intestine of a dog. Reproduced with permission of P. Stevenson.

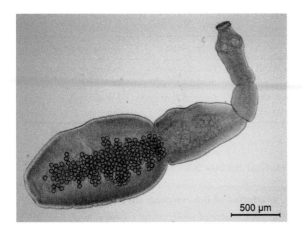

Figure 5.17 A complete *Echinococcus* adult. Reproduced with permission of Merial GmbH.

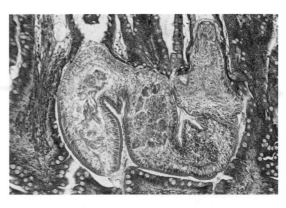

Figure 5.18 Histological section showing the anterior end of an adult *Echinococcus* in the small intestinal mucosa (the scolex is top right). Reproduced with permission of R.C.A. Thompson.

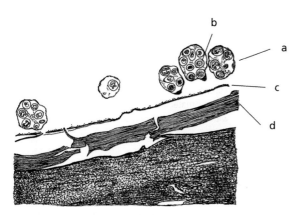

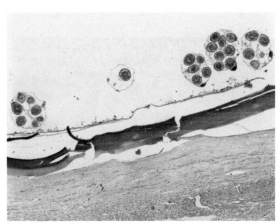

Figure 5.19 Section through hydatid cyst wall: a – brood capsule; b – tapeworm head; c – germinal epithelium; d – laminated layer (broken during preparation of the section).

Metacestodes

Two types of metacestode are associated with *Echinococcus*: the hydatid cyst (*E. granulosus*) and the alveolar cyst (*E. multilocularis*).

Like most taeniid metacestodes, the hydatid cyst is basically a fluid filled bladder lined by a delicate parasitic membrane (see Figure 5.19). It is often encapsulated by host fibrous tissue. Between this and the cyst is a glycoprotein network (the laminated layer) excreted by the membrane to protect itself against host immune attack. The cyst lining is called the 'germinal epithelium' because buds form on its internal surface. These grow into 'brood capsules' which break free and, being

relatively heavy structures, make a sediment (hydatid sand) in the straw-coloured fluid that fills the cyst (see Figure 5.20). Over time, hundreds or even thousands of brood capsules are produced, each containing several inverted tapeworm heads. Each head (protoscolex) can grow into an adult worm if and when the hydatid cyst is ingested by a suitable final host.

The alveolar cyst is similar to the hydatid cyst but with an additional level of complexity – daughter cysts bud off the external surface of the germinal layer. These grow and eventually produce their own external daughter cysts. This proliferation continues with the metacestode infiltrating through host tissues to form an inoperable mass (see Figure 5.21).

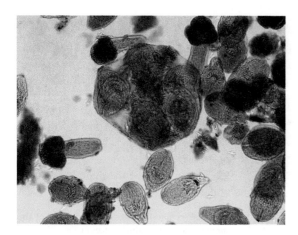

Figure 5.20 Hydatid sand: showing one brood capsule, numerous free inverted tape-worm heads and a few everted protoscolices.

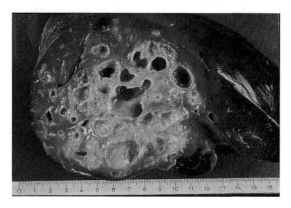

Figure 5.21 Alveolar cyst in human liver. Reproduced with permission of The Institute of Parasitology, University of Zurich.

Life-cycle

Echinococcus has a typical cyclophyllidean life-cycle (see Figure 5.7). The final and intermediate hosts for each species are outlined in following sections. Only one gravid segment is shed by each intestinal worm each week but this meagre reproductive performance is offset by the number of adult tapeworms commonly present (the result of swallowing a metacestode containing many tapeworm heads). This reflects different reproductive strategies adopted by *Echinococcus* and *Taenia* (see Table 5.3).

Echinococcus eggs are identical in appearance to those of *Taenia* (see Figure 5.9).

Table 5.3 Reproductive strategies of *Taenia* and *Echinococcus*

	In final host	In intermediate host
Taenia	Few adult worms; many eggs	Little or no asexual replication
Echinococcus	Many adult worms; few eggs	Massive asexual replication

Practical tip box 5.3

Diagnosis of *Echinococcus* infection in dogs

Echinococcus eggs are not always present in faecal samples from infected dogs and they are, in any case, indistinguishable from other taeniid eggs. Arecoline purges have been used to flush out adult worms for diagnostic purposes, but coproantigen or DNA tests are more satisfactory if available. The adult worm is unlikely to be seen at autopsy as it is very small and has its anterior end buried in the intestinal wall. Microscopic inspection of mucosal scrapings is therefore needed to detect infection.

Beware! *Echinococcus* eggs can infect you! Extreme hygienic precautions are essential when handling any potentially contaminated faecal or autopsy samples. Suspect diagnostic materials should be referred to a laboratory with appropriate expertise and experience.

Hydatid disease

The occurrence of a hydatid cyst in the body is termed 'cystic echinococcosis'. *E. granulosus* can utilise many mammals as intermediate host, but hydatid disease as a clinical entity is usually apparent only in humans. Cysts can occur in any tissue but are most likely to be found in preferred sites. These differ from host to host:

i) sheep: liver and lungs;
ii) cattle: lungs;
iii) horse: liver
iv) human: 70% liver, 20% lungs, 10% other sites

The cysts act as space occupying lesions and can grow to the size of a table-tennis ball in sheep, a tennis ball in horses (see Figure 5.22) and, if left untreated, a football in people. Up to 98% of ewes have been found to carry hydatid cysts in endemic areas where coordinated control measures are not implemented.

Dogs are the main final host but some strains can establish in foxes or other canids.

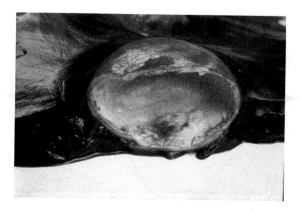

Figure 5.22 Hydatid cyst in horse liver: the liver and cyst have been cut to reveal the thickness of the wall and the appearance of the internal surface. From Jacobs, 1986. Reproduced with permission of Elsevier.

Epidemiology

There are several strains of *E. granulosus* each with biological properties suited to a particular ecological system. Extreme examples include dingo-wallaby, wolf-moose and hyaena-primate cycles. Thus, the detailed epidemiology of *E. granulosus* in any locality will vary according to which strains are present and the availability of the corresponding hosts. Adaptation to particular final and/or intermediate hosts often reduces infectivity of the strain to other potential hosts. In Britain, distinct dog-sheep and dog-horse strains exist. The former has zoonotic potential while the latter has a narrower host-range and is not considered to be infective for humans.

Extra information box 5.2

What's in a name?

The question whether the different biological forms of *E. granulosus* should be described as strains, subspecies or even separate species has been a topic of debate for many years. Molecular techniques are yielding valuable information on relationships and diversity. Hopefully a consensus view will eventually lead to a unified nomenclature. In the meantime, for simplicity, this text regards them as distinct strains within a single species. Readers may, however, come across other nomenclatures – for example, *E. granulosus granulosus* for the British dog-sheep strain and *E. granulosus equorum* for the equine strain.

Dog-sheep strain

The British dog-sheep strain is largely, but not exclusively, associated with upland sheep-rearing regions. It is absent from Ireland. Dogs are more likely than foxes to harbour adult worms. Farm dogs or household pets become infected if fed infected uncooked offal, or by scavenging dead sheep. The prepatent period is 6–7 weeks. Farm dogs are likely to defecate mostly in fields around the homestead. The gravid segments thereby deposited release eggs which are further spread across pastures by rain splash, insect activity, tractor wheels, etc. These eggs are infective particularly for sheep, although cattle and humans (see Section 9.3.2) are vulnerable to a lesser degree. Hill sheep are at greatest risk when the flock is brought down to lower ground for lambing, dipping or other procedures.

Dog-horse strain

This form of *E. granulosus* was once widely distributed throughout the British Isles and Ireland, but fortunately is host specific with cysts developing readily only in horses. Hunt kennels played a major role in disseminating infection when hounds were commonly fed inadequately cooked offal from farm casualties and before effective cestocides had become available.

Extra information box 5.3

Why is the equine strain of *E. granulosus* not considered zoonotic?

There are two main strands of circumstantial evidence:

1. No locally acquired cases of human hydatidosis have been reported in Ireland even though the equine strain of *E. granulosus* is endemic.
2. Attempts to infect primates experimentally with eggs of this strain have been unsuccessful.

Alveolar hydatid disease

E. multilocularis is of widespread distribution in the northern hemisphere, although not as yet endemic in the UK or Ireland. Dogs, racoon dogs and to a lesser extent cats, can harbour the adult tapeworm. The main epidemiological cycle, however, involves the fox as final host and microtine rodents (such as shrews and voles) as intermediate hosts. The eggs are also infective to some other mammals, including humans. Microtine rodents have a very short life-span and so the alveolar cyst grows rapidly. This and its invasive nature, with daughter cysts budding off its external surface, make this infection a particularly dangerous and often lethal zoonosis.

Epidemiology

Fox populations have been growing throughout Europe and they are becoming increasingly urbanised. Up to 60% of foxes are infected with *E. multilocularis* in some central European countries. From the zoonotic perspective, peri-urban foxes are the most significant as they hunt microtine rodents in the countryside during the day and contaminate the city environment at night when foraging human garbage.

Extra information box 5.4

> **The UK Pet Travel Scheme**
>
> Both foxes and microtine rodents are plentiful in the United Kingdom but fortunately there is as yet no *E. multilocularis*. In order to maintain this situation, all dogs entering (or reentering) the UK must, at the time of writing, be treated with an effective cestocide.

5.3.5 Other cyclophyllidean tapeworms

We now leave the taeniids to consider other common cyclophyllidean cestodes of veterinary significance (see Figure 5.6). Members of the family Anoplocephalidae can be recognised as their segments are much wider than they are long. Two cosmopolitan representatives are described: the horse tapeworm, *Anoplocephala* and the ruminant tapeworm, *Moniezia*. The latter has bile duct-dwelling relatives in the tropics. All have very similar life-cycles involving free-living mites as intermediate hosts.

Two tapeworms have been selected to represent the other families. *Dipylidium* is a ubiquitous parasite of dogs and cats while *Davainea* is the most pathogenic of the many poultry cestodes. The latter are of minor significance in intensive housing systems but can be troublesome in free-range birds.

Metacestode

One feature common to all the tapeworms in this section is that they use invertebrate intermediate hosts. There is only one type of cyclophyllidean metacestode found in invertebrates: the cysticercoid (see Figure 5.23). A cysticercoid is like a cysticercus (see Table 5.1) but is tiny (pinhead sized), so the whole volume of the cyst is occupied by a single tapeworm head (which is not inverted).

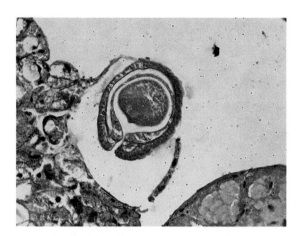

Figure 5.23 Cysticercoid of *Davainea* in tissues of a slug.

Anoplocephala

Three anoplocephalid species occur in equidae but only one, *Anoplocephala perfoliata*, is found commonly. Smaller specimens do not have the ribbon-like appearance typical of tapeworms, but closer inspection reveals a scolex with suckers and an obviously segmented body (see Figure 5.24). There are no hooks on the scolex, but small swellings behind each sucker called 'lappets' confirm species identification.

A. perfoliata typically grows to about 5 cm but can be longer. It is found mainly in the caecum clustered around the ileo-caecal junction (see Figure 5.25), where it causes superficial ulceration, mild inflammation and, in heavy infections, an oedematous swelling. Generally it is of little clinical significance but epidemiological evidence suggests that heavy infections (more than 20

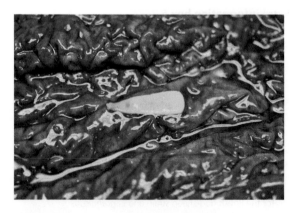

Figure 5.24 An adult *Anoplocephala* (detached from mucosa). Reproduced with permission of M.K. Nielsen.

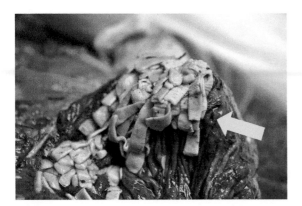

Figure 5.25 A mass of adult *Anoplocephala* at the ileo-caecal junction: note circular ulcer to the right of the tapeworms and the inflammation below. Reproduced with permission of M.K. Nielsen.

tapeworms) can significantly increase risk for spasmodic colic, ileal impaction and some forms of intussusception.

The anoplocephalid egg has an indefinite but nevertheless characteristic shape somewhere between round and triangular (see Figure 5.26). It contains a distinctive chitinous ring with two projections (the 'pyriform apparatus'). The intermediate hosts are oribatid mites. These are ubiquitous, nonparasitic pasture mites. They are most numerous in the summer months on permanent grasslands with soil rich in humus. They feed on fungal hyphae and faecal debris. The life-cycle is completed when mites harbouring cysticercoids are accidentally swallowed by grazing horses.

Moniezia

Moniezia expansa in the small intestine of small ruminants and *M. benedeni* in cattle are of little clinical significance despite their size (up to 2 m), although some believe that there may be an adverse effect on the growth rates of lambs in some circumstances.

Unlike *Anoplocephala*, *Moniezia* has a typical tapeworm appearance (see Figure 5.27). Its presence is usually indicated by white proglottids adhering to the surface of faecal pellets. A spontaneous expulsion often occurs in late summer when long tapeworm fragments can be seen hanging from the tail region. It is a typical anoplocephalid tapeworm and so its segments are much wider than they are long. The eggs resemble those of *A. perfoliata* (see Figure 5.26) and oribatid mites similarly act as intermediate hosts.

Help box 5.3

> ### *Moniezia*
>
> Identification: this is not a problem as *Moniezia* is the only adult tapeworm found in the intestine of farmed ruminants in most regions.
>
> Other cestode infections of ruminants: Other cestodes infections do occur but, with the exception of the tropical bile duct species, these are metacestodes (hydatid cyst, cysticercus or coenurus) and are found in liver, lungs, muscles or cranial cavity.

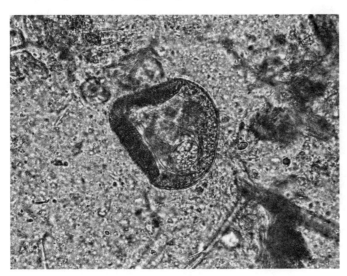

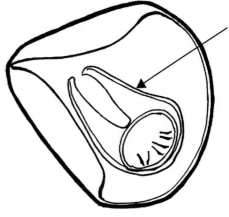

Figure 5.26 An anoplocephalid egg: the 'pyriform apparatus' is arrowed.

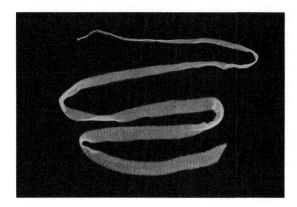

Figure 5.27 *Moniezia*: with scolex top left.

Dipylidium

Dipylidium caninum is a very common parasite of dogs and cats, growing to about half a metre long in the small intestine (see Figure 5.28 and Figure 5.29). The scolex has multiple rows of hooks and the gravid segments can

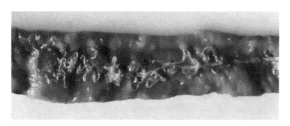

Figure 5.28 *Dipylidium* adults in small intestine of dog. Reproduced with permission of M.J. Walker.

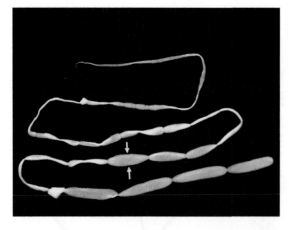

Figure 5.29 *Dipylidium*: with scolex top left, gravid segments bottom right and developing proglottids in between. Arrows point to genital pores on one segment.

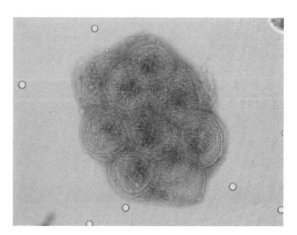

Figure 5.30 A *Dipylidium* egg-capsule: nine eggs are in view; hooks can be seen in some.

be differentiated from those of *Taenia* as they are oval in shape (rather than rectangular) and have two lateral genital pores (rather than one).

It is usually of minor clinical significance causing no more than occasional anal irritation, although diarrhoea can result if the tapeworms are present in large numbers. The proglottids are motile and can upset pet owners when they drop onto furniture or carpet.

The life-cycle of *D. caninum* is intricately intertwined with that of its intermediate host, the flea. Gravid segments and flea eggs are likely to drop from infected dogs and cats onto the same surfaces (see Section 2.2.2). The proglottids eject characteristic capsules ('egg nests') each containing several eggs (see Figure 5.30). Flea larvae have to supplement their staple ration of flea dirt to ensure a balanced diet. *Dipylidium* egg-capsules are eaten along with other organic materials. By the time the hatched oncospheres have transformed into infective cysticercoids, the flea larva has metamorphosed to a host-seeking adult. Flea infestation provokes exaggerated grooming behaviour which increases the chances of a cat or dog swallowing an infected flea and thereby acquiring *Dipylidium*.

Practical tip box 5.4

Control of *Dipylidium* infections

If *Dipylidium* is identified in a dog or cat, then reinfection can be avoided only by persuading the owner that a flea control programme is necessary.

Poultry cestodes

Davainea proglottina is a tiny (~3 mm) tapeworm with only 4–9 segments. It is found in poultry and pigeons attached to the duodenum. It has hooks on its suckers and many more over the rest of the scolex, which is perhaps why this parasite provokes haemorrhagic enteritis if present in large numbers. The intermediate hosts are slugs and snails.

Other poultry tapeworms are less damaging although they may affect productivity. Each species has its own intermediate host. Indoor birds are affected mostly by those utilising flies, as these can be very abundant inside buildings on some farms. Those using earthworms, beetles, ants or other invertebrates are more likely to be found in free-range birds.

5.4 Pseudophyllidean tapeworms

As noted previously, the biology of the two major tapeworm groups differs fundamentally. In contrast to the cyclophyllidean biology described in Section 5.3.1, mature pseudophyllidean proglottids expel eggs while remaining an integral part of the tapeworm chain in the intestine. In place of the metacestode, there is a succession of motile larval stages.

5.4.1 Pseudophyllidean life-cycle

The human fish tapeworm, *Diphyllobothrium*, is used to illustrate the pseudophyllidean life-cycle (see Figure 5.31):

a – Eggs are voided with the host faeces and a ciliated embryo, the coracidium, forms inside each.

b – The coracidium is released as a free-swimming organism, but only when light and moisture conditions are right.

c – If eaten by a copepod (its first intermediate host), the coracidium loses its cilia and develops into a larval stage called the procercoid.

d – When the infected copepod is in turn eaten by a suitable vertebrate (the second intermediate host), the parasite invades the somatic tissues of its new host and transforms into an elongated larva, the plerocercoid. This now ascends a carnivorous food-chain, transferring

to successive vertebrate predators or omnivores as each is devoured by the next.

e – Eventually, if and when it fortuitously finds itself in the intestine of an animal it can use as final host, it can at last grow into an adult tapeworm.

Practical tip box 5.5

Faecal examination and tapeworm infections

Faecal examination is more reliable for demonstrating infection with pseudophyllidean than cyclophyllidean tapeworms. This is because pseudophyllidean eggs are extruded from proglottids within the intestine and so are voided with the faeces (whereas cyclophyllidean gravid segments are generally expelled whole from the host before they start to release eggs). Pseudophyllidean eggs are oval with a 'trapdoor' (operculum) at one end. They look very similar to trematode eggs (see Figure 5.38) and careful laboratory examination is needed to tell them apart.

Avoid common mistakes!

Don't confuse the pseudophyllidean tapeworm *Spirometra* with *Spirocerca* (an oesophageal nematode of dogs).

5.4.2 Important pseudophyllideans

Only two pseudophyllidean genera are relevant in the context of this textbook: *Diphyllobothrium* and *Spirometra*. Both are primarily of zoonotic significance (see Section 9.3.1).

Diphyllobothrium latum is found mostly in colder northern regions. Humans are the main definitive host with fish acting as second intermediate host (see Figure 5.31). The adult tapeworm can establish in other fish-eating mammals, including dogs, but they are not considered to be a major factor in the epidemiology of the human infection.

Cats, and to a lesser extent dogs, may harbour *Spirometra mansonoides* in parts of North America. Other species occur in South America, Asia and Australasia. The adult tapeworm is about 0.5 m long but is generally asymptomatic. It has a complicated life-cycle passing firstly through copepods and then infecting various classes of vertebrates (although not fish). Humans become involved as occasional intermediate hosts. The resulting infection is known as 'sparganosis'.

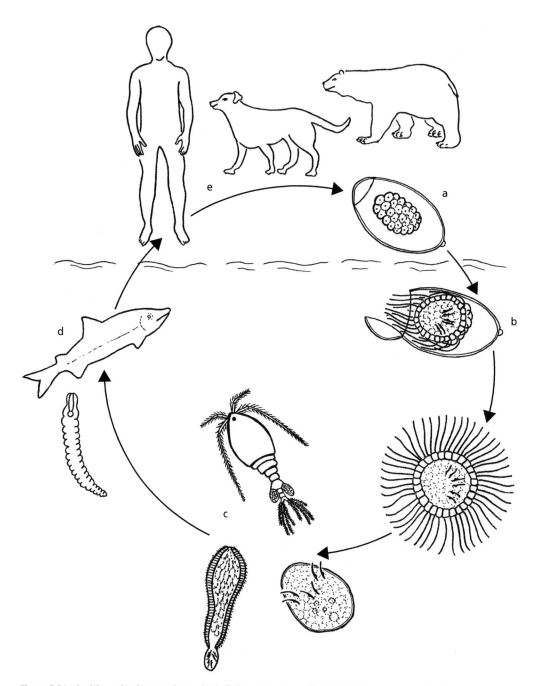

Figure 5.31 The life-cycle of a typical pseudophyllidean tapeworm, *Diphyllobothrium*: a – egg voided in faeces; b – coracidium develops and hatches; c – procercoid forms in copepod; d – plerocercoid develops in second intermediate host; e – adult tapeworm grows in final host (details in text). Immature stages redrawn and life-cycle based on Roberts and Janovy., 1996 with permission of McGraw-Hill Education and Eckert *et al.*, 2008 with permission of Enke Verlag.

5.5 Cestocidal drugs

Treatment options for tapeworm infections are limited. Older drugs such as dichlorophen, niclosamide and nitroscanate are still in use in some countries, but have been largely replaced by praziquantel and its analogue, epsiprantel, which have a broader spectrum of activity (see Table 9.7). Praziquantel is particularly useful against *Echinococcus* as it kills adults at all stages of growth in the intestine. Some benzimidazoles (see Section 7.3.3) have useful activity, but only against a limited range of tapeworm species. Pyrantel (see Section 7.3.1) has moderate activity against *Anoplocephala* in horses.

Therapy is directed almost exclusively against adult tapeworms as effective treatments for metacestodes are usually prohibitively expensive for veterinary use. A possible exception is oxfendazole (a benzimidazole) which has been employed against porcine cysticercosis in public health campaigns.

5.5.1 Praziquantel

Praziquantel and epsiprantel act by inducing a Ca^{2+} influx across the parasite tegument. This causes an immediate muscular spasm so that the adult tapeworm is unable to maintain its position in the intestine and is swept away by peristalsis. Disruption of tegumental defence mechanisms quickly follows, allowing attack by antibodies, immune cells and enzymes. The dead tapeworms are therefore mostly digested before being passed in faeces.

Extra information box 5.5

Destrobilation

Some old-fashioned cestocidal drugs cause the body of the tapeworm (the strobila) to break off at the neck but leave the scolex alive *in situ*. This then starts to bud off new segments. So, even though an impressive amount of cestode material is expelled, the tapeworm quickly regrows.

Contrast this with the action of praziquantel which expels the scolex but is less likely to impress the pet owner as the strobila is digested so little is seen to be passed after treatment!

5.6 Trematodes

Adult trematodes (flukes) are usually easy to recognise because of their flat leaf-like shape and the obvious presence of suckers. There are two trematode groups of veterinary interest: those found as ectoparasites on fish (monogenean trematodes) and those that are endoparasites in vertebrates (digenean trematodes).

Monogenean trematodes have a single oral sucker plus multiple suckers mounted on a prominent posterior attachment organ (the haptor) (see Figure 5.32). They have direct life-cycles and, as there is no intermediate host, infections can spread rapidly by direct transmission in aquaculture systems. This is, however, a highly specialised topic and the interested reader is referred to aquaculture or fish pathology texts for more information. The following sections focus on the digenean flukes of greatest importance in mainstream veterinary practice.

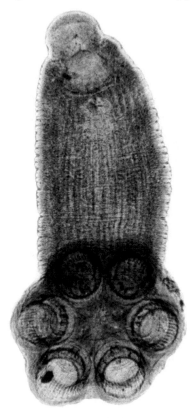

Figure 5.32 A monogenean trematode. Reproduced with permission of L.F. Khalil.

5.6.1 Digenean trematodes

Body structure

Digenean trematodes have just two suckers – ventral and oral (see Figure 5.33). The mouth leads from the latter to a muscular pharynx which pumps food into two blind-ending caeca. In some genera, such as *Fasciola*, these are branched to increase surface area. There is no anus, so they have to regurgitate waste materials through the mouth. There is an ovary, two testes and vitelline glands which produce the eggshell.

Digenean trematodes are covered by a metabolically active tegument (see Figure 5.34) which is important for evading host immune responses. In the liver fluke, *Fasciola*, for example, the several types of tegmental cell that donate cytoplasm to form the outer layer are switched

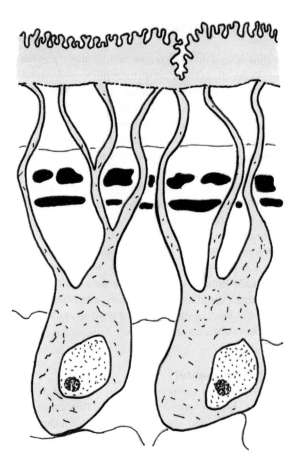

Figure 5.34 Diagrammatic representation of the tegument of a trematode showing tegumental cells donating cytoplasm (depicted in yellow) to the outer surface layer. Modified from Smyth, 1994.

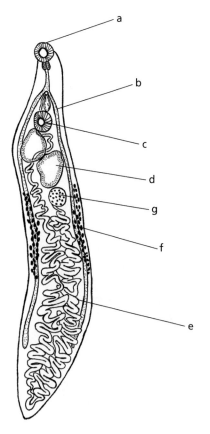

Figure 5.33 A typical trematode (*Dicrocoelium*): a – oral sucker; b – blind ending caeca; c – ventral sucker; d – testes; e – uterus; f – vitelline (egg-shell secreting) gland; g – ovary. Redrawn after Skrjabin and Evranova, 1952 with permission of Nauka from Bray *et al.*, 2008 with permission CAB International.

on and off sequentially. Host immune responses are thereby rendered ineffective as different surface antigens are presented to the host during successive phases of the parasitic life-cycle.

Other strategies used by flukes include:

a – rapid surface turnover: antibodies and hostile host cells are sloughed off before they cause damage;

b – molecular disguise: expressed surface antigens mimic host molecules so the parasite is not recognised as 'foreign';

c – immunomodulation: factors are released that down-regulate or otherwise modify host responses;

d – antibody cleavage: enzymes destroy antibodies as they attach to the parasite.

Life-cycles

Digenean life-cycles are complex with a succession of larval stages and enormous replication occurring in a molluscan intermediate host. The liver fluke, *Fasciola*, is used as an example (see Figure 5.35):

a – The egg is passed in faeces and needs warmth and moisture for development of the first larval stage, the miracidum.

b – When fully formed, the miracidium is ready to hatch out of the egg, but will only do so if in a film of water and exposed to the correct light intensity.

c – The miracidium finds its intermediate host with the help of cilia for swimming, light sensitive spots for orientation and chemotactic responses that are highly sensitive to molluscan chemical signals. It attaches to the surface of the snail and secretes enzymes that enable it to penetrate into the body.

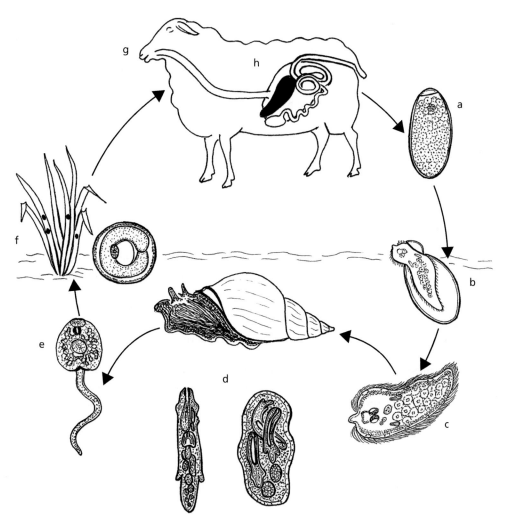

Figure 5.35 The life-cycle of a digenean trematode, *Fasciola hepatica*: a – egg voided in faeces; b – miracidium develops and hatches; c – miracidium seeks snail intermediate host; d – three phases of asexual reproduction produce sporocysts, rediae, then cercariae; e – cercariae leave snail; f – metacercariae form on vegetation; g – metacercaria eaten by final host; h – fluke migrates to its predilection site and matures (details in text). Adapted from FAO, 1994 with permission of FAO; immature stages after J. N. Oldham's drawings in RVC collection.

d – Within the snail's 'liver' (hepatopancreas), the miracidium transforms into a second larval stage, the sporocyst. This sac-like structure is a cloning machine producing more sporocysts and, eventually, rediae (the third larval stage). These are cylindrical and give birth to numerous cercariae (the fourth larval stage). One miracidium entering a snail can give rise to 600 or more cercariae. The speed at which this happens is temperature dependent.

e – The cercaria is heart-shaped with a tail. This is the stage that leaves the snail, but it will only do so in moist conditions.

f – The cercaria swims through water and moves along films of moisture before adhering firmly to vegetation. It sheds its tail and secretes a tough protective wall around itself to become a metacercaria.

g – The final host is infected by ingesting the metacercaria.

h – The immature fluke inside the metacercaria is released in the small intestine and migrates to its predilection site (the bile-duct) where it grows to maturity and eventually starts to lay eggs.

Important digenean trematodes

The classification of trematodes is complicated and of little obvious benefit to understanding veterinary field problems. Figure 5.36, therefore, does no more than list the most significant of the many flukes that infest domesticated animals.

In the liver, *Fasciola* causes production losses worldwide in ruminants with access to wet pastures, *Dicrocoelium* is less damaging and found in drier environments, while *Fascioloides* is harmless in wild ruminants but lethal to sheep. Adult amphistomes are generally benign but their immature stages can have severe and sometimes lethal consequences in warmer, wetter regions. The

schistosomes are serious pathogens, mostly confined to the tropics. Some occur exclusively in humans, some in animals, while a few are capable of transfer from animals to people or visa-versa. *Alaria* and *Nanophyetus* are encountered in North American small animal practice while a number of other genera are found in pet animals in other regions, e.g. *Opisthorchis* in Central and Eastern Europe.

5.6.2 *Fasciola*

The adult liver fluke, *Fasciola hepatica* (see Figure 5.37), grows to a length of 2–5 cm in the bile ducts of a wide range of animals, including sheep, cattle, rabbits and, less often, horses. It can infect humans causing a painful abdominal disease. Its distribution is mostly confined to wetter temperate regions. It is replaced by a similar but slightly larger species, *F. gigantica*, in more tropical climates.

Preparasitic life-cycle

The life-cycle of *Fasciola* was described in broad outline in Figure 5.35. Aspects of particular significance in determining the epidemiology and clinical outcome of fasciolosis are now considered in more detail.

Fasciola eggs are relatively large (140 µm), oval, golden-brown in colour, with a visible operculum (trapdoor) at one end (Figure 5.38). The development of all preparasitic life-cycle stages is temperature dependent with a minimum requirement of 10°C. Consequently, eggs dropped onto the pasture during the spring months in Britain will not be ready to hatch before June at the earliest.

Fluke development within the snail intermediate host takes several weeks and so cercariae are released in the UK from late August into the autumn months. This explains the seasonality of the associated disease with the worst outbreaks of acute fasciolosis in sheep occurring in October and November (see Figure 8.9).

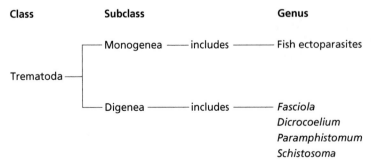

Figure 5.36 The major groups of trematodes.

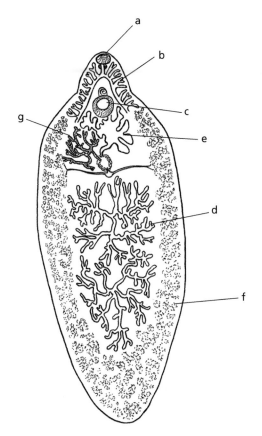

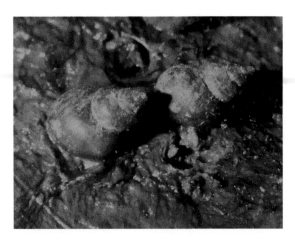

Figure 5.39 *Galba truncatula*, the intermediate host of *Fasciola hepatica* in the British Isles and parts of Europe. From Jacobs, 1986. Reproduced with permission of Elsevier.

Intermediate hosts are lymnaeid snails (see Figure 5.39) and this determines the distribution of fasciolosis. *Galba truncatula* (also known as *Lymnaea truncatula*), which plays this role in the British Isles, lives on wet and muddy terrain. Thus, the greatest economic losses due to fasciolosis occur in the wetter, western parts of the region where this snail is abundant.

Figure 5.37 An adult liver fluke, *Fasciola hepatica*: a – oral sucker; b – blind ending caeca; c – ventral sucker; d – testes; e – uterus; f – vitelline (egg-shell secreting) gland; g – ovary. Adapted from Jones, 2005 with permission of CAB International and A. Jones.

Extra information box 5.6

Things can change!

Climate change, new agricultural practices and other factors can modify long-existing patterns of parasitic disease. For example, new foci of fluke transmission have recently appeared in eastern England due to the re-establishment of wet-lands for nature conservation coupled with local restocking after the 2001 foot-and-mouth epidemic with livestock from fluke-endemic areas. The clinician must be aware that diseases can evolve faster than textbooks can be rewritten.

Snail biology

The muddy habitats of *G. truncatula* are either permanent (e.g. river banks, ditches, low-lying badly drained fields etc.) or temporary (adjacent areas which may be wet or dry depending on season and rainfall). Acid conditions are unfavourable and so fewer snails will be found in peaty areas. The snails feed on green slime (microalgae) and multiply rapidly if food is abundant. The population

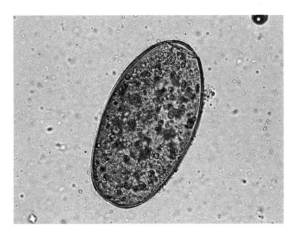

Figure 5.38 *Fasciola hepatica* egg: note the operculum ('trap-door') top right.

will expand to cover all the wet ground available, but dry conditions lead to overcrowding, competition for food and heavy mortality.

Practical tip box 5.6

Fluke habitats

Fluke habitats can be identified by demonstrating the presence of the snail intermediate host. *G. truncata* can be recognised (see Figure 5.39) as it is 5–10 mm long; has a brown-black shell with 5–6 spirals, the first of which is greater than half the total shell length; also, the shell opens to the right when positioned with the opening pointing towards the observer.

The density of metacercariae on pasture is obviously determined by the number of fluke-infected snails and this in turn depends on the extent to which the snail population has been able to multiply and colonise the grazing area. Disease risk is therefore dependent on rainfall patterns during the warmer months of the year when fluke development is taking place inside the snail.

Help box 5.4

Why is risk of fasciolosis dependent on rainfall?

Wet summer conditions:

- ideal for hatching of fluke and snail eggs
- snail habitats expand and food supply abundant

Therefore:

snail population increases rapidly
- many infected snails
- eventual shedding of many cercariae
- high density of metacercariae on herbage
- increased risk of disease for grazing animals.

The opposite happens in a dry year, leading to a reduced risk of disease.

Other aspects of snail biology may influence the pattern of disease outbreaks. For example, British winters are generally cold enough to kill most hibernating lymnaeids. Consequently, the next clinically important epidemiological cycle cannot start until June when a new generation of snails hatch from eggs laid by the few overwintering survivors. This leads to acute disease

in sheep in the autumn followed by chronic fasciolosis in the winter, a process called the 'summer infection of the snail'.

Help box 5.5

What is meant by the 'summer infection of the snail'?

Fluke eggs that are passed in spring (e.g. on mainland Britain):

- hatch in June (coincident with first snail hatch)
- miracidia infect newly hatched snails
- develop and multiply in snail during summer
- cercariae shed from late August onwards
- metacercariae ingested by sheep
- immature flukes migrate through liver
- acute disease September–November
- adult flukes in bile ducts of surviving sheep cause chronic disease January onwards.

A different epidemiological pattern is often seen in the west of Ireland where winters are milder. Under these conditions, snails may survive in sufficient quantity to shed potentially dangerous numbers of cercariae during the following summer. Potentially pathogenic pasture contamination in this case is due to a 'winter infection of snails'.

Help box 5.6

What is meant by the 'winter infection of the snail'?

Fluke eggs dropped late summer (e.g. in western Ireland):

- infect snails
- development in snail halted when temp <10°C (i.e. flukes trapped in hibernating snails through the winter)
- development resumes in spring when temp >10°C
- cercariae shed from July
- disease from August.

The general principles outlined above can be applied in other parts of the world but patterns of disease will vary according to local climate, topography and which lymnaeid species is/are responsible for transmission (some are more aquatic than others). Computer models are used in some countries to forecast disease risk based on field and/or meteorological data.

Parasitic migration

After the metacercaria has been swallowed by a suitable host, the immature fluke (measuring just 0.1 mm) takes about a week to penetrate through the wall of the small intestine and migrate across the peritoneal cavity to the liver. It now meanders through the liver substance for 6–7 weeks eating, growing and becoming ever more destructive. Having reached about a centimetre in length, it enters a bile duct where it feeds by grazing the mucosa and by sucking blood. After 3–6 weeks it starts to lay eggs. The prepatent period is therefore 10–12 weeks.

Disease manifestations

Fasciolosis is a seasonal disease with more serious outbreaks occurring in some years than in others. Deaths, acute, subacute, chronic and subclinical disease occur in sheep of all ages but disease in cattle is almost always chronic or subclinical and confined to younger stock. Species and age susceptibilities are related to the proportion of flukes surviving the journey to the bile ducts. This in turn depends on the relative fibroblastic potential of the liver parenchyma to obstruct the migrating flukes and the degree of protection afforded by immune responses. Both these mechanisms are considerably more effective in cattle than they are in sheep.

Pathogenesis of acute disease

Large numbers of metacercariae ingested over a short period of time give rise to acute disease. Initially, young immature flukes are very small and damage is negligible, but marauding flukes half a centimetre in length destroying liver tissue and rupturing blood vessels provoke serious trauma. Consequently, there is a delay of 2–6 weeks between infection and the onset of clinical signs. Death can occur in sheep with little warning. Autopsy will reveal a pale swollen liver with dark-red parasitic tracts and haemorrhages (see Figure 5.40). A fatal outcome is also likely if damaged liver tissue gives the anaerobic bacterium *Clostridium novyi* type B opportunity to multiply and generate Black Disease toxin.

Sheep with heavy infection (>500 flukes) that survive the initial acute phase of disease may nevertheless start to lose weight rapidly later in the autumn or early winter. They become anaemic and may die. This is known as subacute disease and autopsy reveals both immature and adult flukes in the liver. Large subcapsular haemorrhages are often present (see Figure 5.41).

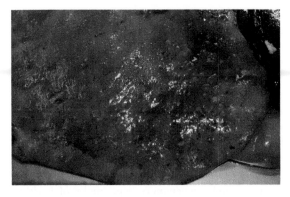

Figure 5.40 Acute fasciolosis: pale liver with haemorrhagic tracts. Reproduced with permission of AHVLA, Carmarthen © Crown copyright 2013.

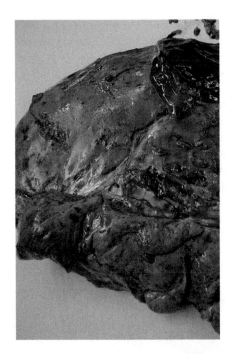

Figure 5.41 Subacute fasciolosis: liver with dark-red parasitic tracts and large subcapsular haemorrhage. Reproduced with permission of AHVLA, Carmarthen © Crown copyright 2013.

Pathogenesis of chronic disease

Smaller numbers of metacercariae ingested over a longer period of time lead to chronic fasciolosis. Hosts surviving the migratory phase of the life-cycle are likely to show long-term economic effects such as suboptimal weight-gain, milk or wool production even if overt signs of weight-loss, anaemia and oedema are not obvious. As with many parasitic infections, chronic fasciolosis tends to depress appetite. This is particularly unfortunate for animals grazing on marginal land as chronic fasciolosis exerts its effects in the winter when the pasture has little nutritive value.

Animals with chronic fasciolosis are further disadvantaged by extensive liver fibrosis caused by a number of mechanisms including postnecrotic scarring of tissues damaged by migrating flukes and peribiliary fibrosis due to the ongoing activities of adult flukes (see Figure 5.42). The bile ducts become calcified in cattle. Shrinkage of scar tissue and compensatory hypertrophy of healthy parenchyma gives the liver an uneven shape.

Of much greater importance, however, is the constant physiological stress due to the feeding behaviour of the adult fluke. Sheep with overt clinical signs are likely to be harbouring at least 250 flukes which equates to a daily haemorrhage into the bile duct of some 50 ml of whole blood (compared to a total blood volume of 1500 ml). The lost blood is digested in the small intestine but the released iron is in a form that cannot be re-absorbed. A ten-fold increase in erythropoiesis is needed to compensate for the continuing loss of red blood cells, but many animals nevertheless slip into a state of normochromic anaemia, which becomes hypochromic when their limited iron reserves are exhausted.

Plasma proteins are also lost into the bile duct, partly due to fluke feeding but also because of increased epithelial permeability (by a mechanism similar to that illustrated in Figure 6.22). The daily breakdown (catabolic rate) of albumin in affected sheep can be increased by a factor of 2.5, with a commensurate loss of nitrogen

in urine. Depending on nutritional status, this may put the animal into negative nitrogen balance giving rise to production losses and welfare issues. In severe cases, hypoalbuminaemia may become clinically evident as oedema.

Help box 5.7

Definition of some physiological terms

Erythropoiesis: The production of new red blood cells (RBCs) in the bone marrow.

Normochromic anaemia: Anaemia due to too few circulating RBCs but with a normal amount of haemoglobin in each RBC.

Hypochromic anaemia: Anaemia associated with RBCs containing insufficient haemoglobin.

Negative nitrogen balance: The animal's dietary nitrogen intake is insufficient to compensate for that being excreted or otherwise lost from the body.

Hypoalbuminaemia: A suboptimal plasma albumin concentration.

Oedema: Excess tissue fluid due to abnormal blood osmotic effects; it manifests as a watery submandibular swelling in sheep ('bottle-jaw').

5.6.3 Other digenean trematodes

This section highlights the most important digenean trematodes, other than *Fasciola*, affecting domesticated animals around the world.

Paramphistomum

Although cosmopolitan, amphistomes are most troublesome in warmer climates, particularly Australia, Africa and India. Historically, they have been diagnosed only rarely in the UK but recently one genus (*Calicophoron*) has been reported with increasing frequency. There are several amphistome genera containing many species, but *Paramphistomum cervi* is the most widespread worldwide. They occur mostly in ruminants (with one tropical genus in horses and pigs).

Amphistomes do not look like other flukes as they are plump and cylindrical but they have the suckers and internal structure typical of a digenean trematode (see Figure 5.43). Adults attach to the wall of the rumen without causing significant damage (see Figure 5.44). The eggs are like those of *Fasciola* (see Figure 5.38) except that they are colourless. The preparasitic life-cycle is also very similar except that the

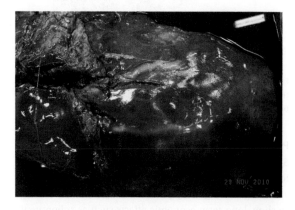

Figure 5.42 Chronic fasciolosis: bovine liver showing distended and thickened bile ducts and liver fibrosis. Reproduced with permission of T. de Waal.

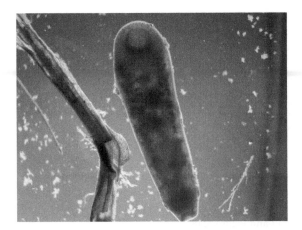

Figure 5.43 An adult paramphistome. Reproduced with permission of AHVLA, Carmarthen © Crown copyright 2013.

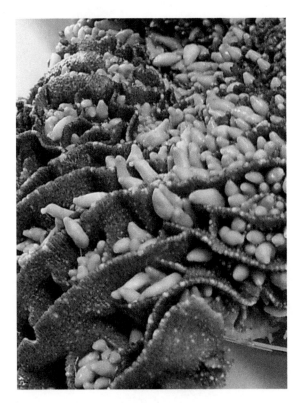

Figure 5.44 Paramphistomes on inner wall of rumen. Reproduced with permission of J. Vercruysse.

intermediate hosts are water snails (planorbids) and this is why clinical outbreaks are usually associated with locations such as the edges of lakes and rivers, swamps or recently flooded terrain. Metacercariae accumu-late on vegetation and, after ingestion, excyst in the jejunum of the final host. Immature flukes have to migrate anteriorly along the duodenum as they head towards the rumen. Since peristalsis forces intestinal contents in the opposite direction, they migrate by burrowing into the mucosa. If sufficiently numerous, they can provoke severe and sometimes fatal enteritis and diarrhoea.

Dicrocoelium

Although of worldwide occurrence, the distribution of this trematode in Britain and North America is restricted to particular localities. It is relatively nonpathogenic but has an amazing life-cycle involving two intermediate hosts: a land snail and an ant. Both require relatively dry habitats and so *Dicrocoelium* infections are usually associated with well drained farms and heathland.

Dicrocoelium dendriticum (see Figure 5.45) is smaller (<1.5 cm) than, and lacks the 'shoulders' which are a prominent feature of adult *Fasciola* (see Figure 5.37). The adult is found in the bile ducts of ruminants and some other herbivores. In contrast to migrating *F. hepatica* (which burrow through liver parenchyma), immature *D. dendriticum* take an easier and less damaging route from the small intestine to their predilection site – they go directly up the common bile duct. Immune responses provide little protection and large numbers of *D. dendriticum* can accumulate. Fortunately, most infections are asymptomatic. Clinical signs are associated with liver cirrhosis and occur only if many thousands of flukes are present.

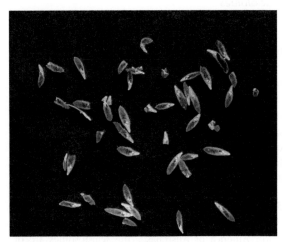

Figure 5.45 *Dicrocoelium*: adult worms.

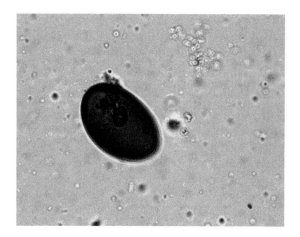

Figure 5.46 *Dicrocoelium* egg: note the two dark eye-spots within the egg.

The small (45 μm) dark brown eggs (see Figure 5.46) already contain a miracidium when passed in faeces. They have to be ingested by the first intermediate host, which can be any of a wide range of land snails. Here, the fluke larvae develop in the usual way. Cercariae are excreted from the snails in slime-balls. These are collected by the second intermediate host, brown ants of the genus *Formica*, taken to their nest and eaten. Metacercariae encyst inside the ants, impacting various anatomic sites including nerve ganglia. This makes the ants revert to a primitive behaviour whereby they climb up and cling onto vegetation overnight instead of retreating to the nest. This enhances the likelihood of them being eaten the following morning by grazing or browsing herbivores.

Fascioloides

Fascioloides magna is big (up to 10 cm long and 3 cm broad). It is endemic in parts of North America and has been introduced into some European countries. The life-cycle is similar to that of *Fasciola* with lymnaeid snails as intermediate host and moose and deer as final hosts. In these, the adult flukes are harmlessly confined within hepatic cysts, eggs escaping via the bile ducts. Sheep and goats are accidental (aberrant) hosts in which the cyst does not form and so there is nothing to stop the fluke from causing massive liver trauma and haemorrhage. This usually has a fatal outcome.

Schistosoma

Although not endemic in domesticated animals in Europe, North America or Australasia, the schistosomes are of enormous importance to animal production and human

health in the tropics. They live in blood vessels and are known collectively as the 'blood-flukes'. *Schistosoma bovis* and *S. mattheei* infect ruminants in Africa and the Middle East, while *S. nasale* causes problems in India. These species are associated with hepato-peritoneal, urogenital and nasal venous networks, respectively. *S. japonicum*, another visceral species, is a serious zoonosis throughout Asia. It affects millions of people and has an enormously wide host-range including both domesticated and wild animals.

Unlike other trematodes of veterinary importance, *Schistosoma* has separate males and females. They are usually found as couples with the smaller cylindrical female in the embrace of a leaf-shaped male (see Figure 5.47 and Figure 5.48).

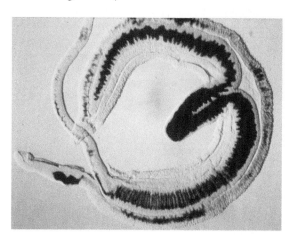

Figure 5.47 A pair of adult schistosomes: the cylindrical female is in the embrace of the leaf-shaped male. Reproduced with permission of J. Vercruysse.

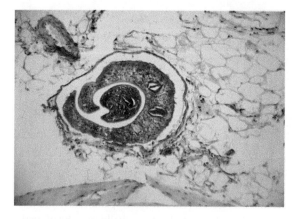

Figure 5.48 A pair of adult schistosomes cut in transverse section showing the cylindrical female (centre) enveloped by the male. Reproduced with permission of J. Vercruysse.

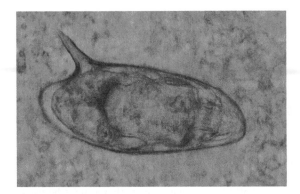

Figure 5.49 A schistosome egg containing a miracidium. Reproduced with permission of J.R. Stothard.

Schistosome eggs vary in size and shape according to species. Most have a spike or spine to assist their passage through the blood vessel wall and into surrounding tissues (see Figure 5.49). They are propelled passively by host tissue movements, ultimately reaching bile, faeces, urine or nasal discharge to access the outside world. If dropped into water, the miracidium hatches out and seeks its intermediate host, an aquatic snail, which will later release cercariae. These swim to locate a final host and enter by skin penetration. Thus, there is no meta-cercarial stage in the life-cycle.

Clinical signs in the final host are associated with pathology accumulating from the entrapment of metabolically active eggs in granulomatous lesions (see Figure 5.50). A separate condition, 'swimmer's itch', is a cutaneous hypersensitivity reaction suffered by some

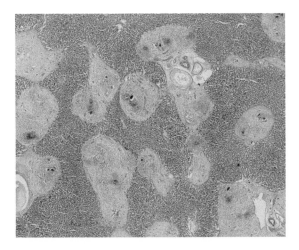

Figure 5.50 Liver showing schistosome eggs within granulomatous lesions.

people when exposed to the cercariae of a schistosome species that cannot establish in humans.

The transmission of schistosomes depends on prolonged contact between the final host and contaminated water, e.g. when grazing marshy pasture, drinking from or wading through ponds, irrigation systems or rivers. Environmental manipulation, such as the building of a hydro-electric dam, can have a profound influence on local epidemiology and disease prevalence by altering the nature and extent of snail habitats.

Extra information box 5.7

Immunity to tissue-dwelling helminths

In the case of tissue-dwelling helminths, infections can invoke stage-specific cytokine profiles (see Help box 1.4). For instance, Th1-reactions are associated with the early invasive stages of *Schistosoma* but these switch to Th2-modulated immune responses once the worms mature and start passing eggs into the blood-stream. This switch seems to be an essential step in the development of protective immunity against such parasites.

Trematodes of dogs and cats

Dogs and cats around the world with the opportunity to catch and eat amphibians or fish may be exposed to a wide range of trematode infections affecting the liver, gastro intestinal tract or lungs. They are very rarely diagnosed in Britain, but in North America typically operculate trematode eggs of at least two genera, *Alaria* and *Nanophyetus*, can sometimes be seen during routine faecal examination. Both are small (< 6 mm) intestinal flukes. Neither is very pathogenic, although *Nanophyetus* can transmit *Neorickettsia salminicola*, the aetiological agent of the disease known colloquially as 'salmon poisoning'. Both have snails as first intermediate host. *Alaria* has frogs and toads as second intermediate hosts and rodents eating these can act as paratenic hosts. This parasite migrates extensively around the body of the final host before settling in the small intestine. Fish act as second intermediate host for *Nanophyetus*.

5.7 Flukicidal drugs

Praziquantel (see Section 5.5.1) is used in the treatment of human schistosomosis and some small animal trematode infections (such as *Alaria*) but it has no useful activity against *Fasciola*. For this, benzimidazoles or salicylanilides are generally employed, but care is needed in the choice of compound as they are not all equally effective against migrating immature flukes. For this reason, only some can be used for treating or preventing acute fasciolosis in sheep grazing contaminated pasture while others are suitable only for treating chronic infection (see Table 8.2).

5.7.1 Benzimidazoles

The benzimidazoles and pro-benzimidazoles are used primarily for their effect against nematodes (see Section 7.3.3.), but some members of the group such as albendazole have activity against adult *F. hepatica* in the bile ducts. Netobimin is reported to be particularly useful against *Dicrocoelium*.

One benzimidazole, triclabendazole, has a different molecular configuration from other members of this class of chemicals. This imparts a unique spectrum of activity. It is inactive against nematodes or cestodes but highly potent against *F. hepatica* of all stages of maturity

in the final host. Thus, it is often the drug of choice for liver fluke control, but it must be used responsibly as resistant strains are starting to appear. It would be disastrous if this drug were to become widely ineffective before a replacement had been discovered.

5.7.2 Salicylanilides

Examples of salicylanilides and halogenated phenols with flukicidal activity are closantel, nitroxynil and oxyclozanide. Greatest flukicidal potency is seen in those that bind most strongly to plasma proteins. A prolonged plasma half-life, however, means they cannot be used in animals providing milk for human consumption. This chemical group has little useful activity against younger flukes migrating through the liver. The stage of maturity at which useful activity starts varies with compound and between host species, so care is needed in selecting an appropriate product to suit each clinical situation.

Closantel also has useful activity against blood sucking nematodes such as *Haemonchus* (see Section 8.2.1).

CHAPTER 6

Nematoda ('roundworms') part 1: concepts and bursate nematodes

6.1 Introduction

As most nematode roundworms are tiny and unpretentious, they escape public attention and are generally ignored by wild-life filmmakers. Nevertheless, they are one of the most numerous and diverse metazoan life-forms on this planet. The great majority are free-living, with species adapted to virtually every habitable aquatic or terrestrial ecological niche. A small minority are parasitic on plants and an even smaller proportion exploit animals for part or all of their life-cycle. Even so, the number of animal parasitic nematodes can be daunting for the student. Luckily, a detailed knowledge of every pathogenic species is unnecessary. This is because closely related nematodes tend to have similar life-cycles, epidemiology, pathogenesis and drug susceptibilities. An appreciation of group characteristics therefore saves a lot of repetitive learning. In this context, the best taxonomic level for our consideration is the superfamily (with names ending in –oidea; see Section 1.2.2). This chapter and the next provide an overview of these shared traits and outline the biology of an illustrative selection of important nematode parasites within each category.

6.2 Key concepts

Nematodes are unique in the animal world as the fluid in their body-cavity is maintained at a relatively high pressure. Movement is governed by muscle bundles working against this inner hydrostatic tension and the

Principles of Veterinary Parasitology, First Edition. By Dennis Jacobs, Mark Fox, Lynda Gibbons and Carlos Hermosilla.
© 2016 John Wiley & Sons, Ltd. Published 2016 by John Wiley & Sons, Ltd.
Companion website: www.wiley.com/go/jacobs/principles-veterinary-parasitology

elasticity of the tough outer layers of the body (the 'cuticle'). These internal forces make swallowing difficult and so a large muscular pharynx (oesophagus) is needed to pump food into the intestine. All these functions are synchronised by a nerve ring around the pharynx which is connected via longitudinal nerves to various ganglia. Many anthelmintic drugs work by disrupting neuromuscular coordination, thereby rendering the worm incapable of feeding or maintaining its position within the host.

6.2.1 Recognition features

Although apparently featureless at first sight (see Figure 6.1), many nematodes are easily identified when placed under the microscope. Memorising the diagnostic characteristics of every species would be a pointless exercise since descriptions and identification keys are readily available. However, the useful employment of such aides is dependent on an ability to recognise a few basic morphological features.

Surface structures

The cuticle which covers the surface of a nematode is not a featureless membrane but a complex structure with microscopic landmarks such as small pits containing tiny finger-like sensory organs (sensory papillae). More prominent diagnostic features are sometimes present, e.g. wing-like protrusions ('alae') and cuticular swellings that encompass the whole circumference of the body (see Figure 6.2 and Figure 6.3).

The position of a diagnostic feature along the body is often indicated by an appropriate descriptive word, for example:

a – cephalic: at the head-end;

b – cervical: behind the head;

c – caudal: at the tail-end.

Accessory sexual structures

Nematodes have separate sexes. The posterior end of the female worm tapers to a blunt point, which is rarely of diagnostic value (see Figure 6.4). The male tail, in contrast, often has accessory sexual structures useful for identification.

Spicules

Spicules are rod-like structures that can be protruded from the cloaca of the male to assist with the transfer of sperm during mating (see Figure 6.5). As they are

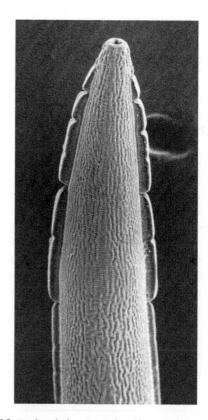

Figure 6.2 Head-end of a nematode with cervical alae. (SEM of *Passalurus*, a nematode of rabbits and hares.) From Gibbons, 1986 with permission of CAB International.

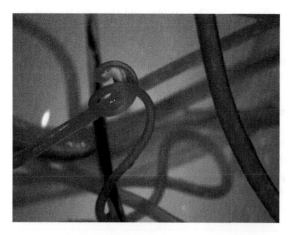

Figure 6.1 Nematodes: gross appearance (*Dirofilaria immitis* from the pulmonary artery of a dog). Reproduced with permission of L. Venco.

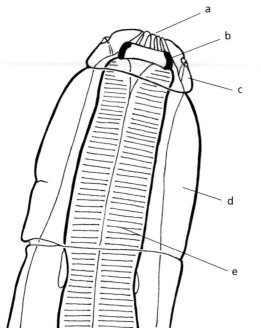

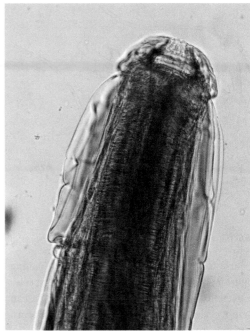

Figure 6.3 Head-end of a nematode (*Oesophagostomum*): a – leaf crown; b – buccal capsule; c – oral collar; d – cervical inflation; e – oesophagus.

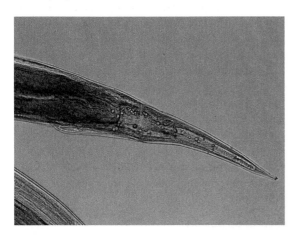

Figure 6.4 The tail-end of a female nematode (*Haemonchus*).

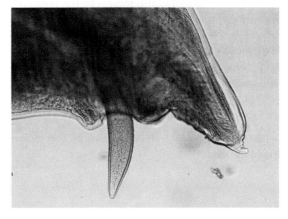

Figure 6.5 Tail-end of a nonbursate nematode (*Toxocara*) showing one spicule protruding from the cloaca.

made of chitin they show up well in prepared specimens under the microscope. They are usually paired and their shape and size is often diagnostic.

Bursa

The bursa (see Figure 6.6) is a very distinctive clasping organ situated at the posterior end of male worms belonging to particular superfamilies. The presence or absence of a male bursa enables a distinction to be made between 'bursate' and 'nonbursate' nematodes, which is a useful first step in worm identification. In some species the bursa is big enough to be seen with the naked eye, appearing as a terminal globule. It is formed of large expansions of the body wall within which are finger-like projections ('bursal rays') that have a sensory function.

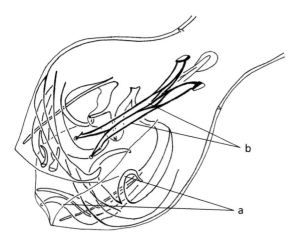

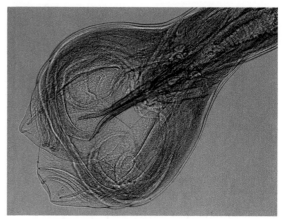

Figure 6.6 Tail-end of a male bursate nematode (*Haemonchus*) illustrating the bursa: a – bursal rays; b – spicules.

The bursa is used to hold the female during mating (see Figure 6.7). This process is aided in some species by the excretion of a cementing substance which can sometimes be seen as a brown 'blob' on female worms. Unfortunately, this is of no diagnostic value.

Nonbursate males achieve a mating posture by using sensory papillae near their cloaca for accurate alignment. Some are helped in this process by the presence of caudal alae which function like a miniature bursa.

Head, mouth and associated structures

Many nematode species have a simple head with a small mouth, which provides little diagnostic assistance, but others have useful distinguishing features (see Figure 6.8), including:

a – leaf crown: rows of leaf-shaped structures arranged around the mouth;

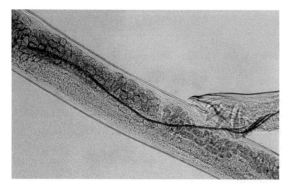

Figure 6.7 Male bursate worm (to right) using its bursa to clasp a female (diagonal).

b – buccal cavity: a large space behind the mouth;

c – teeth: which may be around the mouth and/or at the base of the buccal cavity;

d – cutting plates: which serve the same function as teeth.

The mouth leads, directly or via the buccal cavity, to the muscular pharynx. This is a prominent internal feature when nematodes are viewed under the microscope. The basic form, seen in most free-living and plant parasitic nematodes, is known as a 'rhabditiform oesophagus' and has two thickenings along its length separated by a distinct constriction (see Figure 6.9). This form also occurs in preparasitic life-cycle stages of many animal nematodes.

In contrast, the parasitic stages of animal nematodes need to employ highly specialised feeding techniques and so the shape of the pharynx differs between groups. This can sometimes provide extra information to assist in the identification process.

Practical tip box 6.1

Free-living nematodes

Diagnostic samples (e.g. faecal samples collected from the ground) are often contaminated with free-living adult nematodes. They can be recognised by their 'rhabditiform oesophagus' as illustrated in Figure 6.9.

Appearance in histological sections

When a tissue sample taken at necropsy or by biopsy is sectioned for microscopic examination, it is almost

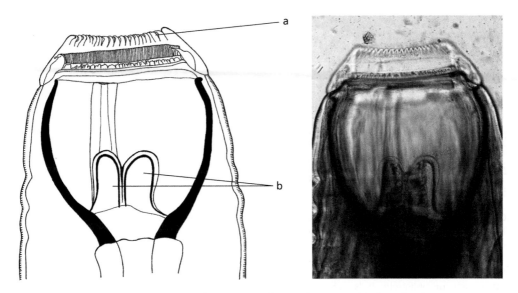

Figure 6.8 Head of a nematode (*Strongylus vulgaris*) showing: a – leaf crown; b – two teeth in buccal cavity.

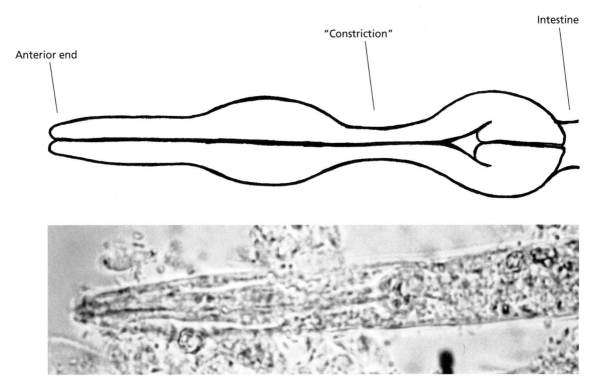

Figure 6.9 Pharynx of a free-living nematode. Photograph reproduced with permission of L.F. Khalil.

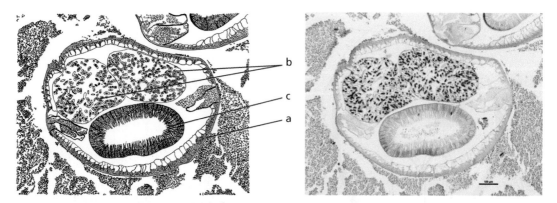

Figure 6.10 Transverse section through a female nematode (*Spirocerca*) in a tissue section: a – cuticle; b – uteri filled with eggs; c – intestine. Photograph reproduced with permission of R.C. Krecek and K. Snowden.

inevitable that any nematode contained therein will be cut transversely or obliquely. It is very unlikely, therefore, that any resemblance of a worm-like shape will be retained. Nevertheless, a nematode in section can be recognised as it is surrounded by a cuticle and the internal organs are often distinctive. The detailed appearance will, of course, vary depending where, along the length of the worm, the cut has been made. A typical example is displayed in Figure 6.10.

6.2.2 General biology

Feeding mechanisms

Many gastrointestinal nematodes, particularly those with small mouths, are found closely applied to the mucosal surface where oxygen tension is highest. Some

swallow part-digested alimentary contents, but most feed on host secretions and may even stimulate the host to provide an abundant supply of modified mucus for them. Some may take in desquamated epithelial cells while others actively graze on mucosal lining cells.

Plug feeders are more aggressive. They suck a mouthful of mucosa into their buccal cavity (see Figure 6.11). Teeth and enzymes reduce host tissue to a pulp which is swallowed. The worm then releases its grip and moves to a fresh site to repeat the process, leaving behind a small bleeding ulcer. Still more vicious are the species that bury their heads deep into the mucosa so they can suck arterial blood.

Thus, there is a range of feeding mechanisms each provoking a different type of pathogenicity. This complexity is increased still further as nematodes also

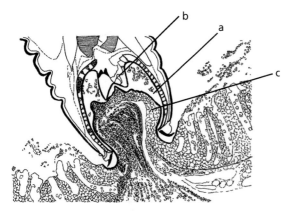
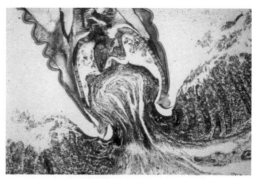

Figure 6.11 Histological section of intestinal mucosa with a plug feeding nematode: a – buccal cavity; b – teeth; c – mucosal plug. Photograph from Jacobs, 1986. Reproduced with permission of Elsevier.

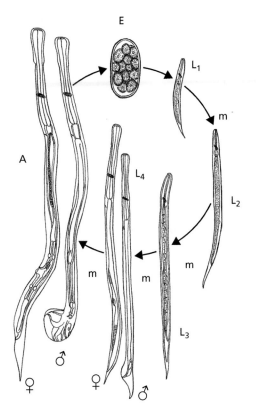

Figure 6.12 Nematode life-cycle stages: E – egg; L_1 - first-stage larvae; m – moult; L_2 – second-stage larva; etc.; A – adult. Larvae redrawn after Stewart, 1954, with permission of Allen Press Publishing Services.

produce excretory and secretory (ES) substances, sometimes in copious quantities, which may be pharmacologically active or which may have immunogenic or immunomodulatory properties.

Life-cycle

The basic nematode life-cycle is very straightforward (see Figure 6.12), although many variations on this simple theme will become apparent as this chapter and the next unfold. Typically, parasitic females produce eggs that pass out of the host, usually in faeces. There follows a succession of four larval stages. These are conveniently called the first-stage larva, second-stage larva and so on, or alternatively: the L_1, L_2, etc. The stage that hatches out of the egg and the stage that is infective for the next host vary between nematode groups. Each larval stage develops until it outgrows its cuticle which is then discarded. This process is called 'moulting'. When

it emerges from its final moult, the nematode is an immature adult, either male or female. After a maturation period, mating occurs and egg-laying commences.

The whole progression can be summarised as follows:

$$\text{Egg} \Rightarrow L_1 \Rightarrow L_2 \Rightarrow L_3 \Rightarrow L_4 \Rightarrow \text{Adult.}$$

Note that asexual multiplication does not take place during larval phases (in contrast to digenean trematodes, for example). So, each nematode egg has the potential to produce just one adult worm.

Nematode eggs vary greatly in appearance and so are useful for diagnosing parasitic infections as they can easily be detected and counted in faecal samples (see Section 1.5.1).

Practical tip box 6.2

Identifying worm eggs

Microscopic identification of nematode eggs and other parasitic structures depends initially on a visual appraisal of their relative size. Select low power first; then move onto high power, if necessary. If this simple routine is not followed, it is easy to confuse, say, a nematode egg and a protozoan cyst.

It would be tedious to memorise the dimensions of all eggs and cysts. Such data are easily accessible when needed. A more useful strategy is to adopt a convenient yardstick for making comparisons. In this textbook we use the typical strongyle egg (see Figure 6.14), which is about 80 μm long, for this purpose. It is easier to remember that a taeniid egg is about half the size of a strongyle egg and that a liver fluke egg is about double, than to remember exact measurements for each.

6.3 Bursate nematodes

As noted earlier in this chapter, animal parasitic nematodes are divided into two major groups: bursate and nonbursate nematodes. When identifying parasitic nematodes, therefore, the first step is to look at the tail-end of the male worms. The presence of a bursa (see Figure 6.6) will narrow the choice down to the bursate superfamilies.

6.3.1 Bursate superfamilies

There are four bursate nematode superfamilies (see Figure 6.13). Three of these, the Trichostrongyloidea, Strongyloidea and the Ancylostomatoidea (hookworms) are closely related, and are known collectively as 'the strongyles' (or

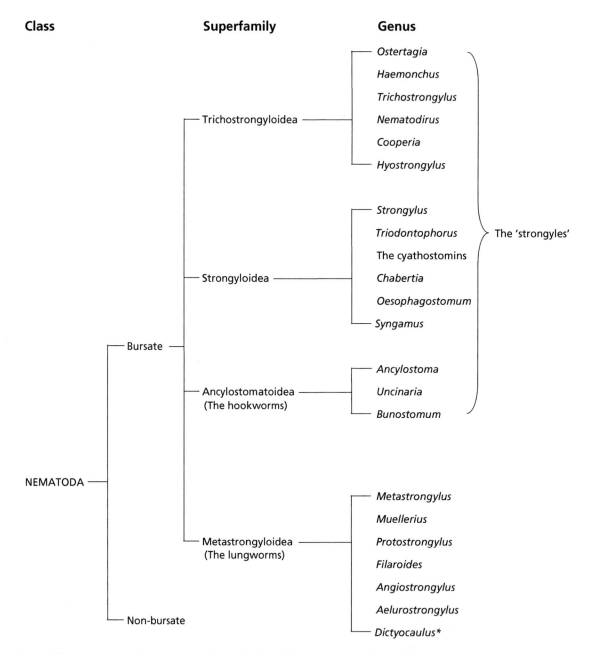

Figure 6.13 Overview of the bursate nematode superfamilies. (*The taxonomic position of *Dictyocaulus* is unclear but is included here as it occurs in the lungs.)

'strongylate worms' in some texts). They are predominantly gastrointestinal parasites with direct life-cycles. Members of the fourth bursate superfamily, the Metastrongyloidea, are associated with the respiratory tract and typically utilise an intermediate host in their life-cycle.

The 'strongyles'

The colloquial term 'strongyle' has no zoological validity but is very useful in Veterinary Parasitology since trichostrongyloid, strongyloid and hookworm species have much in common with respect to their biology,

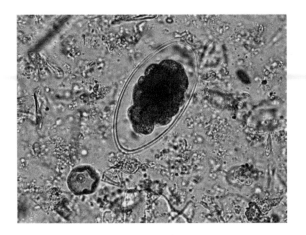

Figure 6.14 Strongyle egg surrounded by faecal debris including a pollen grain (below left).

epidemiology and pathogenicity and because they are associated with an important animal welfare problem: parasitic gastroenteritis (PGE). Also, their eggs (with a few exceptions) are indistinguishable and so laboratory diagnostic reports will often report the number of 'strongyle eggs per gram faeces'. A 'typical strongyle egg' is approximately 80 µm long, oval, thin shelled and generally contains 4–16 cells when passed in faeces (see Figure 6.14).

General strongyle life-cycle

The life-cycles of the strongyle worms have many similarities and follow the general pattern shown in Figure 6.15:

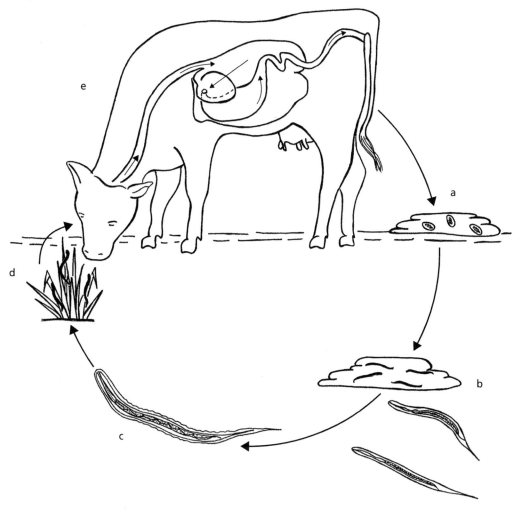

Figure 6.15 General strongyle life-cycle: a – eggs voided in faeces; b – L_1 hatch and develop to L_3; c – ensheathed L_3 climb grass; d – L_3 ingested by host; e – larvae travel to predilection site and develop to adults (details in text which uses the same lettering as shown above). Larvae after Eckert *et al.*, 2008 with permission of Enke Verlag.

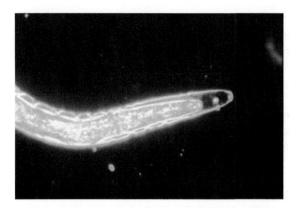

Figure 6.16 Head-end of an ensheathed third stage strongyle larva showing the anterior part of the L_3 within the retained L_2 cuticle. Reproduced with permission of M.J. Walker.

a – The strongyle egg leaves the host with the faeces.

b – The L_1 develops within the egg and hatches. It feeds on bacteria, moults and sheds the cast-off cuticle to become an L_2. The L_2 also feeds on bacteria and moults to become the L_3, but this time the shed skin is retained as a protective envelope (see Figure 6.16). It is now called an 'ensheathed third-stage larva' (see Figure 6.17).

c – The L_3 cannot feed but use stored glycogen to provide energy for locomotion. They have to leave the dungpat, cross the surrounding 'zone of repugnance' (the soiled herbage around a faecal deposit that is normally left ungrazed) and climb onto more distant vegetation. They do this by swimming along films of moisture, although

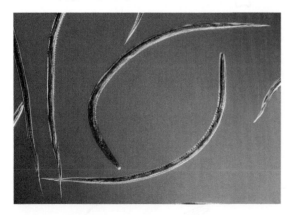

Figure 6.17 Ensheathed third stage strongyle larvae (*Ostertagia*): the L_3 tail can be seen within the retained L_2 cuticle of some larvae (bottom left); note the characteristic 'crinkling' of the sheath where it bends.

rain-splash, insect activity etc. may provide assistance. This process is termed 'translation'.

d – The ensheathed L_3 is the infective stage and has to be swallowed by a suitable host to continue its life-cycle.

e – On reaching its predilection site within the alimentary tract, the L_3 burrows into the mucosa, loses its sheath, starts feeding again and moults. The L_4 or immature adult (depending on species) breaks out of the mucosa (a damaging process called 'emergence') and spends the rest of its life lying on the luminal surface. Egg-laying starts once adult worms have grown to maturity and mated. The prepatent period (i.e. the time from infection to egg-laying) varies between superfamilies.

Some strongyles have added extra steps to this basic pattern. For example, some can enter the host by skin penetration as well as by ingestion and some migrate through body tissues before settling in their predilection site. Where clinically relevant, these variations will be described in the text dealing with individual worms or groups.

General strongyle epidemiology

The condition most commonly associated with strongyle worms is parasitic gastroenteritis, characterised by diarrhoea and weight-loss or suboptimal weight-gains (see Section 8.2.1). PGE is a seasonal disease driven by climatic factors. Ambient temperature is the dominant force in temperate regions, while rainfall patterns are of greater significance in the tropics.

Strongyle eggs and larvae will not develop at temperatures below about 8–10°C but, above this threshold, growth and development accelerate with increasing warmth. The ensheathed third-stage larvae, which are entirely dependent on stored glycogen, become more active at higher temperatures and use up their energy reserves more quickly. Thus, warmer conditions encourage infective L_3 to accumulate more quickly but also shorten their life-span.

Consequently, the disease risk for susceptible animals grazing contaminated pasture depends on a balance between:

a – **the rate at which new infective larvae are developing** (and moving away from faecal deposits onto the grass); and

b – **the rate at which the L_3 are dying** (by succumbing to desiccation or by exhausting their glycogen reserves).

This dynamic determines the overall density of third-stage larvae on the herbage (measured as L_3/kg dry matter) which, in turn, governs the level of exposure of grazing animals to parasitism (since their daily dry matter intake is fairly constant for a given age, weight and class of livestock).

The preparasitic life-cycle functions most efficiently in humid conditions. The L_3 is the most robust larval stage (presumably because the retained sheath provides protection), but it will nevertheless succumb to desiccation or extreme temperatures. Dung pats and snow cover both provide insulation against adverse conditions.

In temperate climates

Since levels of pasture contamination are determined by climate, they follow an annual pattern typical for each locality, although this stereotype can be modified by short-term weather anomalies (e.g. an unusually cold spring or a summer drought). The precise timing of events is also influenced by the composition of the strongyle population as there are subtle differences in threshold temperatures and rates of development between species (*Trichostrongylus* tends to peak later than *Teladorsagia*, for example).

An example of the seasonal fluctuation that typically occurs in the number of L_3 per kg grass on a permanent calf pasture in a temperate climate is depicted in Figure 6.18:

a – During the winter, L_3 surviving from the previous year are inactive and this prolongs their life-span. Temperatures are below the threshold for newly deposited eggs to develop. Pasture contamination therefore remains at a constant, usually low, level.

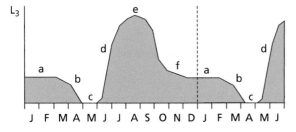

Figure 6.18 Epidemiology of parasitic gastroenteritis (PGE) in the northern hemisphere: numbers of infective third stage larvae on pasture throughout year: a – overwintering L_3; b – L_3 die in spring; c – eggs hatching but larvae not yet at L_3 stage; d – new L_3 accumulating ('autoinfection peak'); e – new recruits outnumbered by dying L_3; f - overwintering survivors (details in text).

b – When temperatures start to rise, overwintered L_3 become active and soon die as their remaining food-stores are exhausted. Larval densities are further diluted by spring grass growth. This is the time of year when live-stock housed over the winter are turned out to pasture. Susceptible animals will become infected with the last of the overwintered L_3 and, after the prepatent period has elapsed (three weeks in the case of the trichostrongyloids), they will start to drop eggs onto the pasture. These will eventually hatch, but development remains slow while ambient temperatures are still relatively cool.

c – There is a short interlude with very few L_3 on the herbage. New larvae are developing in large numbers but they have not yet reached the infective stage.

d – As ambient temperatures continue to rise and larval development accelerates, infective larvae accumulate to reach potentially pathogenic densities after mid-summer. (This is called the 'autoinfection peak' because it is the animals that earlier contaminated the pasture that are now at risk of succumbing to the disease.)

e – At the hottest (and often driest) time of year, the L_3 lifespan on grass is very short and larval densities will eventually decline. This downward trend accelerates when cooler autumnal conditions slow the development of hatched larvae and rainfall encourages new grass growth.

f – When cold weather returns, any surviving infective larvae become inactive and overwinter to restart the epidemiological cycle the following year. Any eggs, L_1 or L_2 stages, being less robust, will most likely perish during this period.

In tropical climates

Temperature is not a limiting factor in warmer regions. Strongyle eggs and larvae, like those of most other nematodes, need a humid microclimate in which to survive. During the dry season, viable infective larvae are mostly confined to faecal deposits as any L_3 on herbage are likely to become desiccated. The onset of rain releases large numbers of L_3 onto pasture. Larval development and translation continue throughout the wet season increasing disease risk still further.

Type I and Type II disease

Once the L_3 has infected a susceptible host, it finds itself in a consistently warm environment with an abundant food supply and so the parasitic phase of the life-cycle can proceed without interruption. If this provokes clinical signs, the process is termed 'Type I' disease.

Many strongyle and other nematode species are capable of pausing parasitic development for a period of weeks (or in some cases many months). This phenomenon is known variously as 'arrested' or 'inhibited' development, or 'hypobiosis'. It is a mechanism for optimising chances of survival for the next generation by synchronising the parasitic life-cycle with external events. In the tropics, for example, parasitic larvae of some species may develop normally within their host during the wetter months but may undergo arrested development during the dry season. In this way, developing worms will not attain maturity and start laying eggs until the humidity of the external environment is favourable for the survival of their off-spring. Similarly, in temperate regions, worms may overwinter in a hypobiotic state to delay egg-production during the cold season.

Arrested development is genetically based and there may be strain variation within a species, so populations may behave differently in different localities. The mechanism may be switched on while the L_3 is still on pasture (e.g. cold autumnal nights influencing *Ostertagia* larvae in Scotland), although in most cases the trigger factor is still unknown. Arrested larvae can accumulate in host tissues over time but, in some cases, may 'wake up' almost simultaneously. If large numbers of larvae emerge from the alimentary mucosa together, the damage they cause can be extensive. This is known as 'Type II' disease.

Help box 6.1

Type I and Type II disease

Gastrointestinal disease associated with nematode larvae often occurs when large numbers of larvae break out of the mucosal wall over a short period of time.

Type I disease is caused by larvae that have developed through their parasitic life-cycle stages without interruption. In temperate climates, Type I disease is seen most often in late-summer or autumn.

Type II disease happens after larvae that have been arrested in their parasitic development resume their life-cycle. In temperate climates, Type II disease is seen most often in late winter or spring; in the tropics, it is most likely to happen around the start of the wet season.

Avoid common mistakes!

Arrested development (hypobiosis) occurs when larvae are within the host – not when they are on the grass.

Immunity

Cattle and sheep are able to develop protective immunity against many strongyle parasites, although this generally occurs only after prolonged exposure. Consequently, calves and lambs remain vulnerable throughout their first grazing season but disease is relatively uncommon later in life. Goats, on the other hand, remain susceptible throughout their lives. Horses occupy an intermediate position on this scale.

The epidemiology of PGE in sheep has an extra component as the immunity of breeding ewes to gastrointestinal nematodes declines significantly over a period of several weeks starting shortly before lambing. During this time, known as the 'periparturient relaxation of immunity', patent trichostrongyloid infections are able to establish. As a result, faecal egg-output increases enormously (see Figure 6.19). The mechanism for this 'periparturient egg-rise' is unclear but it could be associated with the diversion of IgA (which is normally secreted with gastrointestinal mucus) to the udder for colostrum production.

Help box 6.2

How do strongyle larvae overwinter?

Larvae can overwinter in two ways:

i) as preparasitic L_3 on grass; or
ii) as arrested larvae within host tissues.

The proportion of the parasite population overwintering as preparasitic or parasitic larvae depends on the worm species and their susceptibility to local climatic conditions. In the United Kingdom, for example, *Haemonchus* larvae are confined almost exclusively to the host as those on the grass die in winter, while *Teladorsagia* larvae survive on the grass as well as in their host.

What triggers the PGE epidemiological cycle each year?

Cattle: There is normally only one significant source of pasture contamination: calves that ingest small numbers of overwintered L_3 at spring turnout and start dropping eggs onto the pasture three weeks later.

Sheep: There are two sources of pasture contamination:
i) eggs from lambs that have ingested overwintered larvae (as described above for calves);
ii) eggs dropped by ewes during the periparturient egg-rise.

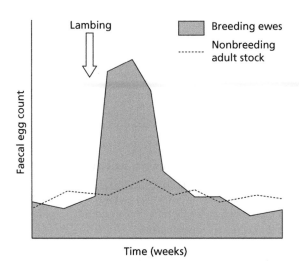

Figure 6.19 The faecal output of strongyle eggs by ewes around lambing time (the 'periparturient egg-rise').

6.3.2 Trichostrongyloidea

Most trichostrongyloids are small worms, 0.5–2 cm long. They look like short lengths of cotton (see Figure 6.20). Each has its own predilection site in the host, usually the stomach, abomasum or small intestine. The head end has no distinctive features and so the male tail is used for identification, the size and shape of the spicules being particularly useful. The life-cycle is typically 'strongyle' (see Section 6.3.1). The parasitic L_3 and L_4 stages develop within the lumen of a gastric gland or intestinal crypt before they emerge from the mucosa. The prepatent period is typically about 3 weeks.

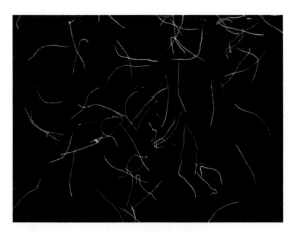

Figure 6.20 A typical trichostrongyloid (*Ostertagia*).

Table 6.1 Some important trichostrongyloids of ruminants

Genus*	Site	Pathogenicity
Ostertagia/ *Teladorsagia*	Abomasum	▼▼▼ (esp. temperate regions)
Haemonchus	Abomasum	▼▼▼ (esp. warm, wet regions)
Trichostrongylus	Small intestine (most species)	▼▼▼
Cooperia	Small intestine	▼
Nematodirus	Small intestine	▼▼▼ (*N. battus*, mostly UK)

*More information in Section 8.2.1.

Important trichostrongyloids

The trichostrongyloids are mostly of importance in ruminants although some occur in other hosts (such as *Hyostrongylus*, which is an occasional cause of gastritis in pigs, and species of *Trichostrongylus* that occur in horses and poultry). Table 6.1 lists the commonest genera although others may be of local significance. All contribute to PGE except *Haemonchus*, which is a blood-sucker provoking anaemia rather than diarrhoea. Some are primary pathogens, e.g. *Ostertagia* and *Teladorsagia*. Others (e.g. *Cooperia*) are less pathogenic and their role in PGE is usually no more than that of making a bad situation worse.

Ostertagia and *Teladorsagia*

Ostertagia ostertagi in cattle and *Teladorsagia circumcincta* in sheep and goats behave very similarly (as does the closely related *Hyostrongylus* in pigs). Adult worms on the abomasal surface are brown and about 1 cm long. Grazing systems in temperate regions must take account of these parasites or serious losses will occur, particularly in younger animals kept at high stocking rates.

Epidemiology

The epidemiology of ostertagiosis follows the pattern illustrated in Figure 6.18, with Type I disease (diarrhoea, weight loss and reduced appetite) occurring mostly after mid-July in the northern hemisphere. Infective third-stage larvae ingested in the autumn become arrested within abomasal glands at the L_4 stage with Type II disease seen 5–6 months later in winter housed yearlings.

Pathogenesis

On gaining access to a gastric gland, the larva grows rapidly. Its increasing bulk stretches the surrounding tissue (see Figure 6.21) and cells lining the gland have

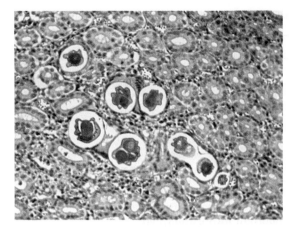

Figure 6.21 Sections through *Ostertagia* larvae in gastric glands.

to multiply to keep pace. In this way, specialised epithelium becomes replaced by undifferentiated cuboidal cells (see Figure 6.22). These divide so rapidly that the

tight junctions linking adjacent cells fail to form properly. If large numbers of glands are affected, abomasal function will be compromised with the following consequences:

a – Loss of acid secreting (parietal) cells: this causes the pH of the abomasum (or stomach in the case of *Hyostrongylus* in pigs) to rise from a pH of 2 up to 7 in heavy infections.

b – Reduction of enzymatic activity: this happens for two reasons. Firstly, pepsinogen-secreting (zymogen) cells are being lost and, secondly, pepsinogen is a precursor molecule that is only converted to the active enzyme, pepsin, in an acid environment.

c – Absence of fully formed tight junctions: This allows macromolecules to pass through the epithelial sheet. In one direction, proteins such as albumin will leak from the body into the abomasal contents (thereby

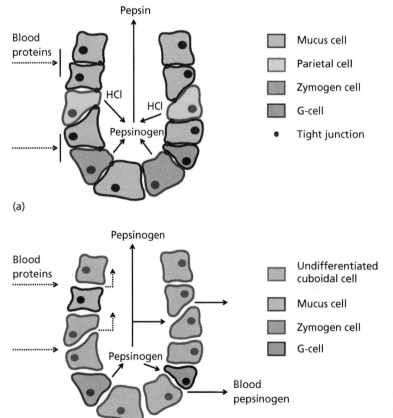

Figure 6.22 Pathogenesis of ostertagiosis: comparison of (a) a normally functioning gastric gland, and (b) one from an affected abomasum (details in text). After Urquhart and Armour, 1973 with permission of the University of Glasgow.

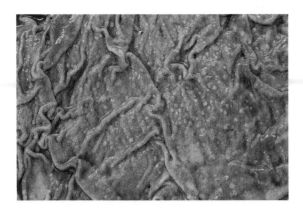

Figure 6.23 Severe case of ostertagiosis: nodules on abomasal mucosa. Reproduced with permission of J. McGoldrick.

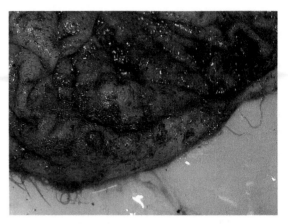

Figure 6.24 *Haemonchus* on the abomasal mucosa of a lamb. Reproduced with permission of AHVLA, Carmarthen © Crown copyright 2013.

producing a protein-losing enteropathy), while pepsinogen can pass the opposite way into tissue fluids and blood.

While the larvae are each contained within an individual gastric gland ('primary nodules'), the overall volume of tissue involved is relatively trivial. When they emerge from the mucosa, however, the proliferation of epithelial cells spreads to surrounding glands. The reason for this is as yet unknown but the result is an enormous amplification of the physiological disturbances. The lesions ('secondary nodules') are now easily visible at autopsy (see Figure 6.23). In severe cases, the nodules coalesce to form the so-called 'Morocco leather appearance'.

Haemonchus

Haemonchus is primarily a parasite of tropical and subtropical regions, although its geographical range is expanding into cooler regions (such as northern Britain and Canada). *H. contortus* is the species found in small ruminants, while *H. placei* is the bovine equivalent. *Haemonchus* is a major constraint on animal production, particularly in hot, humid regions. At 2–3 cm in length, it is larger than other abomasal trichostrongyloids (see Figure 6.24). The fourth-stage larvae and adults both have a small tooth ('lancet') which enables them to suck blood. In females, the intestine with its red contents twists around the lighter coloured egg-filled uterus to give a so-called 'barber's pole' appearance (see Figure 6.25). The appetite of the worms is so great that heavy infections cause a potentially fatal haemorrhagic anaemia.

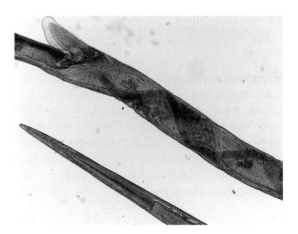

Figure 6.25 Close-up of a female *Haemonchus*: the dark-coloured intestine can be seen twisting around the lighter egg-filled uterus. Also visible are the vulval flap (top left) and (below) the head-end of the worm. Reproduced with permission of Merial GmbH.

Haemonchus is a prolific egg-layer. In warm, humid conditions L_3 develop from eggs within a few days. Thus, pathogenic numbers can appear on pasture very quickly, presenting a sudden and serious disease risk. Several cycles of infection can be completed within a single wet season. Arrested larvae accumulate in the abomasal wall prior to the dry season in the tropics or the winter in cooler regions and these can later give rise to Type II disease.

Temperate areas provide less favourable conditions for the survival of the preparasitic life-cycle stages. Most *Haemonchus* larvae on the pasture die during the winter and so ewes carrying arrested larvae become the primary source of infection for the following summer. Larval development on pasture is slow at cooler temperatures and there is normally only one cycle of infection annually.

Extra information box 6.1

The 'self-cure' reaction

Haemonchus, and sometimes other gastrointestinal trichostrongyloid populations, are sometimes abruptly expelled 2–4 days after sheep are exposed to a high level of pasture challenge with the same parasitic species. This phenomenon, known as 'self-cure' is unpredictable and is most frequently observed in tropical environments. It is associated with Th2 responses (see Extra information box 1.1).

Trichostrongylus

Trichostrongylus is a thin featureless worm less than 1 cm long. There are many species affecting a variety of hosts. These include *T. axei* in the ruminant abomasum and the equine stomach, and *T. tenuis* in the intestine and caeca of poultry and other birds. *T. tenuis* is a contributory factor in the cyclical population crashes that occur on grouse moors. In sheep and goats, the small intestinal species *T. colubriformis* and *T. vitrinus* are major causes of diarrhoea ('black scour') and weight-loss worldwide.

The adult worms lie closely applied to the mucosa of the anterior small intestine, often deeply entwined between villi or even forming superficial tunnels. Cells from the tops of adjacent villi are sloughed off faster than they can be replaced by dividing stem cells at the base of the crypts (see Figure 6.26). This leads to villi becoming flattened (villous atrophy) reducing the surface area available for the absorption of nutrients (amino acids, fats and minerals). Inflammatory and immunological reactions may complicate the process. The integrity of the epithelium is lost and tissue proteins, including albumin, leak into the lumen. If the disease is not too severe, normally functioning regions of the small intestine can largely compensate for these dysfunctions. Nevertheless, even in the absence of obvious clinical signs, chronic malabsorp-

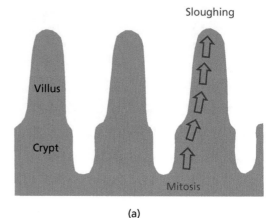

(a)

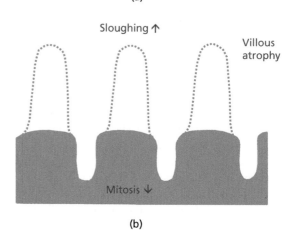

(b)

Figure 6.26 Villous atrophy: a comparison of villi in the small intestine of (a) normal and (b) parasitized animals.

tion together with poor nitrogen retention can affect skeletal growth and mineralisation as well as weight-gain and fleece quality.

Nematodirus

Several species of *Nematodirus* occur in the small intestine of ruminants. They are slender worms up to 2.5 cm long which tangle together if present in large numbers (see Figure 6.27). Only one species (*N. battus*) is a serious pathogen, causing sudden, profuse and often fatal diarrhoea in young lambs (and occasionally in first season grazing calves). *N. battus* is mainly a problem in the British Isles, although it has become established locally in some other sheep rearing regions.

Nematodirus eggs are much larger than those of other strongyles (see Figure 6.28). *N. battus* eggs can be distinguished from those of the less pathogenic species as they

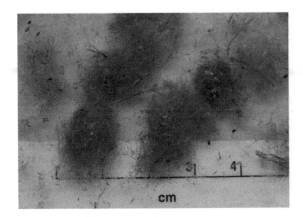

Figure 6.27 Tangled masses of *Nematodirus* recovered from a lamb. Reproduced with permission of AHVLA, Carmarthen © Crown copyright 2013.

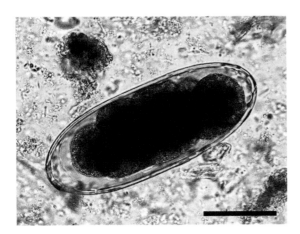

Figure 6.28 A *Nematodirus battus* egg. (Scale-bar = 50 μm.)

have flatter sides and a darker brown colour. The size of the egg gives a clue that *Nematodirus* behaves differently from related genera. Unlike other trichostrongyloids, development from L_1 to L_3 takes place inside the egg. Hatching only occurs after the egg has been exposed to a sequence of stimuli. *N. battus* has the most stringent set of requirements – prolonged exposure to cold followed by a definable period with mean day/night temperatures >10°C. Consequently *N. battus* eggs tend to hatch simultaneously in the spring, leading to sudden, massive and potentially dangerous pasture contamination. This sequence of events has sufficient predictability to allow local meteorological data to be used each year for forecasting the likely timing and severity of disease. *N. battus* usually affects lambs between 6 and 10 weeks

of age. If the mass-hatch occurs early in the season, the risk is reduced as lambs will be suckling and eating relatively little grass. If the mass hatch is late, the lambs will be older, more robust and may perhaps have already acquired some immunity by ingesting larvae of other *Nematodirus* species. The main danger period lies between these extremes.

Hatching stimuli for the less pathogenic *Nematodirus* species are less precise and so larvae appear in smaller numbers over a longer period of time. *Nematodirus* is highly immunogenic and infected lambs quickly acquire a solid immunity. Lambs thereby have opportunity to develop protection before dangerous numbers can accumulate on the pasture. Once immune to *Nematodirus*, protection is life-long and even persists through the period of periparturient relaxation of immunity to other trichostrongyloids. Consequently, the ewe plays no role in the epidemiology of this condition.

Nematodirus persists by being passed from one generation of young lambs to the next as illustrated in Figure 6.29:

a – Infective third-stage larvae survive winter inside their egg.

b – Eggs hatch in spring and the pasture larval count rises. If not eaten by a suitable host, these larvae die when ambient temperatures rise and their food stores are depleted.

c – Meanwhile, susceptible lambs have become infected and, after the prepatent period, they drop new eggs

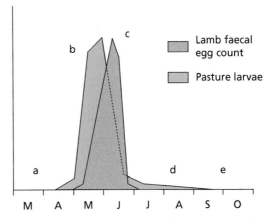

Figure 6.29 Epidemiology of nematodirosis: a – L_3 overwinter inside eggs; b – mass hatch in spring followed by death of larvae; c – faecal egg-counts rise until lambs become immune; d – L_3 develop inside eggs; e – a few may hatch in autumn (details in text). Modified after Thomas, 1959.

onto the ground. Egg output falls rapidly as the lambs become immune.

d – Larvae develop within the eggs but they do not hatch and so are not available to infect animals before the spring of the following year.

e – While the above statements are generally true, there does seem to be some biological variation within *Nematodirus* populations and there is an increasing trend, perhaps associated with changes in climate or sheep husbandry, for L_3 to be seen in the autumn of the same year that eggs are deposited on pasture.

The eggs, which can survive two years or more, are well adapted to live through even the coldest winters as the larvae secrete a protective antifreeze substance.

6.3.3 Strongyloidea

Strongyloid worms are often longer (1–5 cm) and always stouter than the trichostrongyloids (see Figure 6.30). In contrast to the latter, they have elaborate head structures useful for identification. Most reside in the caecum or colon. The life-cycle is generally very similar to that of the trichostrongyloids except that incoming L_3 penetrate more deeply into the tissues of the intestinal wall where they provoke the formation of nodules, the size of which depends on species and the immune status of the host. A strongyloid species is said to be 'nonmigratory' if its larvae return directly to the lumen of the intestine. The larvae of some species, however, are 'migratory' and travel on a predetermined route around the body before returning to the alimentary tract. As might be expected from these different patterns of behaviour, the prepatent periods of strongyloid species differ widely (from three weeks to a year).

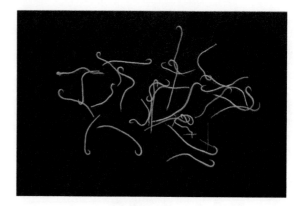

Figure 6.30 A typical strongyloid (*Oesophagostomum*).

Important strongyloids

Horse owners around the world are familiar with the 'large and small strongyles' (also called 'red-worms'). These are colloquial terms for, respectively, the migratory genus *Strongylus* and a large group of nonmigratory strongyloids from several genera within the subfamily Cyathostominae (Table 6.2). Another equine genus, *Triodontophorus*, is also nonmigratory, but is regarded as a 'large strongyle' because of its size.

Species of the 'nodular worm' *Oesophagostomum* are commonly found in ruminants and pigs, sometimes causing diarrhoea. Ruminants also harbour *Chabertia* which is remarkable for having a particularly big buccal cavity, but it is nevertheless of minor clinical significance.

It is not unusual for a parasitic group to contain outliers that, despite a close taxonomic affinity, have nevertheless followed a divergent evolutionary pathway. In this category, the Strongyloidea has two related genera: *Syngamus*, the poultry gapeworm, and *Stephanurus*, the swine kidney worm.

Table 6.2 Some important strongyloid parasites

Genus (or subfamily*)	Host	Site	Pathogenicity	More information in Section:
Strongylus	Equidae	Caecum or colon	▼▼▼ (esp. *S. vulgaris*)	9.1.1
Triodontophorus	Equidae	Colon	▼	
Cyathostominae*	Equidae	Caecum and/or colon	▼▼▼	9.1.1
Oesophagostomum	Ruminants, pig	Large intestine	▼	8.3.1
Chabertia	Ruminants	Large intestine	▼	
Syngamus	Birds	Trachea	▼▼▼	8.4.1
Stephanurus	Pig	Kidney	▼	

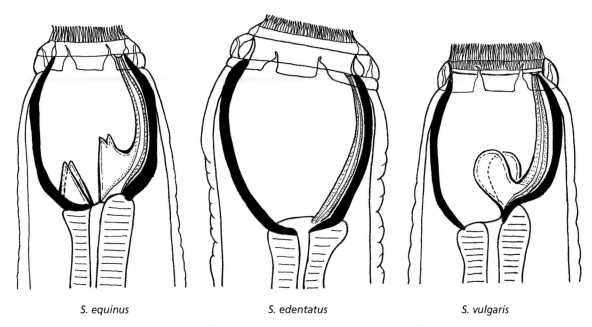

S. equinus   *S. edentatus*   *S. vulgaris*

Figure 6.31 Head-ends of the three equine *Strongylus* species. Drawn from photomicrographs by Lichtenfels, 1975.

Strongylus

Strongylus species are deep red in colour and can be identified and differentiated by their size, site, and the number of teeth in their large buccal capsule (see Figure 6.31). The main features of this genus are summarised in Table 6.3.

S. vulgaris is the most pathogenic of the three equine species. It also used to be the most common, although its prevalence has declined markedly in well-cared-for horses since the introduction of regular deworming programmes incorporating macrocyclic lactone anthelmintics.

The adults of all three species are plug feeders. They erode the intestinal wall down to the muscularis mucosa leaving behind small but clearly visible circular bleeding ulcers (see Figure 6.32). If present in large numbers

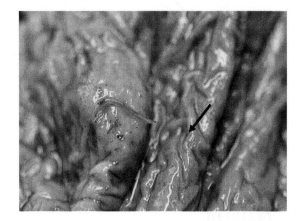

Figure 6.32 Adult *Strongylus* on intestinal mucosa: note small red feeding site to right of worm (arrow). Reproduced with permission of M.K. Nielsen.

Table 6.3 Important features of the three equine *Strongylus* species

Species	Size (cm)	Teeth	Main site	Migration	Prepatent period (months)	Pathogenicity
S. vulgaris	1.5–2 (shortest)	2 ('ear-shaped')	Caecum	Cranial mesenteric artery	6–7	▼▼▼ (larvae) ▼ (adult)
S. edentatus	2–4.5	None	Right ventral colon	Liver (via portal vein)	11–12	▼ (adult)
S. equinus	3–5 (longest)	3 (one with 2 points)	Caecum and right ventral colon	Liver (via peritoneal cavity)	9	▼ (adult)

they contribute to the unthrifty appearance and malaise typical of the 'wormy horse'.

The preparasitic life-cycle is typically strongyle (see Section 6.3.1), but once within the host each species embarks on its own unique journey around the abdomen before returning to the large intestine to mature and lay eggs.

Strongylus vulgaris

The migratory route used by *S. vulgaris* exposes its host to considerable risk through a complex sequence of events outlined in Figure 6.33 and the next paragraphs:

a – Grazing horses ingest ensheathed L_3 which invade the intestinal wall.

b – The larvae penetrate into arterioles and ascend the arterial tree using their mouthparts to hold on to vessel walls to avoid being swept back by the blood flow. In about two weeks they reach their destination, the cranial mesenteric artery. Here they grow and develop for 3–4 months.

c – The larvae return down the arterial tree and become enclosed within large mucosal nodules, finally emerging after 6–8 weeks into the lumen of the caecum as fourth-stage larvae.

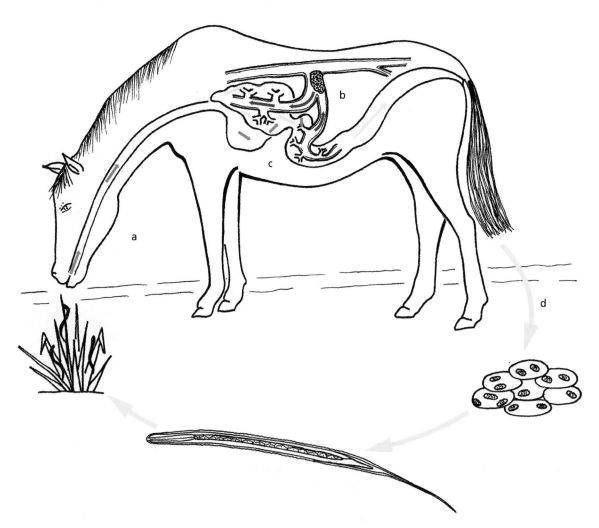

Figure 6.33 Life-cycle of *Strongylus vulgaris*, the cause of verminous endarteritis: a – L_3 ingested and penetrate intestinal arterioles; b – larvae develop in cranial mesenteric artery; c – larvae return to caecum; d – egg-output starts after 6½ months (details in text). L_3 after Poluszynski, 1930.

d – Egg production commences approximately 6½ months after infection.

Verminous endarteritis

Migrating *S. vulgaris* larvae injure the endothelial lining of the arteries and their progress is marked by sinuous fibrin tracts (see Figure 6.34). Damage to the cranial mesenteric artery where larvae accumulate can be considerable. The wall becomes progressively thickened and distorted due to persistent thrombus formation and organisation (see Figure 6.35). Despite the result-

ant disruption in blood flow dynamics, many cases of verminous endarteritis are asymptomatic and are only discovered incidentally as an abnormal abdominal mass during rectal palpation or at autopsy.

Sometimes, however, a piece of thrombus can be dislodged from the arterial lesion and swept along with the blood-flow until trapped in an intestinal arteriole or capillary. In many cases this is of little consequence as the equine intestine is well endowed with collateral circulation. If a large embolus blocks a critical arteriole, however, the tissues supplied by that vessel will become ischaemic and eventually necrotic (see Figure 6.36). The likely clinical outcome is colic and death.

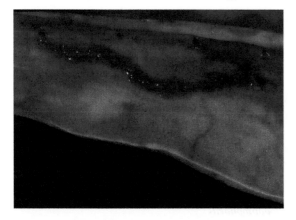

Figure 6.34 Tract on arterial wall produced by migrating *Strongylus vulgaris* larva. Reproduced with permission of T.R. Klei.

Help box 6.3

Verminous endarteritis: terms used

Cranial mesenteric artery: This is the main branch off the aorta that carries oxygenated blood to the intestines.
Thrombus: A blood clot that forms inside a blood vessel.
Organising thrombus: The organisation of a thrombus is the process whereby blood flow is restored by the breakdown of fibrin (from an initial fibroblastic response) and its replacement by a network of new capillary channels.
Collateral circulation: An alternative blood supply route that can be used if the main supply channel is impeded.
Embolus: A piece of thrombus that has broken away from its point of origin.

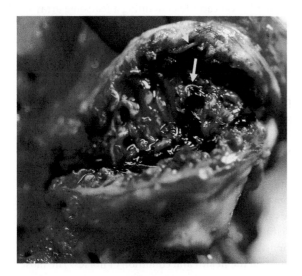

Figure 6.35 Verminous endarteritis: organising thrombus causing thickening and distortion of cranial mesenteric artery: parts of several larvae can be seen on close inspection (arrowed). Reproduced with permission of M.K. Nielsen.

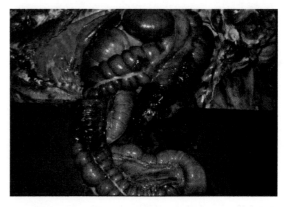

Figure 6.36 Necropsy of a pony that had died of colic. Note the dark red discolouration indicating necrosis at the tip of the caecum and on parts of the colon. Reproduced with permission of T.R. Klei.

Strongylus edentatus

S. edentatus larvae penetrate the intestinal wall and are carried via the hepatic portal venous system to the liver where they grow and develop inside nodules for several months (see Figure 6.37). Becoming active again, they travel beneath the liver capsule in search of the hepatic ligament which they follow to subperitoneal tissues on the horse's right flank (see Figure 6.38). A second period of nodule formation and growth takes place before the worms use the mesentery to guide them back to the alimentary tract to be enclosed once again within nodular lesions before breaking free to complete their life-cycle in the lumen.

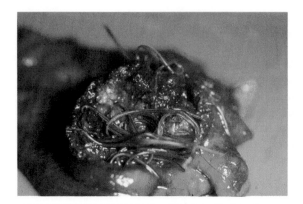

Figure 6.39 *Triodontophorus* adults in an ulcer they have created. From Jacobs, 1986 with permission of Elsevier.

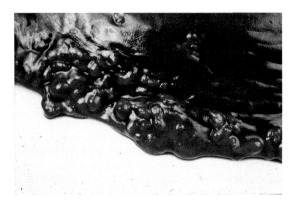

Figure 6.37 Nodules in horse liver probably caused by migrating *Strongylus* larvae. From Jacobs, 1986 with permission of Elsevier.

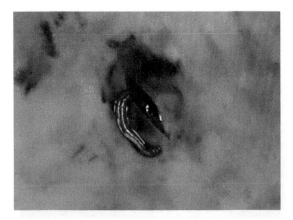

Figure 6.38 *Strongylus* larva migrating beneath peritoneum (which has been cut to release larva). Reproduced with permission of T.R. Klei.

Strongylus equinus

The migratory pathway of *S. equinus* is not well understood but seems to be basically similar to that of *S. edentatus* except that nodule formation is less marked and it travels to the liver and back to the intestine across the peritoneal cavity.

Triodontophorus

Although about the same size as *S. vulgaris*, this non-migratory genus can be recognised as it has a much smaller buccal capsule containing a fearsome array of teeth. Although individual worms cause only superficial damage, they tend to be gregarious and, by feeding in groups ('herds'), form large ulcers (see Figure 6.39).

The cyathostomins

Fortunately, the 40+ cyathostomin species are sufficiently similar to be regarded as a single clinical entity. Most species are no more than 1.5 cm in length (see Figure 6.40). They are easy to overlook at autopsy amongst the fibrous debris covering the intestinal mucosa. The adult worms have shallow buccal cavities and would be relatively innocuous but for the fact that they can be present in tens or hundreds of thousands. Their cumulative effect can have a detrimental effect on the health and condition of horses. The most serious consequences of infection are, however, associated with the mucosal larvae.

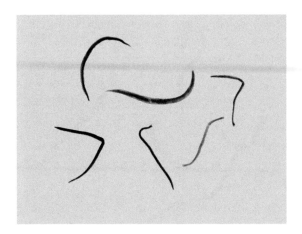

Figure 6.40 Adult cyathostomins.

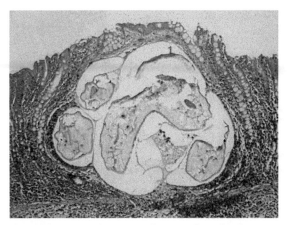

Figure 6.41 Section showing cyathostomin larva developing in intestinal mucosa. From Jacobs, 1986 with permission of Elsevier.

Help box 6.4

The term 'cyathostomin'

'Cyathostomin' is a convenient word used to include all the constituent genera and species belonging to the subfamily Cyathostominae. Other terms currently in scientific or colloquial usage for this group of worms include: cyathostomes, trichonemes, small redworms and small strongyles.

Larval cyathostominosis

The cyathostomins have a typically strongyle life-cycle. They are nonmigratory and so parasitic larvae are confined to small nodules in the wall of the large intestine. Some species remain in superficial tissues (see Figure 6.41), while others burrow down into the submucosa (see Figure 6.42). Fourth-stage larvae appear as brown flecks in the mucosa (the so-called 'pepperpot lesion'; see Figure 6.43) before emerging into the lumen. The prepatent period varies from 8 to 12 weeks depending on species.

Cyathostomin larvae can develop in the host without interruption or they can become arrested during the early parasitic third larval stage (EL_3). This can happen at any time of the year, but mostly in the late summer and autumn. The EL_3 can remain in a hypobiotic state for years and they often accumulate in their millions. Resumption of activity is usually seasonal, in late winter or spring, but other factors such as the removal of adult worms by anthelmintic treatment can trigger a similar event.

If massive numbers of EL_3 restart development together, the subsequent emergence of fourth-stage larvae from the mucosa can result in catastrophic damage. Generally, however, only a small proportion of encysted EL_3 are triggered at any one time and Type II disease is therefore sporadic in occurrence.

Epidemiology

The clinical effects of the cyathostomins are most apparent in young horses (< 5 yr), but can occur at any age as immunity gives incomplete protection. There is no

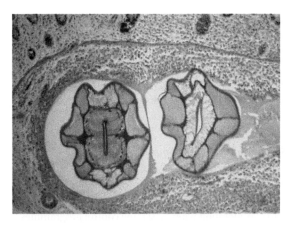

Figure 6.42 Section showing cyathostomin larva developing in intestinal submucosa. From Jacobs, 1986 with permission of Elsevier.

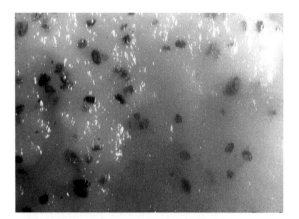

Figure 6.43 The 'pepperpot lesion' (cyathostomin larvae in intestinal mucosa). From Jacobs, 1986 with permission of Elsevier.

periparturient relaxation of immunity, but the seasonal reactivation of arrested larvae ensures a rise in faecal egg-counts in spring. The long-tailed preparasitic L_3 (see Figure 9.1) is robust and generally survives winter on pastures in large numbers.

Practical tip box 6.3

Identifying horse strongyle eggs and larvae

Anthelmintic resistance is a growing problem in cyathostomin populations and so faecal egg-counts are an essential part of equine health programmes. *Strongylus* spp. eggs tend to be rounder than those of the cyathostomins, but reliable differentiation depends on microscopic examination of L_3 cultured from the faeces – a job for the expert. The risk associated with particular pastures can be assessed by counting larvae washed off representative grass samples. Ensheathed horse strongyle larvae are easily distinguished from those of other host species by their long tails (see Figure 9.1).

Syngamus and *Stephanurus*

The use of earthworms as paratenic hosts differentiates *Syngamus* and *Stephanurus* from other strongyloid genera. This additional reservoir of infection has to be taken into consideration when designing control programmes. *Syngamus* occurs in the trachea of birds while *Stephanurus* adults are found in the perirenal fat of pigs.

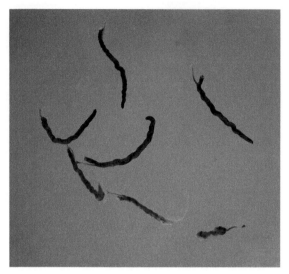

Figure 6.44 *Syngamus trachea*: note the smaller males attached to females giving a 'Y' shape. Reproduced with permission of AHLVA, RVC Surveillance Centre © Crown copyright 2013.

Syngamus

Syngamus is deep red in colour and is easily recognised because it seems to be 'Y'-shaped (see Figure 6.44). This bizarre appearance is due to each female worm being permanently accompanied by an attached smaller male. The length of the female varies from 0.5 to 2 cm depending on the size of the host. *Syngamus* infects many wild birds as well as poultry and pheasants. It lives in the trachea and can cause respiratory distress.

The *Syngamus* egg is like a typical strongyle egg except that it has an operculum at each end. The larva develops to the L_3 stage inside the egg. Birds can become infected by ingesting either: an egg containing an L_3, an L_3 that has hatched out of its egg, or an earthworm that has previously swallowed an L_3 (free or within an egg). The earthworm acts as a paratenic host and so the following scenario commonly occurs where pheasants are reared in outdoor pens with earthen floors:

a – infected wild birds: crows, blackbirds etc. contaminate the soil with droppings containing *Syngamus* eggs;

b – earthworms: accumulate L_3 in their tissues and become a potent reservoir of infection;

c – susceptible pheasant poults: acquire infection by eating the earthworms.

Stephanurus

The adult swine kidney worm, found in many warmer regions, is a stout worm, up to 4.5 cm long, with a transparent cuticle. It forms a cyst close to the kidney and its eggs are passed via a channel to the renal pelvis or ureter to be expelled in pig urine. *Stephanurus* L_3 can penetrate skin, so pigs can acquire infection by lying on contaminated damp ground, as well as by ingesting the L_3 or eating an infected earthworm. Transplacental infection of unborn piglets is also possible. Migrating larvae spend at least three months in the liver parenchyma before moving on to the kidney region. The main deleterious effect, a failure to grow satisfactorily, is due to liver damage.

6.3.4 Ancylostomatoidea (hookworms)

Members of this superfamily are similar in appearance to smaller members of the Strongyloidea except that the head, which has a large buccal cavity armed with teeth and/or cutting plates, is bent dorsally – hence the name 'hookworm' (see Figure 6.45). They all live in the small intestine. Many are blood-suckers with big appetites and are therefore capable of causing anaemia if present in large numbers. The life-cycle is typically strongyle except that the L_3 can enter the host either by ingestion or by skin penetration. In the latter case, it proceeds to its predilection site via the lymphatics and blood-stream. The larvae of some species can become arrested in their development in subcutaneous tissues.

Hookworm dermatitis can occur if L_3 enter the skin of an animal that is not the natural host or a normal host that has been sensitised by previous exposure. It often takes the form of twisting red tracks marking the route of travel (cutaneous *larva migrans*). This can have zoonotic implications (e.g. for people walking barefoot in localities where dogs or cats harbour *Ancylostoma braziliense*).

Animals exposed to hookworms develop an immunity which, as with many parasitic infections, substantially reduces the risk of overt disease without necessarily blocking new infections completely. Hookworm anaemia is therefore seen mostly in young animals, but adults may nevertheless be passing eggs.

Important hookworms

Hookworms are of greatest significance in small animal practice. Species do occur in farm animals but not in the horse (see Table 6.4). The genus *Ancylostoma*, after which the superfamily is named, is important in human medicine and also includes several species parasitizing dogs and/or cats. Most are of relatively low pathogenicity and so the emphasis in this text is on *A. caninum*, a species that can cause severe and sometimes fatal anaemia in puppies.

Hookworm disease is seen mostly in warm humid climates, although one genus, *Uncinaria*, occurs in temperate and even Arctic regions. In North America, the endemic territories of the two canine species, *Ancylostoma caninum* and *Uncinaria stenocephala*, overlap in Pennsylvania. In Europe, *A. caninum* is common in the Mediterranean region but is found only rarely in the UK, where *U. stenocephala* predominates.

Ancylostoma

A. caninum has three teeth on either side of its mouth (see Figure 6.46) as well as teeth in the buccal cavity. It uses these to bite deeply into the intestinal mucosa so the pharynx can pump copious volumes (0.1 ml/worm/

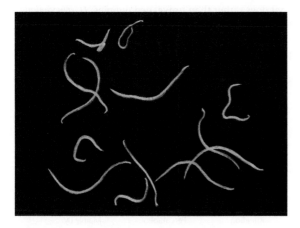

Figure 6.45 A typical hookworm (*Bunostomum*): note the backwardly bent heads.

Table 6.4 Some important hookworms

Genus	Host	Pathogenicity	More information in Section:
Ancylostoma	Dog, cat	▼▼▼ (esp. *A. caninum*)	9.2.1
Uncinaria	Dog, cat	▼	9.2.1
Bunostomum	Ruminants	▼▼ (in warm, wet regions)	

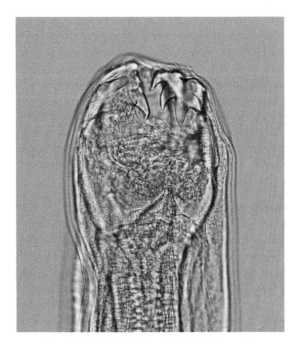

Figure 6.46 Dorsal view of the head of *Ancylostoma*: one of the two sets of three teeth can been clearly seen (upper right).

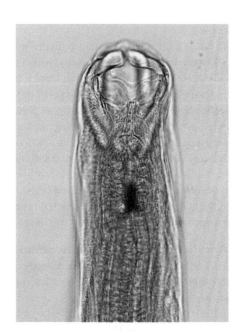

Figure 6.47 Dorsal view of the head of *Uncinaria* showing the cutting plates on either side of the mouth.

day) of arterial blood through its body. The prepatent period is 2–3 weeks and female worms produce large numbers of eggs. The hatched larvae can develop to the L_3 stage in 5 days under optimal conditions. Percutaneous infection is epidemiologically important in this species as larvae which become arrested in their development in subcutaneous tissues are reactivated around the time of parturition. They then migrate to the mammary gland. Suckling pups are therefore particularly vulnerable to the pathogenic effects of this worm.

Practical tip box 6.4

Identifying hookworms

The microscopic inspection of hookworm mouthparts is sometimes necessary for diagnostic purposes but this can be tricky. Because the head is bent dorsally, the worm tends to flop over onto its side obscuring the mouth opening. Care must be taken therefore to orientate the specimen correctly before examining it.

Uncinaria

U. stenocephala has cutting plates instead of teeth (see Figure 6.47). It is a shallow plug feeder responsible for protein-losing enteropathy. Consequently, heavy infec-

tions are associated with poor growth and intermittent diarrhoea rather than anaemia. Third-stage larvae entering the skin can provoke a hypersensitivity reaction, particularly in the skin between the toes, and generally fail to reach their predilection site in the intestine. Ingestion of the L_3 is therefore the main route of infection. There is no direct vertical transmission from the bitch to her offspring and so clinical signs are commonest in adolescent dogs rather than unweaned puppies. *U. stenocephala* is seen most often in greyhounds and rural dogs.

Help box 6.5

Key features of the dog hookworms *Ancylostoma* and *Uncinaria*

	A. caninum	*U. stenocephala*
Endemic zones	Warm, hot, humid	Cool, cold
Recognition	Teeth in and around mouth	Cutting plates only
Pathogenicity	Blood sucker → anaemia	Protein leak → diarrhoea
Infection	Percutaneous important	Mainly by ingestion
Vertical transmission	Via colostrum and milk	Does not occur
Pedal dermatitis	Yes	Yes

6.3.5 Metastrongyloidea (lungworms)

The Metastrongyloidea are bursate nematodes but are not included in the 'strongyle' category as they behave differently in many ways. Most, for example, inhabit the respiratory tract or associated blood vessels – hence the colloquial term 'lungworm'. In a wider zoological context, the superfamily is a reasonably cohesive grouping but seen from a veterinary viewpoint it appears wildly anarchic as several clinically important lungworms break the metastrongyloid ground-rules.

Extra information box 6.2

The *Dictyocaulus* enigma

It looks like a lungworm; it lives in the upper respiratory tract; and at least one molecular phylogeny study suggests an affinity with the Metastrongyloidea; but its life-cycle is different and other aspects of its biology suggest a closer kinship with the Trichostrongyloidea! Further consideration of this controversial issue is beyond the scope of this book and is probably of little relevance for clinicians so, for convenience, *Dictyocaulus*, the cattle lungworm, is included in this section along with the other lungworms.

General life-cycle

The typical metastrongyloid life-cycle, as illustrated by the cat lungworm *Aelurostrongylus* (see Figure 6.48), involves a molluscan intermediate host:

a – Female worms in the lungs lay eggs which quickly hatch. Eggs and hatched L_1 are wafted up the bronchi and trachea by epithelial cilia to the throat and are swallowed.

b – L_1 are passed with the faeces.

c – The L_1 penetrates the foot of a terrestrial gastropod (slug or snail) and develops to the infective L_3.

d – The gastropod may be eaten by a vertebrate which is not its final host, which then acts as a paratenic host.

e – The final host is infected by ingesting either the gastropod intermediate host or the vertebrate paratenic host. The L_3 then migrates from the intestine via mesenteric lymph nodes to enter the blood-stream and reach the lungs.

It will be apparent from this life-cycle description that it is the L_1 and not an egg that appears in faeces. Larvae can be recovered for diagnostic purposes using the Baermann technique (see Section 1.5.1). Most, but not all, metastrongyloid L_1 can be recognised by the presence of an indentation on the dorsal side of the tail which gives

it a characteristic 'wavy' appearance. Some species also have a small peg-like protrusion just before this indentation (see Figure 6.49).

Important lungworms

Metastrongyloids vary greatly in size from a few mm to several cm in length. The larger ones resemble pieces of string. Their pathogenicity depends largely on their position in the respiratory tree (see Table 6.5). *Aelurostrongylus* and *Muellerius* are tiny worms living in terminal alveolar ducts. They are easily walled off by host responses and cause insignificant damage even if present in large numbers. This is fortunate as the greenish nodules associated with *Muellerius* infection are commonly found in sheep at slaughter. At the other end of the spectrum, *Dictyocaulus* and *Metastrongylus* are much larger and inhabit the lumen of the upper respiratory tract. Eggs, larvae and fragments of worms killed by immune attack can be aspirated to set up a foreign body pneumonia that can, in heavy infections, affect considerable volumes of lung tissue. *Protostrongylus* holds an intermediate position, but *Oslerus osleri* (also called *Filaroides osleri*) is an anomaly since the adults are embedded in the walls of the airways and are therefore less likely to cause pneumonia. *Angiostrongylus* in dogs presents a different clinical picture from the other lungworms for reasons explained in the following paragraphs.

Angiostrongylus

A. vasorum has a typically metastrongyloid life-cycle except that the 2 cm long worms do not reside in the lung but in the pulmonary artery and right side of the heart. The white reproductive tract of the female worm twists around its red intestine giving a 'barber's pole' appearance (see Figure 6.50). Eggs are swept by arterial blood-flow to the lungs where they are trapped in capillaries. On hatching, the larvae break into pulmonary alveolae, ascend the respiratory tree and pass along the alimentary tract. The L_1 are very active and generally easy to recover from faecal samples. The intermediate hosts are slugs, such as the orange-grey *Arion rufus,* which feeds on faecal deposits.

In Europe, *A. vasorum* used to be restricted to regions with mild winters such as southern parts of Ireland and France, but the endemic area is expanding and now covers most of the UK with foci of infection in southeast England and south Wales. Possible reasons include: the influence of global warming on slug populations, the

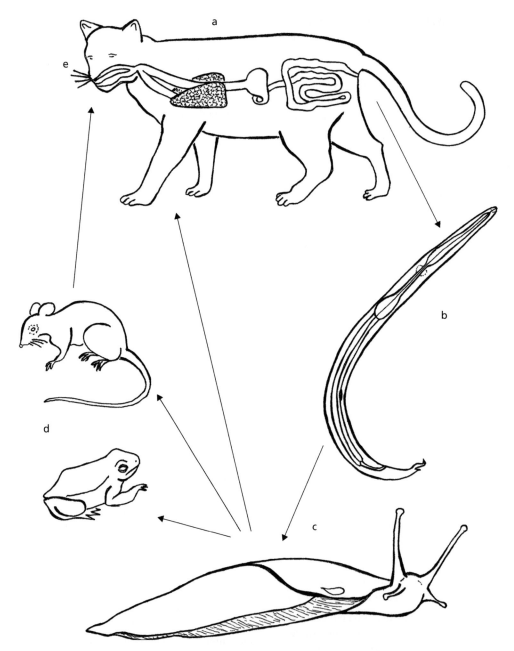

Figure 6.48 Life-cycle of a typical metastrongyloid, *Aelurostrongylus abstrusus*: a – eggs laid in lungs hatch and larvae swallowed; b – L_1 passed in faeces; c – L_3 develops in molluscan intermediate host; d – L_3 may be taken up by paratenic host; e – cat eats intermediate or paratenic host (details in text). L_1 after Gerichter, 1949 with permission of Cambridge University Press.

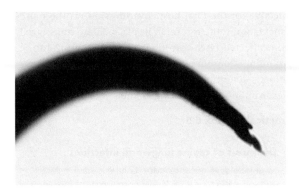

Figure 6.49 Tail-end of a first stage metastrongyloid larva (*Angiostrongylus vasorum*).

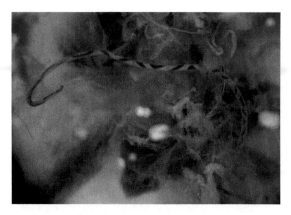

Figure 6.50 *Angiostrongylus vasorum*: female worm in pulmonary artery. Reproduced with permission of the Institute of Parasitology, Justus Liebig University, Giessen.

increase in dog movements around the country, and an expanding fox population providing a reservoir of infection. It has been predicted that *A. vasorum* could spread similarly in North America from its current endemic focus in eastern Canada.

There are two main contributory factors to the pathogenicity of *A. vasorum* and these are caused by different life-cycle stages. The adult worms, seeking to prevent excessive thrombus formation in the pulmonary artery, secrete a powerful anticoagulant. This serves its purpose well but makes the host vulnerable to bruising and internal haemorrhages. Another pathological process is initiated every time an L_1 enters an alveolus. Each such event causes a trivial microinjury but if thousands of eggs are being produced week after week, accumulating damage (see Figure 6.51) will eventually give rise firstly to exercise intolerance and then respiratory distress (dyspnoea).

Oslerus (Filaroides)

At least three species of *Oslerus* or *Filaroides* affect dogs, but *O. osleri* is the only one seen regularly in small animal practice.

O. osleri has evolved a highly specialised lifestyle which sets it apart from other metastrongyloids. Clusters of worms coil together within fibrous nodules that can be a few mm to 2 cm in diameter (see Figure 6.52). These protrude into the respiratory tract at the distal extremity of the trachea or sometimes at the upper end of the two major bronchi. They are easily seen on endoscopy. The lesions are not normally large enough to interfere with airflow, but there can be a dry cough.

There is no point in describing the adult worm as they are only ever seen in histological section. The number of eggs they produce is small. Emerging larvae

Table 6.5 Some important lungworms

Genus	Host	Site	Pathogenicity	More information in Section:
Aelurostrongylus	Cat	Alveolae/terminal bronchioles	▼	
Angiostrongylus	Dog, fox	R heart/pulmonary arteries	▼▼▼	9.2.2
Oslerus (*Filaroides*)	Dog	Bifurcation of trachea	▼▼	9.2.2
Muellerius	Sheep, goat	Alveolae/terminal bronchioles	Ubiquitous but normally nonpathogenic	
Protostrongylus	Sheep, goat	Small bronchioles	▼	
Metastrongylus	Pig	Bronchi/trachea	▼▼▼	
Dictyocaulus	Ruminants, equidae	Bronchi/trachea	▼▼▼	8.2.2, 9.1.2

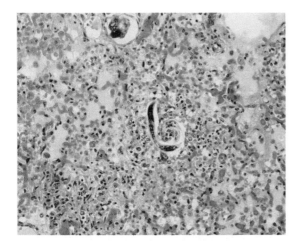

Figure 6.51 Angiostrongylosis: section of first stage larva in damaged lung. Reproduced with permission of B. Smyth.

are sluggish and short-lived. This is because they do not need to find an intermediate host. Unlike other metastrongyloids, *O. osleri* has a direct life-cycle and, uniquely for the bursate nematodes, it is the L_1 that is

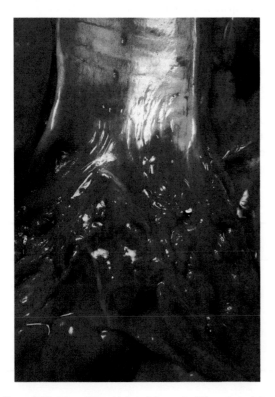

Figure 6.52 *Oslerus* (*Filaroides*) nodules at the bifurcation of the trachea of a greyhound.

infective for the final host. Transmission via the more usual faecal route is rare. In its place, L_1 are transferred from infected bitches to their pups in sputum during grooming. Consequently, the epidemiology of this condition is determined largely by the distribution of puppies from infected breeding kennels.

Practical tip box 6.5

Diagnosis of canine lungworm infections

Most but not all metastrongyloid L_1 have a 'wavy' tail and some also have an associated peg-like structure (see Figure 6.49). The larvae of the various lungworm species can be distinguished on the basis of tail morphology, but this is a job for the expert. When examining dog sputum or faeces, it is fairly safe to assume that finding a few sluggish L_1 suggests an *O. osleri* infection, while a large number of vigorous larvae indicates *A. vasorum*. To complicate matters, foxes harbour other lungworms (e.g. *Crenosoma*) which can infect dogs. Don't forget that hookworm larvae and free-living nematodes may also be present if the faecal sample was not fresh when collected. These will not have a 'wavy' tail.

Avoid common mistakes!

Filaroides (the alternative name for *Oslerus*) belongs to the Metastrongyloidea and has nothing to do with the filarial worms discussed in the next chapter.

Dictyocaulus

Dictyocaulus is a white thread-like worm, up to 8 cm long, found lying in frothy mucus in the trachea and larger bronchi (see Figure 6.53). *D. viviparus* is responsible for

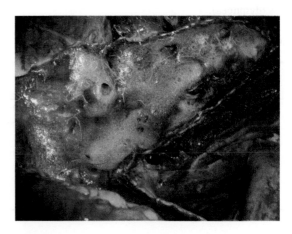

Figure 6.53 *Dictyocaulus viviparus* adults in trachea. Reproduced with permission of B. Smyth.

bovine parasitic bronchitis, a major disease of cattle in temperate regions, particularly in parts of the British Isles and Western Europe. A closely-related species is sometimes responsible for deaths in farmed deer, while other members of the genus cause sporadic disease in horses and small ruminants.

Extra information box 6.3

Bovine parasitic bronchitis

This disease is also known as dictyocaulosis or verminous pneumonia and has a number of local onomatopoeic names like 'husk' (England) and 'hoose' (Scotland) depicting the cough and respiratory sounds commonly associated with the condition.

Dictyocaulus viviparus

Bovine lungworm is responsible for reduced weight gain, coughing, respiratory distress and deaths in young stock and abruptly lowered milk yield in dairy cows. There are serious welfare implications if affected animals are left untreated. *D. viviparus* is the only nematode infection for which a commercial vaccine is currently available (see Section 1.6.5).

Life-cycle

Unlike most other lungworms, *D. viviparus* has a direct life-cycle (see Figure 6.54):

a – Eggs laid in the upper airways are coughed up, swallowed and hatch during their passage through the alimentary tract.

b – L_1 are passed in faeces. Development to L_2 and L_3 occurs within the dungpat.

c – L_3 are distributed over surrounding pasture by *Pilobolus* fungi (as explained later in this section).

d – L_3 are ingested by grazing cattle.

e – Larvae penetrate the intestinal wall and take a week to migrate via the lymph and blood circulation to the lungs. They ascend via alveolae and bronchioles to reach their final destination in the larger bronchi and trachea. The prepatent period is 3½ weeks.

The *Dictyocaulus* life-cycle has a number of distinctive features. The L_1 does not have the 'wavy' tail typical of other lungworms. Preparasitic larvae do not feed but retain both cuticular sheaths as they moult from L_1 to L_2 to L_3. To enable them to do this, the intestinal cells of the L_1 are packed with glycogen. This shows up microscopically as greenish refractile granules, providing a useful diagnostic indicator (see Figure 6.55).

The larvae conserve energy by being very lethargic and by engaging the services of a faecal-dwelling fungus, *Pilobolus*, to spread them beyond the zone of repugnance and onto the pasture beyond. Fungal hyphae proliferate within the dung-pat and send stalks carrying 'fruiting bodies' to the surface (see Figure 6.56). *Dictyocaulus* larvae climb onto the fruiting bodies which swell with water until they burst, sending the fungal spore with its hitchhiker larva flying through the air onto fresh grass, where both can be eaten by a grazing animal. *Dictyocaulus* larvae can be transported 3 m in this way and further still with wind assistance.

Epidemiology

Parasitic bronchitis is a seasonal condition occurring in summer and autumn months. Where calves are grazed separately from older stock, infection persists from one year to the next by the survival of low numbers of L_3 on pasture through the winter. The low-grade infections that establish in calves after spring turn-out can lead to a rapid build-up of pasture contamination as L_1 dropped onto the grass can develop to the infective L_3 in about a week in favourable conditions.

Although *D. viviparus* induces a solid, protective immunity relatively quickly, the rate at which this happens depends on the level of exposure. Disease occurs when infective larvae accumulate on grass faster than the calves grazing that pasture can acquire protection. Conversely, a slower build-up of larvae enables grazing stock to become immune before larval densities reach a critical threshold. Such animals will remain healthy even though the pasture would be damaging or lethal to newly introduced susceptible stock. Parasitic bronchitis is therefore a sporadic disease and farmers may not realise that it is endemic on their property until the ecological balance is disturbed (e.g. by unusual weather conditions or a change in grassland management).

Older cattle are generally immune but a few carry a patent infection. These can excrete larvae in sufficient numbers to initiate a new epidemiological cycle if susceptible calves graze that pasture.

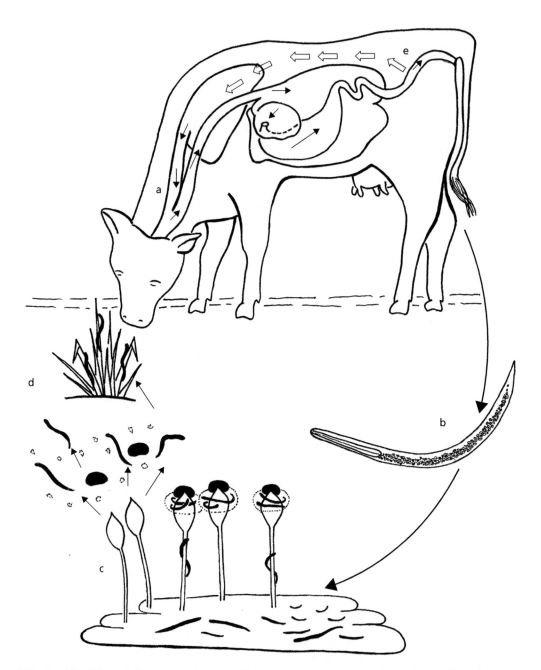

Figure 6.54 Life-cycle of the cattle lungworm, *Dictyocaulus viviparus*: a – eggs pass up the trachea and are swallowed; b – L_1 passed in faeces develop to L_3; c – L_3 dispersed by fungal spores; d – L_3 ingested by host; e – L_3 migrate to lungs and establish in trachea (details in text).

Dictyocaulus larvae can be dispersed by *Pilobolus* across boundaries onto adjacent fields. They can also be carried on tractor wheels, farm workers' boots, etc.

Recently, outbreaks have been occurring with greater frequency in adult dairy cows. This shift in the epidemiological pattern may be due to climate change, altered farming practices, inadequate immunity as a result of the overuse of anthelmintics in young stock or to a failure to vaccinate during calfhood.

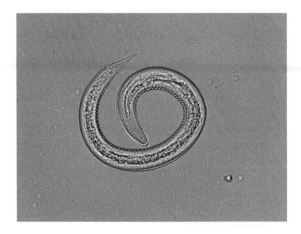

Figure 6.55 *Dictyocaulus viviparus* infective third stage larva.

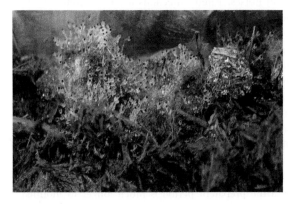

Figure 6.56 The fungus *Pilobolus* growing on horse dung: black spores can be seen sitting on top of 'fruiting bodies' at the tips of the hyphae. Reproduced with permission of D.E. Jacobs and C.N.L. Macpherson.

Help box 6.6

Sequence of events leading to an outbreak of parasitic bronchitis in calves

1. Small numbers of L_3 survive the winter on the pasture.
2. After turnout, a few calves in the group become infected and after 3½ weeks (the prepatent period) start shedding L_1.
3. L_1 develop to L_3 in about a week.
4. The remaining calves become infected and start shedding L_1 after 3½ weeks.
5. Thereafter, one, two or more waves of infection establish in the calves while more and more L_3 accumulate on grass until:
   either   disease breaks out
   or   the calves become immune and the worms are expelled from the lungs.

Pathogenesis

The lungs of calves that die of parasitic bronchitis appear swollen with large volumes of collapsed or consolidated tissue, especially in the distal part of the diaphragmatic lobes (see Figure 6.57). The pathology is complex with different processes at play during each stage of the disease. An understanding of these is necessary when managing an outbreak in order to predict the likely outcome.

Migrating larvae in the bronchioles induce copious amounts of mucus (see Figure 6.58). This blocks air flow to downstream alveolae and stimulates coughing. The reduced surface area available for gaseous exchange leads to faster and deeper breathing (tachypnoea) and, in severe cases, dyspnoea. Nevertheless, there is no physical injury and no lasting damage once the infection is terminated. Early diagnosis and anthelmintic treatment will therefore ensure a rapid clinical response. The prognosis is favourable provided patients are protected from reinfection.

Blockage ceases to be a problem once the worms reach wider air-passages, although bronchitis is a continuing feature. More importantly, eggs, newly hatched larvae, and fragments of adult worms killed by immune responses are aspirated into the bronchioles and alveolae. This sets up a parasitic pneumonia with intense cellular infiltration. Such lesions resolve only slowly following removal of the worm population. A long period of convalescence will be needed before normal lung function is restored.

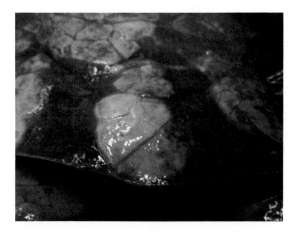

Figure 6.57 Bovine parasitic bronchitis: part of lung showing consolidated lobules (red) between more normal tissue (pink). Reproduced with permission of B. Smyth.

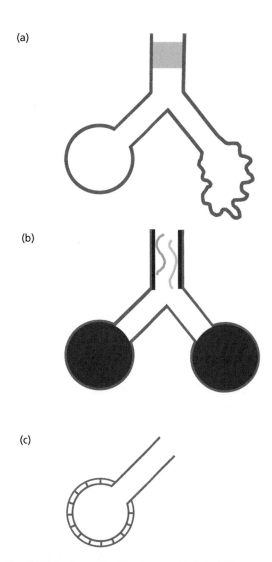

(a)

(b)

(c)

Figure 6.58 Pathogenesis of bovine parasitic bronchitis: a – prepatent disease; b – patent disease; c – postpatent disease.

But the situation can get even worse. A small proportion of calves apparently recovering from *D. viviparus*-induced parasitic pneumonia will relapse and die. This happens even though most adult worms have already been expelled by anthelmintic treatment or immunity. A poorly understood trigger causes the ultra-thin lin-

ing of the alveolae to be replaced with cuboidal cells (epithelialisation), thereby rendering oxygen uptake impossible.

Reinfection syndrome

Immune cattle only display clinical signs if exposed to massive challenge. When this happens, large numbers of larvae reach the bronchioles and become trapped in grey-green granulomatous reactions measuring ~5 mm. This results in coughing and a sudden fall in milk-yield. As very few adult worms establish, faecal larval counts are low or zero.

Dictyocaulus arnfieldi

D. arnfieldi seems better adapted to living in donkeys than horses. Patent infections are more common and longer-lasting in donkeys but are usually without ill-effect. In horses, migrating lungworm larvae mostly die in the lungs inducing a chronic cough. The epithelium lining air passages in affected parts of the lung becomes hyperplastic and the bronchioles are surrounded by a thick band of lymphoid tissue (peribronchial cuffing). This combination acts as a valve which traps air in the alveolae, producing discrete raised patches of overinflated lung tissue which can be several cm in diameter.

The life-cycle is similar to that of *D. viviparus* except that the adult worms tend to be in smaller bronchi and the prepatent period is much longer (3 months). Embryonated eggs are voided in the faeces, although they hatch very soon after being passed.

Metastrongylus

There are three species of *Metastrongylus* in pigs but they all behave alike, inhabiting the larger bronchioles and smaller bronchi in the distal part of the diaphragmatic lobe of the lung. They superficially resemble *Dictyocaulus* and can cause severe lung damage. Even low-level infections check live-weight gain, but immunity develops quickly. The life-cycle is typically metastrongyloid except that larvated eggs are passed in faeces and earthworms act as intermediate hosts. Hence, lungworm infections are most likely to be seen in outdoor pigs.

CHAPTER 7

Nematoda ('roundworms') part 2: nonbursate nematodes and anthelmintics

7.1 Nonbursate nematodes

DNA evidence suggests that over the long evolutionary history of the nematodes, the transition from a free-living lifestyle to animal parasitism may have taken place on several separate occasions. Consequently, the parasitic nematodes are a very diverse group. Chapter 6 described one cluster of related superfamilies (the 'bursate' nematodes). These are characterised by the presence on the male tail of a prominent cuticular structure, the bursa. The story now moves on to the nematode superfamilies of veterinary importance that do not display this feature – the 'nonbursate' nematodes. Most are only distantly related to one another and so their biological characteristics are correspondingly disparate. This chapter also includes a brief description of the Acanthocephala ('thorny-headed worms') which are unrelated to the Nematoda but are included in the vague colloquial term 'roundworm'. Reference is also made to another worm-like group that does not fit comfortably into the structure of this book: the leeches, which are more closely related to earthworms than to nematodes.

Principles of Veterinary Parasitology, First Edition. By Dennis Jacobs, Mark Fox, Lynda Gibbons and Carlos Hermosilla.
© 2016 John Wiley & Sons, Ltd. Published 2016 by John Wiley & Sons, Ltd.
Companion website: www.wiley.com/go/jacobs/principles-veterinary-parasitology

7.1.1 Nonbursate superfamilies

There are six nonbursate superfamilies of particular interest (see Figure 7.1), although others may be encountered less commonly in veterinary practice. The Spiruroidea and Filarioidea are related but other nonbursate superfamilies are so different from each other that each is best considered as a separate entity.

7.1.2 Rhabditoidea

This superfamily is a transitional group in which the majority of species are free-living but some have started to exploit opportunities provided by parasitism. Most members of the group spend their whole life-cycle in inanimate habitats such as soil or decaying vegetation. Some are parasitic on or in plants (the potato eel-worm, for example). A few are basically free-livers but will parasitize animal tissues if a chance arises (i.e. they are facultative parasites). *Pelodera* and similar genera can invade the skin of dogs or other animals lying on damp bedding and may cause dermatitis. The usually saprophytic *Halicephalobus* is particularly dangerous as it can penetrate through the skin of immunocompromised animals to breed prolifically in kidney, CNS and other tissues, forming tumour-like lesions. It is an occasional cause of ataxia in horses and, rarely, a human infection. There is just one genus that has adopted parasitism as an essential (obligatory) component of its life-cycle: *Strongyloides*. This must have proved a successful strategy as there are many *Strongyloides* species affecting a wide range of hosts.

Strongyloides

Humans and domesticated animals each have their own *Strongyloides* species (e.g. *S. westeri* in horses, *S. papillosus* in ruminants, *S. ransomi* in pigs etc.). Cross-infection between hosts is uncommon, although some strains of a dog species, *S. stercoralis*, are thought to have zoonotic potential.

Strongyloides adults collected from their animal host are small (< 1 cm) and thread-like resembling trichostrongyloids (see Figure 6.20). Closer inspection, however, will fail to detect the presence of any bursate males – in fact, there are no male worms in the animal host, only females (as will be explained below). If confirmation of identity is needed, the *Strongyloides* pharynx, at almost a third of the total body length, is much longer than the trichostrongyloid equivalent. The eggs are thin-shelled and half the size of a typical strongyle egg (see Figure 7.2). Each already contains a first-stage larva when it is passed in faeces.

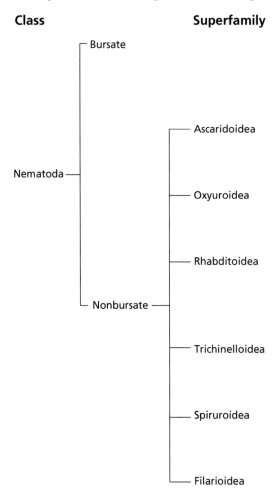

Class   Superfamily

Bursate

Nematoda

Ascaridoidea

Oxyuroidea

Rhabditoidea

Nonbursate

Trichinelloidea

Spiruroidea

Filarioidea

Figure 7.1 Overview of the nonbursate nematode superfamilies.

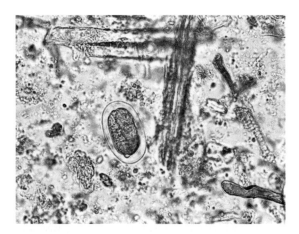

Figure 7.2 *Strongyloides* egg.

Help box 7.1

Avoid common mistakes!

Confusingly, *Strongyloides* is not a strongyle worm, nor does it belong to the Strongyloidea. It would be much better if it could be given a different name but, unfortunately, the laws of international zoological nomenclature do not permit this.

The life-cycle of *Strongyloides* is unique in that it involves a parasitic cycle and a free-living cycle. In some species these alternate; in others external stimuli may influence the route taken by successive generations. Remarkably, free-living adults do not resemble their parasitic siblings, being much stouter and having a differently shaped pharynx (presumably reflecting different food sources and feeding mechanisms). Parasitic adults live close to the mucosa of the small intestine while free-living adults inhabit soiled bedding or other humid, nutrition-rich environments.

The life-cycles of the various *Strongyloides* species vary in detail but are broadly similar. The equine species *S. westeri* is used as an example (see Figure 7.3):

a – Larvated eggs on the ground hatch and the larvae develop via L_1 and L_2 to the L_3 stage.

b – A third-stage larvae is **either** infective **or** noninfective.

Parasitic phase of life-cycle:

c – Infective L_3 can enter the host by skin penetration. If entering an adult mare in this way, the larvae accumulate in subcutaneous tissues and migrate to the mammary gland during lactation.

d – Larvae are acquired by foals either by skin penetration or from the mare via colostrum and milk. They travel to the small intestine where they develop into females that are able to lay fertile eggs even though no males are present in the parasitic phase of the life-cycle (i.e. they are parthenogenic).

e – Larvated eggs are voided with faeces bringing us back to (a).

(In some species, e.g. *S. stercoralis* in dogs, the egg hatches in the intestine and the L_1 is passed in faeces.)

Free-living phase of life-cycle:

f – All hatched larvae that are not predestined to become parasitic females develop via a free-

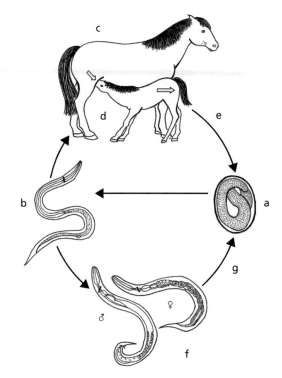

Figure 7.3 Life-cycle of *Strongyloides westeri*: a – larvated egg; b – L_3 (infective or free-living); *Parasitic cycle:* c – infective L_3 infects mare or foal by skin penetration; d – transmammary infection of foal; e – larvated eggs passed in faeces; *Free-living cycle:* f – free-living L_3 develops to adult; g – larvated eggs produced (details in text which uses same lettering as shown above). Redrawn after Jacobs, 1986 with permission of Elsevier; larval and adult stages after Grove, 1989 with permission of Taylor and Francis.

living L_4 stage to become free-living adult males and females.

g – The free-living females produce larvated eggs and, once again, we are back to (a).

Pathogenicity

Patent infections are commonest in very young animals and may be associated with diarrhoea or dysentery, particularly in piglets and puppies. Often, however, infections are symptomless even though faecal egg-counts are high.

Species such as *S. stercoralis*, with eggs that hatch before leaving the host, can give rise to persistent infections, especially if the animal is immunocompromised. In this case, larvae that develop to the infective stage within the host digestive tract penetrate the intestinal wall or perianal skin. This is known as 'autoinfection'.

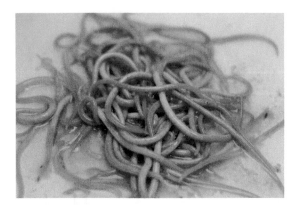

Figure 7.4 Ascarid worms (*Parascaris* from a horse). Reproduced with permission of M.K. Nielsen.

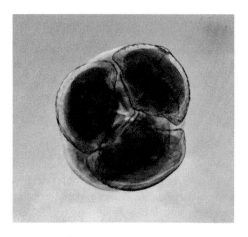

Figure 7.5 *En face* (head-on) view of the head of an ascarid showing three large lips.

7.1.3 Ascaridoidea (ascarids)

When animal owners report seeing a 'roundworm', they are most often referring to an ascarid. This is understandable as ascarids are big fleshy worms (see Figure 7.4) that are very obvious if present in faeces or vomit. On a smaller scale, the larvae of one group of ascarids, the anisakids, are sometimes found in herring and other fish. These are not only unsightly but occasionally cause human health problems (see Section 9.3.1).

General characteristics

Adult ascarids live in the lumen of the small intestine. They are typically between 5 and 40 cm long (depending on species, sex and stage of development) and pinkish-white or ivory-white in colour. Close inspection of

the head reveals three prominent lips around the mouth (see Figure 7.5).

The females are very prolific, each producing hundreds of thousands of eggs per day. The eggs are almost spherical, so they appear round when seen under the microscope (see Figure 7.6). At 85–100 µm, they are just a little bigger than a standard strongyle egg (Practical tip box 6.2). They have a thick protective shell. This is smooth-surfaced, but some species have an additional albuminoid layer which gives the surface a rough or sculptured appearance.

Ascarid eggs are unembryonated when passed into the environment. If conditions are favourable, an infective larva will develop inside each. The egg does not hatch until swallowed by a host.

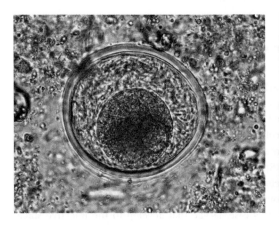
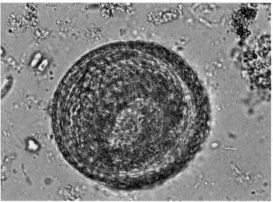

Figure 7.6 Ascarid eggs: left – a smooth-shelled species (*Toxascaris*; unembyonated); right – a rough-shelled species (*Toxocara*; embryonated).

Extra information box 7.1

Ascarid infective stage

The infective stage for ascarids is widely considered to be the L_2. For convenience, this convention is followed in this book, although some experts now believe the infective stage to be an L_3. This controversy does not affect the two important practical points:
i) the egg is not infective until it is fully embryonated;
ii) the infective larva does not hatch until the egg is swallowed by a host.

General life-cycle

The ascarids tend to have complicated life-cycles. An understanding of these is necessary in order to appreciate the epidemiology of associated disease and to design sensible control programmes. The following paragraphs describe the life-cycles of three ascarids in order of ascending complexity.

The first is the poultry ascarid, *Ascaridia*, which is 'nonmigratory' (i.e. the larvae do not migrate around the body). It is one of the simplest of the ascarid life-cycles (see Figure 7.7):

a – Adult female worms in the intestine produce large numbers of colourless smooth-shelled ascarid eggs which pass out of the bird in its droppings.

b – An infective larva develops within each egg.

c – Earthworms can harbour eggs and infective larvae, thereby acting as transport hosts.

d – The avian final host is infected either by swallowing an embryonated egg (i.e. an egg containing an infective larva) or by eating a transport host carrying eggs or larvae.

e – Eggs hatch in the intestine of the bird. The larvae develop through L_3 and L_4 stages to become adult. Some larvae may spend part of this period superficially embedded in the intestinal mucosa.

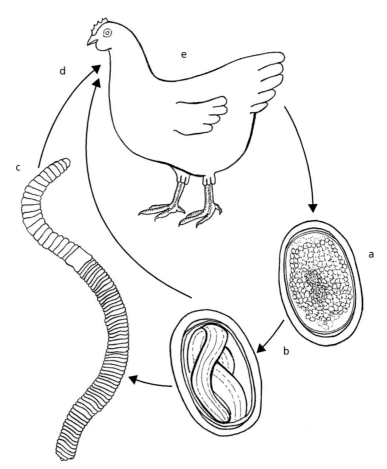

Figure 7.7 Life-cycle of a nonmigratory ascarid, *Ascaridia*: a – eggs passed in faeces; b – infective larva develops inside egg; c – earthworm transport host; d – bird swallows embryonated egg or earthworm; e – larva develops to adult worm in intestine (details in text). Eggs redrawn after Ackert, 1931 from Mozgovoi, 1953 with permission of Nauka.

Extra information box 7.2

Transport and paratenic hosts

There is some ambiguity as to whether the earthworm acts as a transport* or paratenic* host (or both) for *Ascaridia* and other ascarids but the epidemiological outcome is the same, so it is convenient (if not strictly correct) in this context to use the term 'transport host' for the invertebrates that are nonessential (facultative) components in ascarid life-cycles and 'paratenic host' for vertebrates that are similarly involved.

*Reminder: transport host – a casual relationship, the parasite being carried passively;
paratenic host – an intimate relationship where the parasite invades host tissues.

Hepatotracheal migration

After entering the final host, the larvae of some ascarid species undergo an extensive journey through the body, called hepatotracheal migration, before establishing in the small intestine. An example is the equine round-worm, *Parascaris* (see Figure 7.8):

The preparasitic life-cycle of *Parascaris* is very similar to that of *Ascaridia* (see Figure 7.7) except that the egg is brown with an irregular albuminous coating.

a – Eggs passed by an infected horse embryonate on the ground.

b – If ingested by a grazing foal, the larva hatches and invades the intestinal mucosa. It enters the hepatic portal blood system to be transported to the liver.

c – It is then carried by venous blood flow from the liver to the heart and from there to the lung capillary bed.

d – The larva breaks out of a capillary into an alveolus and ascends via bronchioles, bronchi and trachea to the throat.

e – The larva, now an L_4, is swallowed and passes down the alimentary tract to arrive once again in the small intestine where this time it stays to complete its development. The prepatent period is around 3 months.

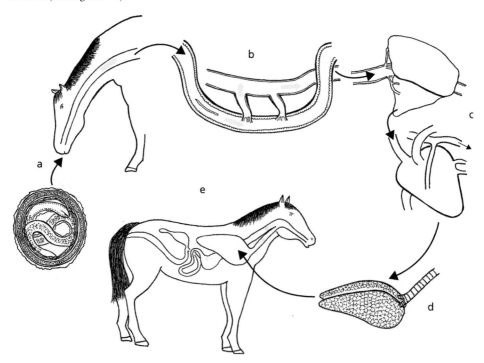

Figure 7.8 Life-cycle of a migratory ascarid, *Parascaris*: a – egg passed in faeces and embryonates on ground; b – infective egg is swallowed and hatched larva enters hepatic portal veins; c – larva carried to liver then via blood to heart and lungs; d – larva ascends trachea; e – larva is swallowed and develops to adult worm in small intestine (details in text). Egg redrawn after Antipin, 1940 from Mozgovoi, 1953 with permission of Nauka.

Somatic infection

The most complex ascarid life-cycles are those that involve 'somatic larvae' as well as migrating larvae. The difference between migrating and somatic larvae is that the former are motile and continue to develop while travelling around the body of their host. Somatic larvae, on the other hand, come to rest in host tissues such as liver, kidney, CNS or musculature and go into a state of arrested development. They do not grow and they do not start to develop until they are reactivated. They are nevertheless metabolically highly active, producing large amounts of excretory/secretory (ES) substances that modulate host immune responses as well as a thick mucin that spreads over the cuticle to protect against cellular and antibody attack. This coating is left behind when the larva moves on. These activities provoke the formation of small granulomatous nodules.

An example of an ascarid that utilises somatic infection as an important component of its life-cycle is *Toxocara canis*, one of the ascarids found in dogs and other canids (see Figure 7.9). The preparasitic development of *T. canis* is similar to that described for *Parascaris* (see Figure 7.8) as is the subsequent hepatotracheal migration that occurs in puppies. Somatic infection occurs when embryonated eggs are swallowed by a paratenic host or a mature dog. The consequences of this are outlined in the following paragraphs.

T. canis in paratenic hosts

In any warm-blooded animal that is not a dog, fox or other canid, *T. canis* eggs hatch and larvae migrate via the liver and heart to the lungs, as happens in the initial stages of hepatotracheal migration (see Figure 7.8). In the lungs, however, they stay in the blood-stream and are returned to the heart to be distributed around the whole body via the general circulation. They settle out in various somatic tissues and become arrested in their development (see Figure 7.10). They now wait for the paratenic host in which they reside to be eaten by a dog, fox, wolf, dingo, etc. If and when this happens, the larvae are released within the digestive tract of their new host and can resume their normal developmental behaviour.

The category 'any warm-blooded animal that is not a dog, fox or other canid' includes humans and somatic infections can establish in people just as in any other paratenic host. *T. canis* is therefore a potentially zoonotic pathogen (see Section 9.3.2).

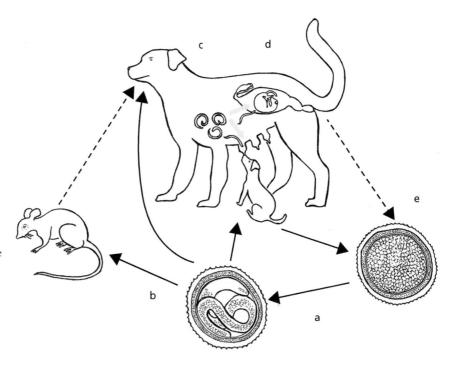

Figure 7.9 Life-cycle of *Toxocara canis* (illustrating somatic infection): a – eggs embryonate on ground; b – embryonated eggs infective for pups, adult dogs and paratenic hosts; c – somatic larvae accumulate in bitch; d - pups infected by activated somatic larvae *in utero* and while suckling; e – adult worms establish in the intestine of pups (and occasionally older dogs) and eggs passed in faeces.

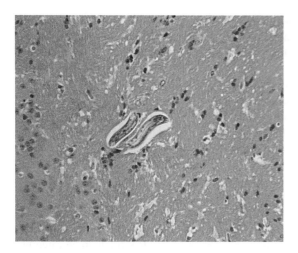

Figure 7.10 A *Toxocara* larva in a brain section from an infected mouse. Reproduced with permission of C. Strube.

T. canis in older dogs

When infection takes place in dogs older than about two months of age, only a very small proportion (if any) of *T. canis* larvae undergo hepatotracheal migration. Most become somatic larvae in the same way they would if they were in a paratenic host. In this case, however, they are waiting for a reactivation stimulus. This happens only after the host becomes pregnant. The greatest numbers of somatic larvae are activated in late pregnancy, some during lactation, but others remain dormant until subsequent pregnancies. Activated larvae migrate to the placenta or mammary glands and are thereby transferred to foetuses *in utero* ('transplacental transmission') or to neonates via colostrum or milk ('transmammary transmission'). Once in the foetus or puppy, the larvae undergo hepatotracheal migration. The first adult worms reach maturity in the small intestine in the third week of independent life.

General epidemiology

The horizontal transmission of ascarid infections within host populations is usually via the faecal-oral route, although paratenic hosts can be an important supplementary pathway for species that parasitize predators (e.g. the feline species *Toxocara cati*). The time taken for eggs passed in faeces to reach the infective (embryonated) stage varies from weeks to months depending on temperature and humidity. Once introduced onto a property, ascarid infection can be very persistent. This is because embryonated ascarid eggs can remain viable for 5 years or more in protected surroundings (e.g. in moist soil or in humid cracks and crevasses). Furthermore, eggs with an albuminoid coat are sticky and will adhere to skin, structural surfaces, boots etc. Consequently, casual cleaning routines will be ineffective, especially as the thick eggshell protects the larva within from most disinfectants. The eggs will, however, succumb to desiccation and direct sunlight.

Ascarid infections induce a protective immunity, although this generally takes many months to develop. Consequently, the proportion of host animals harbouring patent intestinal infection and the number of worms present declines with age. Nevertheless, the fecundity of the worms is so great that just a small number of older carrier animals can ensure perpetual contamination of premises.

Immunity is, however, ineffective against somatic larvae. Thus, somatic infection can persist into adulthood enabling vertical (transplacental and/or transmammary) transmission to take place. This adds an extra dimension to the epidemiology of those ascarid species that include somatic larvae in their life-cycle. The consequences of this will be described in the *Toxocara* section below.

General pathogenicity

Different stages of the ascarid life-cycle provoke different pathological effects. The adults of most species are so big that they can cause catastrophic blockage and even perforation of the intestine if present in large enough numbers. Smaller numbers may provoke diarrhoea and sometimes vomiting. The presence of just a few worms can adversely affect the growth-rate of the host at an early age, but is more likely to be asymptomatic in older animals.

Larval migration is marked by parasitic pathways which attract intense eosinophilic infiltration. Passage through the liver induces fibroblastic responses appearing as white spots. Large numbers of larvae in the lung may induce allergic reactions giving rise to nasal discharge and other respiratory signs. Damage to the lungs may exacerbate preexisting pulmonary bacterial or viral infection or provide a gateway for secondary infection. Finally, the presence of ascarids may interfere with postvaccination immunity to some other pathogens.

Table 7.1 Some important ascarids

Genus	Host	Hepatotracheal migration?	Paratenic host?	Vertical transmission?	Zoonotic importance	More information in Section:
Ascaris	Pig, human	Yes	No	No	▼	8.3.1
Parascaris	Equidae	Yes	No	No		9.1.1
Toxocara	Dogs, cats, cattle	Yes	Yes	Yes	▼▼▼	9.2.1; 9.3.2
Toxascaris	Dogs, cats	No	Yes	No	*	
Ascaridia	Poultry	No	No	No		8.4.1
Heterakis	Poultry	No	No	No		8.4.1

* Probably of little or no zoonotic importance.

Important ascarids

Ascaris and *Parascaris*

Ascaris suum is the most important macroparasite of pigs (swine) worldwide (see Table 7.1). A very closely related species, *A. lumbricoides*, is a significant human health problem wherever public hygiene standards fall below ideal. These two ascarid species are mostly restricted to their own respective hosts but cross-infection can occur. If embryonated *Ascaris* eggs are swallowed by animals other than their natural final host (for example, lambs grazing a former pig pasture), larvae will migrate to the liver and perhaps to the lungs, but will not establish in the intestine.

Adult female *Ascaris* grow to 40 cm long, but *Parascaris equorum*, in horses and other equids, is even bigger – up to 50 cm. *P. equorum* is ubiquitous and can be troublesome in younger horses. The life-cycle of *Ascaris* is very similar to that of *Parascaris* (see Figure 7.8), although the prepatent period is a little shorter. Hepatotracheal migration occurs within the final host, but there is no transplacental or transmammary transmission.

Ascaris suum

Each phase of the parasitic life-cycle can result in economic or welfare problems in pigs, including all the direct and indirect effects described in the 'General pathogenicity' section above. Even small numbers of *A. suum* larvae passing through the liver can trigger a fibroblastic response (see Figure 7.11). The lesions are roughly spherical, except where they meet the liver surface, and they sometimes have a haemorrhagic centre. They vary from several millimetres to a couple of centimetres in diameter with white strands radiating out between adjacent liver lobules. The pathological term for these 'milk-spots' is 'chronic focal interstitial hepa-

titis'. The lesions resolve in about six weeks leaving a very small nodule.

There is a complex relationship between immunity and 'milk-spots'. On exposure to *A. suum*, pigs develop a protective immunity over a period of months. Initially, migrating larvae pass through the liver and lungs, and it is not until they arrive back in the intestine that they succumb to immune attack. Thus, it is not an unusual occurrence in an abattoir to find 'milk-spots' in the livers of younger pigs even though they have no adult worms in the intestine. As pigs become more solidly immune, larvae are killed before they reach the liver, and 'milk-spots' are therefore observed less frequently in slaughtered sows.

Sows nevertheless play an important role in the epidemiology of 'milk-spot' livers. Despite their immunity, a small proportion of sows do carry a small number of adult worms in their alimentary tract. As female *A. suum* are such prolific egg-layers, the farrowing house can quickly become contaminated. As a result, the susceptible piglets acquire infection, carry it with them to the fattening house and perpetuate the problem.

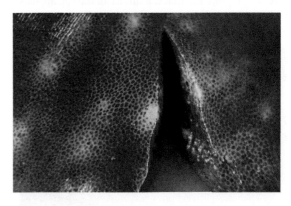

Figure 7.11 Milk-spot lesions in pig liver. Reproduced with permission of A. Daugschies.

Parascaris equorum

As adult horses rarely harbour patent infection, the transmission of *P. equorum* is generally from one year's foals to the next via contaminated pastures. Foals are often infected in their first month of life but eggs do not appear in the faeces for a further 10–12 weeks (i.e. the prepatent period). Light infestations are asymptomatic but perpetuate the transmission cycle by contaminating the pasture anew. In heavier infections, lung damage by migrating larvae may provoke coughing and nasal discharge, while intestinal worms contribute to unthriftiness or weight-loss. As the worms are so large, obstructive impaction or even perforation of the small intestine can occur in extreme cases with severe or fatal consequences.

Toxocara

Toxocara can be severely detrimental to the welfare of young animals. It is also responsible for human disease. There are three major species: *T. canis* in dogs and other canids, *T. cati* in cats and other felids, and *T. vitulorum* in buffalo and cattle. The dog and cat ascarids are cosmopolitan, but the bovine species is found mostly in warmer climates. Although each species can, as a general rule, establish as an adult worm only in its own final host, all are indiscriminate in their choice of paratenic hosts. The pathogenic role of *T. canis* in human tissues is well documented (see Section 9.3.2), but the extent to which *T. cati* and *T. vitulorum* contribute to human disease is ill-defined.

T. canis and *T. cati* adults grow to about 10–18 cm in length (see Figure 7.12) but *T. vitulorum* is longer (up to 30 cm). The deep brown eggs are described as subglobular (i.e. not quite spherical). The sticky albuminous layer is sculptured so that the surface of the egg appears rough under light microscopy (see Figure 7.13).

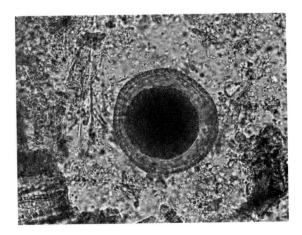

Figure 7.13 *Toxocara* egg.

Toxocara canis

If left untreated, almost all puppies will harbour *T. canis* to a greater or lesser extent. Most of the worms are acquired prenatally, but these are later supplemented by the ingestion of larvae passed with colostrum and milk. Further infection can take place by swallowing embryonated eggs from the environment. Feral canids are exposed to yet another source of infection once they start to take solid food – somatic larvae in the tissues of prey animals such as mice.

The prepatent period of *T. canis* is 4–5 weeks, but eggs start to appear in the faeces of puppies after the second week of life. This apparent anomaly occurs because activation of somatic larvae in the bitch happens during the last three weeks of gestation. Prenatally acquired larvae have therefore started their hepatotracheal migration in the pups prior to whelping. Infected pups excrete (literally) millions of *T. canis* eggs in their faeces during the suckling period.

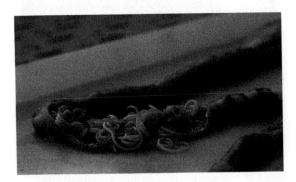

Figure 7.12 *Toxocara canis* in the small intestine of a puppy.

Help box 7.2

Dogs can become infected with *Toxocara canis* in four ways:

1. Transplacental: somatic larvae in the bitch are activated and infect foetuses.
2. Transmammary: activated somatic larvae are transmitted in colostrum and milk.
3. Environmental: by swallowing embryonated eggs.
4. Food-borne: by ingesting somatic larvae in tissues of a paratenic host (e.g. mouse).

From the age of about six weeks, pups start to lose their intestinal *T. canis* population spontaneously, a phenomenon well-known to all dog breeders (see Figure 9.20). During this period, a progressively greater proportion of ingested larvae become arrested in somatic tissues rather than taking the hepatotracheal route. Thus, only a minority of dogs over 4–6 months of age harbour patent infection and they are likely to have no more than a few adult worms. Their *T. canis* egg-output is correspondingly low but sufficient nonetheless to ensure widespread environmental contamination. Higher egg-counts are, however, encountered in suckling bitches as these often experience a temporary increase in their intestinal worm burden. Adult foxes, too, tend to carry greater numbers of intestinal *T. canis* than most domestic dogs.

As with many other ascarid infections, a few worms do no discernible harm, but greater numbers can stunt growth and cause serious, and sometimes fatal, disease (see Section 9.2.1).

Toxocara cati

T. cati infects cats and other felidae. Its biology is in many respects similar to that of *T. canis* but there are only three routes of transmission – transmammary, embryonated eggs and infected paratenic hosts. As there is no prenatal infection, kittens are first infected during suckling and eggs will not appear until the end of the prepatent period (i.e. when the kittens are around 8 weeks old).

Help box 7.3

Cats catching mice are likely to become infected with a

1. Nematode   *Toxocara cati*
2. Cestode   *Taenia taeniaeformis*   (Section 5.3.3)
3. Protozoan   *Toxoplasma gondii*   (Section 4.7.3)

Avoid common mistakes!

The names *Toxocara* and *Toxoplasma* are easily confused, especially as each is associated with parasites of mice and men.

Toxascaris

Toxascaris leonina is 'the other ascarid' of both cats and dogs. It is a little smaller than *Toxocara* but this is not a reliable differential characteristic. In cats, the two genera are easy to tell apart as the cervical alae of *T.cati* are distinctly arrow shaped (see Figure 7.14). In dogs, however, both have similarly shaped heads. There are other minor morphological differences but it is usually easier to look at eggs in a faecal sample or taken from the uterus of a female worm. *T. leonina* eggs are smooth-shelled and transparent in contrast to those of *Toxocara* which are dark and rough shelled (see Figure 7.6).

T. leonina has no hepatotracheal migration in the final host; there is no prenatal infection; nor is there any transmammary transfer of larvae. The only routes of transmission, therefore, are ingestion of embryonated eggs and predation of paratenic hosts. Consequently, infection is first seen in adolescent animals.

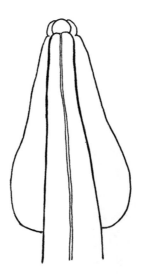 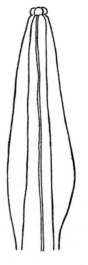 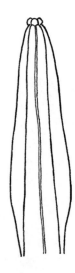

Figure 7.14 The head-ends of a – *Toxocara cati*; b – *Toxascaris leonina*; c – *Toxocara canis*. Redrawn after Morgan and Hawkins, 1953 from Miyazaki, 1991.

Toxocara cati   *Toxascaris leonina*   *Toxocara canis*

This species is not generally considered to be of zoonotic significance but, as somatic *T. leonina* larvae do occur in paratenic hosts, the possibility cannot be totally excluded.

Poultry ascarids

The two poultry ascarids, *Ascaridia* and *Heterakis* both have transparent smooth shelled eggs, and comparable life-cycles (see Figure 7.7), but there the similarities end. *Ascaridia* is typically ascarid in appearance, stout and up to 12 cm long, and lives in the small intestine. In contrast, *Heterakis* lives in the caeca and is only 1.5 cm long. It is slender and has a pointed tail (see Figure 7.15). Despite this appearance, microscopic examination reveals three lips around the mouth and a large posterior bulb on the pharynx confirming its relationship with the ascarids.

The commonest *Ascaridia* species in poultry is *A. galli*, while another species can cause problems in pigeons. Many birds are symptomless carriers, especially in free-range and deep litter systems. Heavier infections can reduce growth-rate in young birds and egg-production in layers. Occlusion of the intestine can occur in severe cases. Occasionally, a member of the public is alarmed by finding an ascarid worm inside a hen's egg and will complain to the supermarket or other retail source. The culprit will most likely be a displaced *Ascaridia* that has mistakenly ascended the uterus from the cloaca.

Heterakis in chickens is itself relatively harmless, yet it plays a remarkable role in the transmission of a protozoan pathogen, *Histomonas meleagridis* (see Section 4.5.2). Another *Heterakis* species, however, is a serious pathogen of game birds.

7.1.4 Oxyuroidea (pinworms)

Pinworms are very common in rabbits, rodents, tortoises and humans. Almost all of us will have harboured *Enterobius* at some time during our childhood. There are, however, no oxyuroids in dogs and cats. This is important to remember as pets are sometimes blamed unjustly as a source of human pinworm infection. Ruminants and horses also have oxyuroid species, but these are mostly overlooked because of their small size and trivial clinical impact. An exception to this statement is the horse pinworm, *Oxyuris equi*, as the female worm is relatively large and can cause discomfort.

General characteristics

Most pinworm species are small (< 1 cm) and all have a distinctive double-bulbed pharynx (i.e. there are two obvious muscular swellings towards the posterior end of the pharynx which are separated by a constriction; see Figure 7.16). The males are unusual in that they have only one spicule. Pinworms gain their name from the fact that females of this superfamily have long, tapering tails. The vulva is not near the tail as it is in most other female nematodes, but is situated towards the anterior part of the body. This reflects the reproductive behaviour of the group. Female oxyuroids push their heads through the host's anus and then lay eggs suspended in a sticky fluid onto the surrounding perineal skin.

Oxyurid eggs are flattened on one side and have an operculum at one end (see Figure 7.17). An infective larva later develops within each. The egg-masses on perineal skin cause pruritus and rubbing or scratching. The eggs eventually drop to the ground and infection occurs when they are accidentally swallowed. After a brief period in the intestinal mucosa, the larvae develop to adult worms in the lumen of the colon and rectum. Pinworms are generally of low pathogenicity.

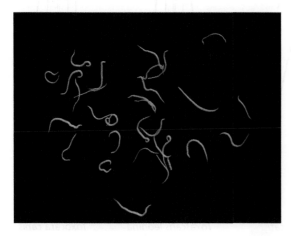

Figure 7.15 *Heterakis*: adult worms.

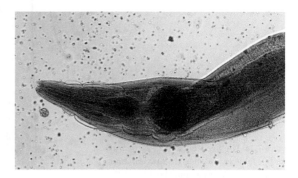

Figure 7.16 Head-end of an oxyurid (*Passalurus*, a nematode of rabbits and hares) illustrating the double-bulbed pharynx.

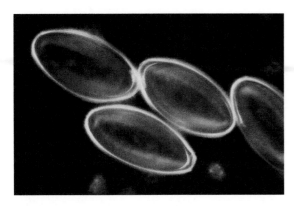

Figure 7.17 Oxyurid (*Oxyuris*) eggs. From Jacobs, 1986 with permission of Elsevier.

Oxyuris

Many equestrian workers will have seen a female *Oxyuris equi* lying in a pile of horse dung. This plump worm, up to 10 cm long, would have been swept from the anus having chosen the wrong moment to lay its eggs. Its tapering tail (see Figure 7.18) differentiates it from *Parascaris*, which may also be expelled in faeces as horses develop immunity. The male *Oxyuris* is rarely seen as it is tiny, like other pinworms.

In heavy infections, *Oxyuris* egg-masses accumulating on the peri-anal skin may appear as grey-white streaks. Otherwise, the only clinical sign is rubbing in response to the associated pruritus (known colloquially as 'seat itch') and consequent loss of hair.

7.1.5 Spiruroidea and Filarioidea

Taxonomists concerned with a broader zoological perspective have redefined the spiruroid and filarial worms as a series of smaller superfamilies but, for veterinary purposes, it is convenient to retain the original division.

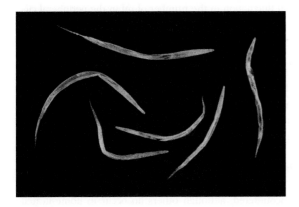

Figure 7.18 *Oxyuris equi*: female worms.

General characteristics

The spiruroid and filarial worms share a number of features but differ fundamentally in other ways. Characters common to both superfamilies include a pharynx divided into a short anterior muscular part and a longer glandular section; and spicules that are unequal in length and dissimilar in shape. The tail end of the male is coiled: flat in the Spiruroidea (see Figure 7.19) and corkscrew-shaped in the Filarioidea (see Figure 7.20).

The spiruroids vary considerably in size and shape. Most inhabit the upper alimentary tract, although a few are associated with the eye. Filarial worms are usually long and filamentous living in connective tissues, blood or body cavities.

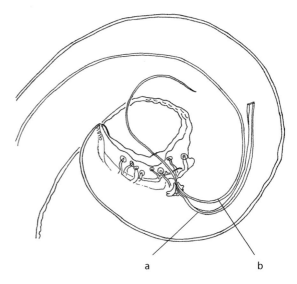

a   b

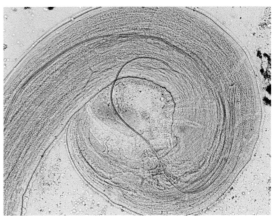

Figure 7.19 Tail-end of a male spiruroid worm showing the coiled tail and unequal spicules typical of this superfamily: a – short, thick spicule; b – long, filamentous spicule (partly protruding from the cloaca).

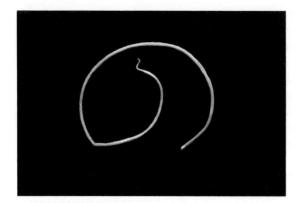

Figure 7.20 A filarial worm (*Setaria*) showing the corkscrew-shaped tail typical of this superfamily.

General life-cycles

The adults of many, but not all, spiruroid and filarial species live in large granulomatous lesions. Some species provoke tumour-like swellings. All have indirect life-cycles. Most use arthropod intermediate hosts.

Spiruroids

Most spiruroids produce narrow, thick-shelled eggs that already contain a larva (see Figure 7.21). They are about

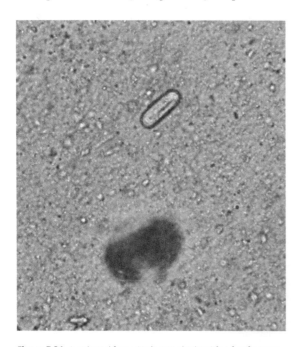

Figure 7.21 A spiruroid egg (*Spirocerca lupi*) with a hookworm egg (below, blurred) for size comparison. Reproduced with permission of R.C. Krecek.

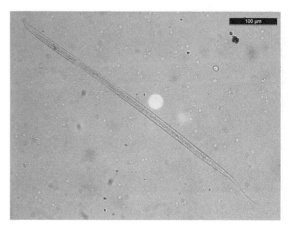

Figure 7.22 Microfilaria of *Dirofilaria immitis*. Reproduced with permission of D. Otranto.

half the length of a typical strongyle egg. Progress to the infective L_3 stage occurs within an intermediate host, often a coprophagic beetle or dipteran larva. Paratenic hosts are often employed to enhance the chances of onward transmission to a final host.

Filarial worms

While some 'primitive' filarial genera produce eggs similar to those of the spiruroids, most members of the superfamily have females that give birth to 'microfilariae' (often abbreviated to 'mf'). These are motile embryos (see Figure 7.22). They have not yet developed an alimentary tract and so are not fully formed L_1. The microfilariae of some filarial species retain the eggshell as a delicate elongated flexible outer sheath. Microfilariae accumulate at the anatomical site or in the tissue most appropriate to the feeding habit of their particular intermediate host, which is always a biting arthropod. With some blood-borne species, a diurnal fluctuation in the number of mf in the peripheral circulation (known as 'periodicity') is similarly coordinated with the feeding behaviour of their host.

Within the intermediate host, the mf develops through L_1 and L_2 stages to become an infective L_3. If this is an insect, the L_3 uses the puncture wound at the next feeding site to enter its new host. If the intermediate host is a tick, the L_3 migrates to the salivary gland and is passively injected into the final host.

Important spiruroids

Table 7.2 highlights those spiruroid genera most widely encountered, although others do occur in domesticated

Table 7.2 Some important spiruroids

Genus	Site	Host	Intermediate host	Paratenic hosts?	Pathogenicity	More information in Section:
Spirocerca	Oesophagus and stomach	Mainly dog	Coprophagic beetles	Major role	▼▼▼	9.2.1
Habronema/ Draschia	Stomach	Horse	Muscid flies	No	▼	9.1.3
Ascarops/ Physocephalus	Stomach	Pig	Coprophagic beetles	Minor role	▼	
Thelazia/ Oxyspirura	Eye	Various	Muscid flies	No	▼	9.2.4

animals, especially in tropical climates. Spirocercosis is top of the list as it is a serious canine welfare problem in many warmer regions. The stomach worms, *Habronema* and *Draschia* in horses and *Ascarops* and *Physocephalus* in pigs are of worldwide distribution (although only the first of these is found in the UK). Several species of the eye-worm, *Thelazia*, occur in mammalian hosts, while *Oxyspirura* is the equivalent avian genus. Impressive numbers of the latter can sometimes be recovered from the conjunctivae of village chickens in the wet tropics, although often with surprisingly little associated pathology.

Spirocerca

Spirocerca lupi occurs in the oesophageal wall of dogs and, rarely, in cats and other animals. Prevalence rates can be high in endemic areas, which include most global subtropical and tropical regions. Adult worms are red, spirally coiled and up to 8 cm long. They are usually only seen in histological section as they lie deeply embedded within nodular lesions (see Figure 6.10).

Life-cycle

The life-cycle of *S. lupi* utilises both intermediate and paratenic hosts (see Figure 7.23):

a – Small larvated eggs (see Figure 7.21) pass from parasitic nodules in the oesophageal wall via narrow fistulae into the lumen. They pass through the alimentary tract and are eventually carried to the outside world in the faeces of their host.

b – The egg is ingested by a coprophagic beetle, which acts as intermediate host, and the larva develops to the infective L_3.

c – A wide variety of vertebrates, from lizards to chickens, can become a paratenic host if they eat an infected beetle.

d – Dogs become parasitized by consuming an infected beetle or a vertebrate paratenic host.

e – The L_3 is released by digestive processes and penetrates into the stomach wall. It migrates via the coeliac artery to the abdominal aorta and from there to the thoracic aorta, which it reaches in about three weeks.

f – After a further three months, the worm crosses from the aorta to the nearby oesophageal wall where it matures. The prepatent period is about six months.

Pathogenicity

Many infections are asymptomatic and diagnosed only fortuitously by radiology or at autopsy. Larval damage can narrow the aperture of the aorta or, less often, weaken the wall with risk of rupture. Granulomatous lesions in the wall of the oesophagus (see Figure 9.19) can grow to the size of a golf ball and may contain dozens of adult worms. Vomiting, difficulty in swallowing and weight-loss may result. The oesophageal nodules have a tendency to become fibrotic and some develop into fibrosarcomas or osteosarcomas. The latter may metastasise to the lungs and hyperplastic pulmonary osteoarthropathy may also occur.

Help box 7.4

Spirocerca: explanation of terms

Fistula: A pathological passage through a tissue that allows fluids to drain away.
Coprophagic: Faeces-eating.
Fibrosarcoma, osteosarcoma: Cancerous growths derived from fibrous connective tissue and bone, respectively.
Hyperplastic pulmonary osteoarthropathy: A thickening of the long bones of the leg that sometimes occurs in dogs with pulmonary disease.

Gastric spiruroids

Habronema and *Draschia*

Habronema and *Draschia* are closely related spiruroids found in the stomach of horses. They are longer (1–3.5 cm) and stouter than *Trichostrongylus axei*, the other

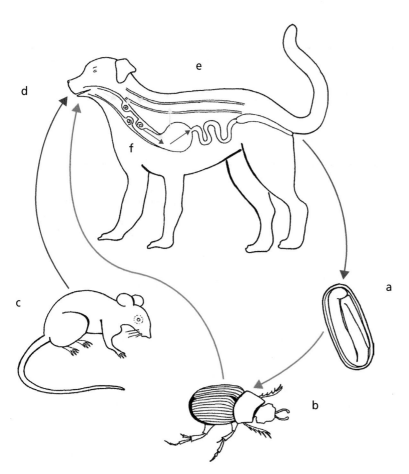

Figure 7.23 Life-cycle of *Spirocerca lupi*: a – eggs passed in faeces; b – coprophagic beetle intermediate host; c – vertebrate paratenic host; d – dog infected by eating intermediate or paratenic host; e – larva migrates to aorta; f – adult develops in wall of oesophagus (details in text). Egg drawn from photomicrograph in Soulsby, 1965 with permission of John Wiley & Sons, Ltd.

nematode found at this site. Adult *Habronema* lie on the mucosal surface and stimulate the production of thick mucus but otherwise do little significant damage. *Draschia* adults penetrate into the mucosa provoking the formation of granulomatous nodules that later become fibrous (see Figure 7.24). These can grow to golf ball size but seem to interfere with gastric function only if situated close to the pylorus.

The eggs of *Habronema* and *Draschia* are narrow, thin-walled and larvated, but rarely seen in faecal samples. The intermediate hosts are muscid flies, such as *Musca* and *Stomoxys*, that lay their eggs on faecal deposits and dung heaps. The spiruroid larva develops inside the fly larva (maggot) and has reached the infective stage by the time the imago fly emerges from its pupa. The L_3 is released when the fly feeds and completes its life-cycle when swallowed by a horse grooming its skin. If larvae are deposited into an open wound, they may delay or prevent healing ('cutaneous habronemosis'; see Section 9.1.3).

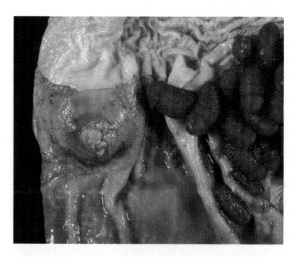

Figure 7.24 Horse stomach opened to show a *Draschia* nodule (on left with concurrent stomach bot infestation on right). Reproduced with permission of T.R. Klei.

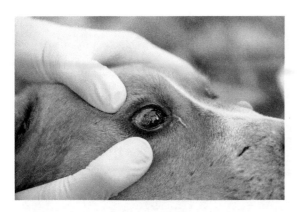

Figure 7.25 *Thelazia* worms on conjunctival mucosa. Reproduced with permission of D. Otranto.

Ascarops and *Physocephalus*

The gastric spiruroids of the pig, *Ascarops* and *Physocephalus*, grow up to 2 cm long. Like *Habronema*, they lie on the stomach mucosa and induce the production of thick mucus. Generally, they are of little economic consequence, although heavy infections can cause a mild gastritis and a check in growth-rate. Pigs are generally infected by eating coprophagous beetles acting as intermediate host, although paratenic hosts may perhaps play a role.

Thelazia

There are at least three *Thelazia* species in the eyes of cattle, two in dogs and one in horses. They are up to 2 cm long but often difficult to see on ophthalmic examination as they are semitransparent (see Figure 7.25) and usually hidden in tear ducts or beneath the third eyelid. The female worms do not lay eggs but eject first-stage larvae directly into the host's lachrymal secretion. The L_1 are then ready to be taken up by muscid intermediate hosts. *Thelazia* infections are mostly nonpathogenic but can cause excessive lachrymation, conjunctivitis,

corneal opacity and, occasionally, ulceration. They can also predispose to other conditions such as infective keratoconjunctivitis ('pink eye') in cattle. Clinical problems are seasonal, related to the feeding activity of the intermediate hosts.

Important filarial worms

The filarial worms are of great importance in human tropical medicine, causing distressing diseases such as elephantiasis and river blindness. Veterinary interest (see Table 7.3) is focused primarily on the canine heartworm, *Dirofilaria immitis*, which is a major cause of morbidity and mortality in dogs, especially in warm, humid climates. There are several other canine filarial worms, such as *Dirofilaria repens* and *Dipetalonema* (also known as *Acanthocheilonema*), which live in subcutaneous and intermuscular connective tissues. These are far less pathogenic but those with blood-borne microfilariae can complicate the diagnosis of canine heartworm disease.

Several *Onchocerca* species occur in different hosts, including horses, cattle and dogs. Human river blindness is also caused by a member of this genus. Fortunately, animal species are generally of minor clinical consequence. Some are very common and their microfilariae may be found fortuitously when examining skin biopsies. A more startling observation is occasionally made during equine abdominal surgery or autopsy – an ivory white worm, up to 13 cm long living in the peritoneal cavity. This is a *Setaria* species which is considered to be harmless (see Figure 7.20).

Parafilaria and *Stephanofilaria* in horses and cattle, respectively, live in subcutaneous tissues and both provoke open lesions to attract their intermediate host, the horn-fly (*Haematobia*). The microfilariae of *Stephanofilaria* congregate at the base of small ulcerations, while the embryonated eggs of *Parafilaria* are present in blood that oozes from ruptured nodules.

Table 7.3 Some important filarial worms

Genus	Site	Host	Intermediate host	Pathogenicity	More information in Section:
Dirofilaria	Heart (*D. immitis*)	Dog	Mosquito	▼▼▼	9.2.2
Onchocerca	Ligaments, tendons	Horse, cattle, dog	Midges, simuliids	▼	9.1.3
Parafilaria/ Stephanofilaria	Skin	Horse/cattle	Muscid flies	▼▼	9.1.3

Extra information box 7.3

Elaeophora

Elaeophora spp. are filarial worms that inhabit blood vessels. Relatively nonpathogenic species occur in horses in southern Europe and cattle in Asia and Africa. Another, in North America, is harmless in its natural host, mule deer, but it causes blindness, deafness and circling when transmitted by tabanid flies to other hosts, including sheep. Developing larvae reduce blood flow in leptomeningeal and other arteries. Later, mf can induce a severe recurrent dermatitis with intense pruritus.

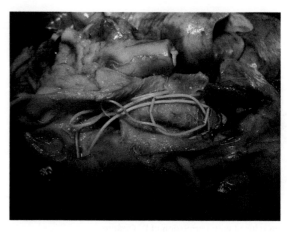

Figure 7.26 *Dirofilaria immitis* in the main pulmonary artery of a dog. Reproduced with permission of L.Venco.

Dirofilaria

Canine heartworm disease (HWD), caused by *Dirofilaria immitis*, is one of the most prominent and challenging conditions experienced in small animal practice in regions with a warm humid climate. This includes parts of the USA, southern Europe (particularly the Po valley in Italy) and Australia, as well as the tropics and subtropics. The presenting signs of chronic HWD are those of chronic heart failure, but sudden collapse may occur in heavily infected dogs.

The endemic zone for HWD is spreading as people and their pets become increasingly mobile. There is as yet no known transmission taking place in the UK, but infected dogs are being brought into the country now that pet-travel regulations have been relaxed. Clinical signs may not become apparent for many months after importation as *D. immitis* has a long prepatent period. Veteri-narians in nonendemic areas need an understanding of this complicated parasite so they can give appropriate advice to dog-owners planning to take their pet into a transmission zone.

Life-cycle

Female *D. immitis* are slender white worms up to 30 cm long, while males are half this size. They live free in the blood in the right side of the heart and in the pulmonary arteries (see Figure 7.26). If left untreated, they have a life-span of 5–7 years. A broad outline of the life-cycle is given in Figure 7.27. Further detail required for successful disease management and prevention is given in the paragraphs that follow.

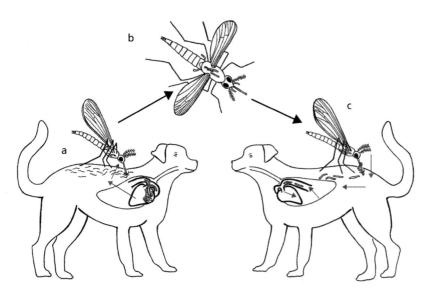

Figure 7.27 Life-cycle of the canine heartworm, *Dirofilaria immitis*: a – microfilariae (mf) circulate in blood and are taken up by mosquito intermediate host; b – mf develop to L_3 in mosquito; c – larvae enter new host when mosquito feeds and migrate through connective tissues to pulmonary arteries and right ventricle of heart. Details of mosquitoes based on Carpenter and Lacasse, 1974.

Microfilariae

Female worms expel microfilariae (see Figure 7.22) directly into the blood-stream. Maximum numbers appear in the peripheral circulation in the evening and after nightfall, coinciding with patterns of mosquito feeding activity. Microfilariae have a life-span of about 2 years.

Intermediate host

There are many species of mosquito that can act as intermediate host for *D. immitis* and many more that do not. The local transmission rate is determined by the mosquito species present in that area, their feeding preferences and their population density.

Development from mf to infective L_3 takes place inside the mosquito over a period of a week at 30°C and a month at 18°C. Normally, there is no development below 14°C, although there is evidence that strains of *D. immitis* are adapting to cooler climates (in southeastern Canada, for example).

The next time the infected mosquito feeds on a dog, up to a dozen L_3 are deposited onto the skin. These enter the body via the puncture wound left behind by the mosquito.

Final host

The principle final hosts of *D. immitis* are the dog and other canidae. Cats and ferrets can also become infected but they are unsuitable hosts and so very few worms establish. Human cases are diagnosed occasionally, but worms do not reach the heart.

On entering a dog, *D. immitis* larvae migrate through connective tissues taking four months to reach the caudal distal pulmonary arteries (see Figure 7.28). By this time they are 1–5 cm long immature adults. They proceed along the arteries towards the right ventricle of the heart and start producing microfilariae 6–7 months postinfection.

The prevalence of infection in unprotected dogs can be very high in endemic areas (up to 45% in some parts of the USA, for example).

Acute prepatent disease

Many clinical signs associated with canine heartworm disease are directly or indirectly attributable to lung damage aggravated by worm-derived substances with pharmacological or immunogenic properties. As these are soluble and can disperse through adjacent tissues,

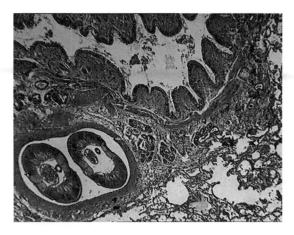

Figure 7.28 Canine heartworm disease: early infection showing two cross-sections of *Dirofilaria immitis* within a pulmonary artery (bottom left). Reproduced with permission of L.H. Kramer.

pulmonary lesions are not confined to the immediate vicinity of the worms. Large numbers of immature adult worms in distal pulmonary arteries provoke an intense diffuse eosinophilic reaction in the lung parenchyma. Coughing becomes apparent on exercise but couch-potato (sedentary) dogs are often asymptomatic.

Chronic disease

Lethargy and exercise intolerance are typical signs of chronic HWD and are due to right-sided heart failure. The sequence of events leading up to this outcome is as follows:

a – Endothelial cells: there is proliferation of the arterial endothelium lining the pulmonary arteries, which can fold to form villi (see Figure 7.29). The permeability of vessel walls increases.

b – Inflammatory processes: result in periarteritis with a proliferation of smooth muscle and a thickening of the media.

c – Thrombi: form within blood vessels.

d – Impairment of blood-flow: the above changes interfere with blood flow, inducing a rise in blood pressure (pulmonary hypertension) and right ventricular strain.

e – All of which leads to: right ventricular hypertrophy and right-sided heart failure.

Post caval syndrome (dirofilarial haemoglobinuria)

In particularly heavy infections (>60 worms), entangled clumps of worms in the heart can impair closure of the

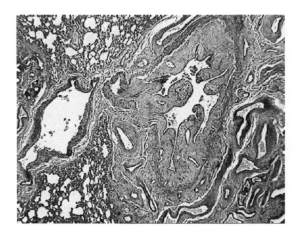

Figure 7.29 Canine heartworm disease: intense endothelial proliferation within a pulmonary artery of a chronically infected dog. Reproduced with permission of L.H. Kramer.

tricuspid valve giving rise to an inadequate inflow of blood from the vena cava. The resulting venous stagnation leads to acute or chronic congestion of the liver, hepatic dysfunction or failure, and increased erythrocyte fragility.

Help box 7.5

Overview of chronic canine heartworm disease

The disease process has three main components:
    Eosinophilic pneumonitis ⟹ lung damage
    Chronic heart failure ⟹ organ damage
    Microfilaria ⟹ immune reactions (in some dogs).
Heart failure leads to multiple system dysfunction.
The clinical signs of HWD are therefore variable and nonpathognomonic.

Onchocerca

The females of some *Onchocerca* species are over 50 cm long but are rarely seen, except in histological sections, as they are very slender and lie hidden in ligaments, tendons and other connective tissues. In general, they have little clinical effect on their host, although some species provoke large subcutaneous nodules which diminish carcase value.

Onchocerca microfilariae can occasionally provoke corneal opacity. Some horses become hypersensitive to dying microfilariae and may develop a localised oedematous reaction along the ventral abdominal midline after macrocyclic lactone therapy for general worm con-

trol. Each *Onchocerca* species utilises a particular species of midge or simuliid as intermediate host.

7.1.6 Trichinelloidea

In evolutionary terms, members of the Trichinelloidea are distant relatives of the other nematodes considered in this book. Consequently, drugs developed primarily for controlling strongyle and ascarid worms often work less effectively against them.

A weird feature of this superfamily is the pharynx. It is formed of a series of doughnut-shaped cells that are stacked on top of each other so the holes through the middle of each match up to form a tube. This is lined by a very thin muscular layer. The 'doughnuts' are secretory cells that replace glands found in other nematode groups.

There are only three genera of veterinary interest in the superfamily Trichinelloidea: *Trichuris* and *Capillaria*, which share a number of common features; and *Trichinella* which has characteristics that are unique amongst the nematodes. *Trichinella* is of major importance as a zoonosis and is an economic burden on the pig-meat industry.

Trichuris and *Capillaria*

Trichuris

The common name for *Trichuris* is the 'whipworm'. This alludes to a long filamentous neck joined onto a relatively short stumpy body (see Figure 7.30). The hind end of the female is gently curved while the male tail

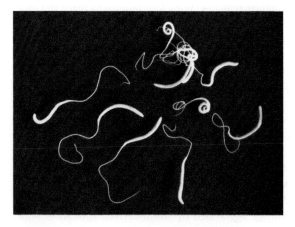

Figure 7.30 Adult *Trichuris*. Reproduced with permission of A. Daugschies.

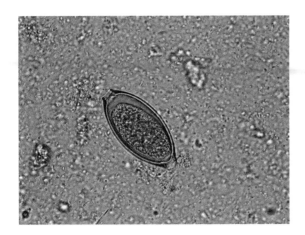

Figure 7.31 *Trichuris* egg.

is coiled terminating in a single spicule protruding from a thick sheath. There are a number of *Trichuris* species including *T. vulpis* in dogs and *T. suis* in pigs. At least two species occur in ruminants. Whipworms are not found in horses or birds.

Trichuris eggs are lemon-shaped, brown, smooth shelled and have a distinctive plug at either end (see Figure 7.31). They can survive for up to 12 years in soil. The infective stage is the L_1 within the egg. This genus is more troublesome in warmer regions as development within the egg occurs only very slowly in temperate climates (so there is less opportunity for large numbers of embryonated eggs to accumulate). The lifecycle is direct. After the embryonated egg is swallowed, the hatched larva develops within an intestinal nodule before reemerging into the lumen.

Practical tip box 7.1

Diagnosis of *Trichuris* and *Capillaria* infections

Although about the same size as strongyle eggs, *Trichuris* eggs are a little heavier and so do not always float as well in saturated salt solution. A flotation medium with a higher specific density is therefore preferred when whipworm infections are suspected. As an additional complication, the output of *Trichuris* eggs tends to be erratic and so a zero egg-count on one occasion does not necessarily rule out whipworm infestation.

As a rough guide, *Capillaria* and *Trichuris* eggs can be distinguished from each other as the former are lighter in colour (often with a greenish tinge), more rectangular in shape and the outer shell has a granular texture (see Figures 7.31 and Figure 7.32)

Whipworms are found in the caecum, although heavy infections spill over into the colon. The neck is inserted superficially into the caecal mucosa with the rest of the body lying free in the lumen. Movement of the neck during feeding disrupts epithelial integrity and opens a portal of entry for other enteropathogenic organisms. Whipworm pathogenicity therefore ranges from intermittent mild diarrhoea to severe dysentery depending on the number of worms and the composition of the gut microflora.

Extra information box 7.4

Possible use of *Trichuris suis* in human medicine

In experimental models, *Trichuris* markedly increases T-regulatory activity thereby suppressing some immune-mediated disease processes (Th2 responses upgraded; Th1 downgraded). Some human immune-mediated diseases are largely restricted to affluent societies (inflammatory bowel disease and Crohn's disease, for example). They are thought to occur because the human immune system, which has evolved in the constant presence of T-regulating helminths, tends to go into overdrive in some worm-free individuals in the absence of this external regulatory influence. The pig and human whipworms are closely related and *T. suis* can establish in small numbers in people. This has lead to the hypothesis that carefully managed infection of selected human patients with *T. suis* might ameliorate the symptoms of chronic inflammatory bowel disease. Clinical trials (placebo-controlled cross-over studies) are in progress at the time of writing to investigate this possibility.

Capillaria

Capillaria species are hair-like worms varying in length from 1 to 5 cm. They are easily differentiated from other nematodes of similar size by the presence of double-plugged light-coloured eggs (see Figure 7.32) within the female uterus. The single spicule of the male provides confirmation, if needed.

There are many species of *Capillaria* in mammals and birds. They are mostly found in the alimentary tract, although there are species in the trachea and bronchi of dogs and urinary bladder of dogs and cats. Another species lives in the liver of rodents and, sometimes, of other animals such as dogs and humans. The eggs of this species accumulate in the hepatic parenchyma (see Figure 7.33) and are not released into the environment until the host dies and decomposes, or is eaten by a predator or scavenger (when the eggs pass through to emerge in their faeces).

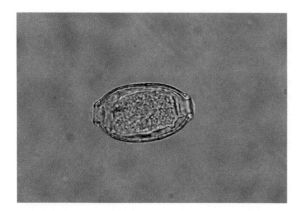

Figure 7.32 *Capillaria* egg. Reproduced with permission of C.A. Tucker and T.A. Yazwinski.

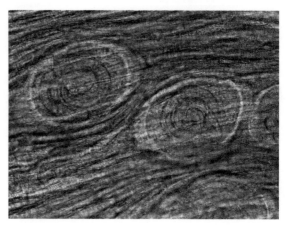

Figure 7.34 *Trichinella spiralis* larvae in a muscle squash preparation.

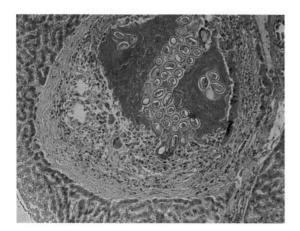

Figure 7.33 *Capillaria hepatica* eggs in liver lesion walled off by fibrous tissue.

Most *Capillaria* species have direct life-cycles, but some avian species use earthworms as intermediate or paratenic hosts. The predilection site varies with species and can be at any level of the digestive system. Their pathogenicity also differs greatly. Most do little harm, but some avian species cause serious enteritis.

Trichinella

Trichinella stands alone amongst the nematodes because:

a – It uses the same individual animal as:

i)   final host

ii)   and then, without exiting the body, as intermediate host.

b – The infective L$_1$ stage: develops as an intracellular parasite within a muscle cell (see Figure 7.34).

There are several closely related but phenotypically distinct forms of *Trichinella*. They differ in their geographic distribution, in their spectrum of infectivity to different mammalian hosts (and, in one case, crocodiles), in their zoonotic potential and in some other biological attributes (for example, tissue cyst formation and larval resistance to freezing). Some are designated as separate species while the taxonomic status of others is less clear. One species is of exceptional importance because of its human pathogenicity and its almost cosmopolitan occurrence. This is *T. spiralis* which is considered a parasite of pigs and rats although it can infect many wild-life hosts as well as domesticated animals and humans. Infections are symptomless in most animals, but humans unfortunately suffer very unpleasant and sometimes fatal consequences. As eating undercooked meat from infected pigs is the most common source of human infection, expensive surveillance and meat inspection procedures are needed even in countries where the prevalence in farm livestock is very low.

Life-cycle of *T. spiralis*

Adult *T. spiralis* are only 1–3 mm long. They are closely applied to the mucosa of the small intestine where they lie entwined between villi, pushing their bodies into intestinal crypts and sometimes penetrating into the mucosa itself. Thus, they are likely to be seen only in histological sections.

The pig is used to illustrate the life-cycle of *T. spiralis* (see Figure 7.35), although many other mammalian species can harbour infection. *T. spiralis* adults have a very short life-span (around two weeks) but during this time

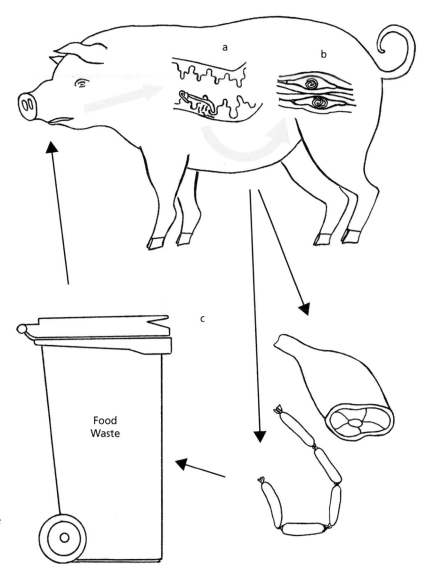

Figure 7.35 Life-cycle of *Trichinella spiralis*: a – adult worms in small intestine produce larvae; b – larvae encyst in striated musculature; c – pig infected by eating meat containing encysted larvae.

each female worm gives birth to hundreds of larvae. These immediately burrow into the intestinal mucosa and enter the lymphatic drainage system or small veins to gain access to the general circulation.

At this stage, the larvae are very immature and less than 100 μm long. Each enters a striated muscle cell and reprograms host genomic expression to meet its physiological requirements. Muscle proteins disappear, collagen genes are upregulated and the cell switches to anaerobic metabolism. The muscle cell has thereby been transformed into a *Trichinella* nurse cell. It even becomes surrounded by a network of blood capillaries supplying nutrients and removing waste products.

Within three weeks the larva has grown ten-fold in size and is now an infective L_1 with recognisable primordial gonads. (*Trichinella* is the only nematode that is sexually differentiated at this early developmental stage.)

By two months post infection, the L_1 has curled up and has become encapsulated within a host-derived membrane. The nurse cell is now called a 'trichinous cyst'. In this state, the L_1 enters a waiting phase and can survive the life-span of many of its host species. It can even persist for days or weeks in the carcase of a host after its death.

The life-cycle of *T. spiralis* can be completed only when the flesh of an infected animal is eaten by another potential host. In the case of pigs this usually occurs when they are fed inadequately cooked kitchen waste containing scraps of infected pork meat (this is sometimes called 'pseudo-cannibalism').

Once released in the intestine of its new host, *T. spiralis* completes its life-cycle with remarkable speed. It completes its four moults to be become adult within 2 days.

Help box 7.6

More common mistakes to avoid

Unlike most other nematodes, there is no free-living larval stage in the *T. spiralis* life-cycle. Transmission occurs only when one animal eats the flesh of another. Thus, faecal examination is futile for diagnostic purposes as neither eggs nor larvae are passed in faeces. In any event, muscle larvae survive much longer than the intestinal adults. Diagnosis therefore relies on microscopic or molecular detection of larvae in muscle samples taken by biopsy or at autopsy, or on the results of immunological tests.

Epidemiology

As most *Trichinella* species infect such a wide variety of mammals, both sylvatic and domestic transmission cycles occur. These may be independent or overlapping, depending on circumstances. Suitable hosts include a wide range of mammalian predators and scavengers. Herbivores may become involved accidentally (e.g. if a horse swallows fragments of a dead mouse in a bale of hay).

An example of epidemiological relationships is given in Figure 7.36:

a – Domestic cycle: The domestic *T. spiralis* cycle centres on the pig. There are three ways in which pigs can become infected:

i **Inadequately cooked swill:** the main route of transmission is by feeding pigs food-waste from processing factories, hotels, restaurants etc. that has not been boiled long enough to kill any *Trichinella* larvae present in meat scraps.

ii **Scavenging:** Pigs may occasionally eat a dead rat or, if allowed to roam around human habitation or rubbish dumps, they may consume garbage containing infected meat.

iii **Pig to pig transmission:** This may occur rarely as a result of tail-biting.

b – Human involvement: People acquire *Trichinella* by eating undercooked meat from an infected

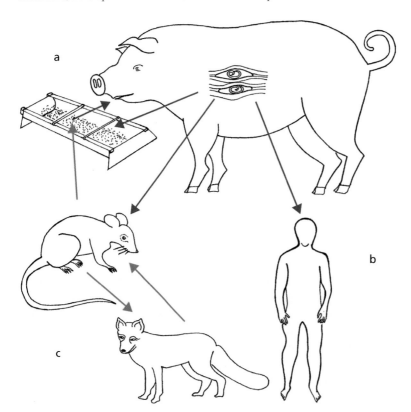

Figure 7.36 A simple overview of the epidemiology of *Trichinella spiralis* infections: a – pigs infected by eating, for example, kitchen waste containing infected pork; b – transmission to humans via infected pork; c – a sylvatic cycle (details in text).

animal. This is most commonly a pork product but meat from other animals can be responsible (see Section 9.3.1).

c – Sylvatic cycle: In sylvatic cycles, scavengers such as rats become infected by eating the remains of dead animals and pass the infection on when they in turn become prey to larger predators. *Trichinella* thereby ascends the food-chain to top carnivores and omnivores (e.g. foxes and bears in the case of *T. spiralis* or walruses and polar bears in the case of the related arctic species).

Extra information box 7.5

> **Dioctophyma**
>
> *Dioctophyma* is the sole representative of veterinary importance in a superfamily related to the Trichinelloidea. It has a wide host range including dogs and mink in cool northern regions. It lives in the kidney and can grow to a metre in length. It is unusual for both kidneys to be affected. Eggs are passed in urine and aquatic annelid worms act as intermediate hosts.

7.2 Other parasitic worms

This section presents two worm-like parasitic groups that have no affinity with nematodes: 'thorny-headed worms' (Acanthocephala) and leeches (Hirudinea). The first is a separate phylum while the latter belongs to the Annelida (the phylum that includes earthworms).

7.2.1 Acanthocephala

The acanthocephalans are easily mistaken for 'roundworms'. Closer inspection, however, shows that the head-end of the worm has an extendable proboscis covered with hooks (see Figure 7.37) – hence the name 'thorny-headed worms'. They have no digestive tract but absorb nutrients through their body surface.

They are encountered mostly in wild-life medicine, particularly in aquatic birds, although canine infections are an occasional finding in the USA. Otherwise, the only acanthocephalan commonly seen in veterinary practice is *Macracanthorhynchus*, which occurs in many regions (but not Western Europe).

Macracanthorhynchus is the thorny-headed worm of pigs and superficially resembles *Ascaris suum*. It grows to 35 cm or more in length (see Figure 7.38). Its proboscis

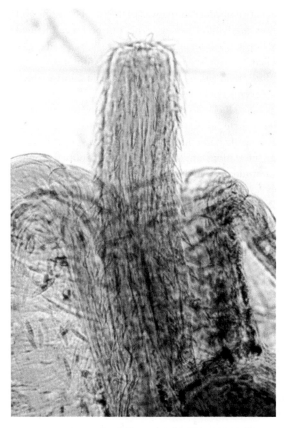

Figure 7.37 An acanthocephalan head showing the retractable proboscis with hooks. Reproduced with permission of A. Jones.

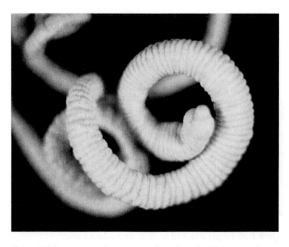

Figure 7.38 *Macracanthorhyncus.* Reproduced with permission of A. Jones.

is deeply embedded in the wall of the small intestine and causes mechanical damage. This can become inflamed and develop into an ulcer. The eggs are brown and thick-shelled, but can be easily distinguished from *Ascaris* eggs as they are larger, more oval and contain a larva which has several hooks and is covered in small spines. The eggs hatch if eaten by beetle larvae (grubs) which act as intermediate hosts. The cycle is completed when a pig eats a beetle harbouring the infective stage of the parasite. Infestations are therefore mostly confined to pigs kept outdoors or in deep-litter yards.

7.2.2 Leeches

Leeches are segmented hermaphrodite worms with a sucker at each end of their elongated body. The majority are predators feeding on small invertebrates but there are also many blood-sucking species. The latter have three cutting blades around the mouth and they make a 'Y'-shaped incision. Depending on the strength of their mouthparts, some species can cut through tough skin (see Figure 7.39), but others have to target softer mucosal surfaces. They maintain their position by suction and secrete a number of powerful substances that aid the feeding process. These include an anaesthetic, which renders the bite painless, and anticoagulants. When replete, the leech releases its hold and will spend the subsequent weeks or months digesting its meal

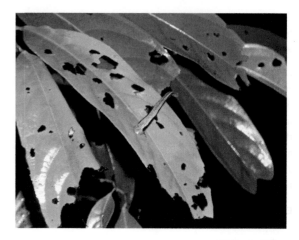

Figure 7.40 Leech seeking a host.

(which can be several times its own body weight) before laying eggs in a cocoon.

Most leeches live in freshwater and feed on amphibians, fish, aquatic birds etc., although some will attack the nasal cavity or pharynx of ruminants, horses and other mammals while they are drinking. Terrestrial leeches are found mostly in wet tropical and subtropical forests. They survive the dry season in soil. When conditions are right, they climb onto vegetation with a looping movement and stretch out to make contact with a passing animal (see Figure 7.40). They are not host-specific.

Leeches take minutes or hours to feed. Often the animal (or human) is unaware of their presence. They will drop off spontaneously if left alone for long enough but, if there is a need, they are best removed by sliding a fingernail or something similar between the skin and mouth to release the suction. Lighted cigarettes, insect repellent etc. may work more quickly but cause the leech to regurgitate with a risk of infecting the wound. Otherwise, leech bites are generally clean but should be washed as a precaution. This also removes leech anticoagulant, thereby reducing the time the wound continues to bleed.

Leeches have been used throughout medical history for removing blood from patients, often for spurious reasons, but there are valid indications in modern practice, e.g. where there are difficulties relating to venous drainage that cannot be easily resolved with more conventional techniques.

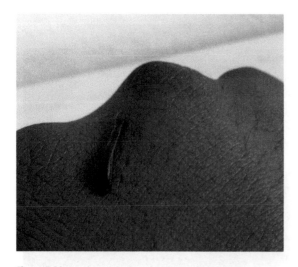

Figure 7.39 Leech attached to skin. Reproduced with permission of M.F. Hassan and C. Panchadcharam.

7.3 Anthelmintics

Anthelmintics are chemotherapeutic agents that kill or result in the expulsion of parasitic worms. Those used to combat tapeworm or trematode infections were described in Sections 5.5 and 5.7. This chapter focuses on anthelmintics which play an important role in the treatment and control of animal parasitic nematodes (see Figure 7.41).

Most modern anthelmintics belong to one of a very limited number of chemical classes. As the range is so limited, it is important to prevent or delay the development of new resistant strains and to manage existing resistance problems appropriately (see Section 1.6.3). To do this, it is necessary to know the chemical nature and mode of action of each product available for use. To assist this process, many countries have a statutory labelling system using symbols and/or colour coding to represent each class of chemicals.

There are three main chemical classes with broad spectrum activity against parasitic nematodes: the levamisole group (tetrahydropyrimidines); the macrocyclic lactones (MLs) and the benzimidazoles (BZDs). These have been in use for several decades. Their excellent performance in conjunction with the upwardly spiralling cost of drug discovery and development resulted in a long period during which little innovative chemistry reached clinical application. More recently, however, the increasing prevalence of nematode strains resistant to one or more of these anthelmintic groups

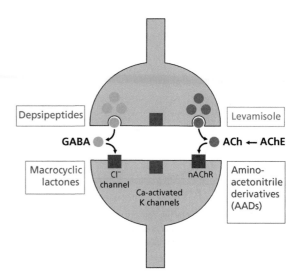

Figure 7.42 Diagrammatic representation of a nematode nerve synapse showing the site of action of four groups of anthelmintics. Modified from I. Denholm with permission.

has stimulated commercial development of compounds with novel modes of action. These include the amino-acetonitrile derivatives (AADs), depsipeptides and spiroindoles.

All except the BZDs disrupt nematode neuromuscular coordination (see Figure 7.42) so that the worm becomes paralysed and is unable to feed or maintain its position in the body. In contrast, the BZDs indirectly affect energy metabolism, leading to starvation and a slow death. The different chemical classes also have characteristic pharmacological properties that influence the way they are used in clinical practice.

Older anthelmintics such as piperazine had a narrower spectrum of activity than modern products and are now largely obsolete. Arsenical compounds are an exception. They are still widely used for the treatment of adult heartworm infection in dogs since there is as yet no equally effective alternative.

As with the ectoparasiticides discussed earlier (see Section 3.5), selective toxicity is achieved in most cases by the compound having a greater affinity for the biochemical target site in the parasite than it has for the equivalent host receptor.

7.3.1 Levamisole group

Levamisole acts at neural and neuromuscular synapses by mimicking the action of acetylcholine (i.e. it is

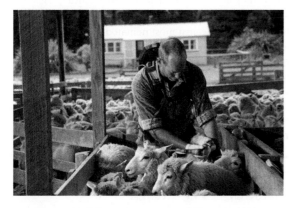

Figure 7.41 Drenching sheep: a reservoir of anthelmintic is held in the knapsack on the operator's back while the handheld device delivers a metered dose. © 2014 Eli Lilly and Company or affiliates.

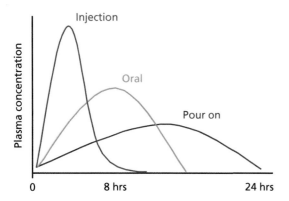

Figure 7.43 Levamisole plasma concentrations following a single treatment given by injection, oral administration or as a pour-on application (notional diagram).

a cholinergic agonist) thereby inducing paralysis (see Figure 7.42). It is absorbed into and excreted from the body rapidly. Nematodes succumb quickly and anthelmintic potency is related to peak plasma concentration.

Levamisole can be given orally, by injection or as a pour-on. Pour-on formulations are absorbed more slowly and higher doses are therefore required to attain the same plasma peak (see Figure 7.43). The safety margin is relatively narrow, particularly in horses and dogs. This limits its use in these species.

Levamisole has a wide spectrum of activity against intestinal and pulmonary nematodes, but has deficiencies against some larval stages, particularly hypobiotic forms (Table 7.4).

Morantel and pyrantel are related compounds with a similar mode of action to levamisole. They have a different pharmacokinetic profile, however, as they are not absorbed from the alimentary tract and therefore have no effect against mucosal larvae or lungworms. Their use is restricted to a few specialised purposes in cattle (morantel) and dogs and horses (pyrantel).

7.3.2 Macrocyclic lactones

The macrocyclic lactones (MLs) are complex macromolecules derived by fermentation processes from different species of moulds (*Streptomyces* spp.). To optimise performance, some MLs are derived from genetically engineered moulds and others are semi-synthetic analogues. The MLs include two closely related chemical groups: the avermectins, including ivermectin, doramectin and eprinomectin; and the milbemycins including milbemycin and moxidectin.

Activity

The MLs open invertebrate-specific glutamate-gated chloride channels in the postsynaptic membrane producing flaccid paralysis in nematodes (see Figure 7.42). Most are extremely potent (with dose-rates measured in micrograms/kg body weight) and have a very wide spectrum of activity including most (but not all) common nematodes in all their developmental stages as well as many blood-sucking and tissue dwelling arthropods (see Table 7.5).

The term 'endectocide' is used for ML parasiticides that are active against both worms and arthropods. Note, however, that trematodes and cestodes are not susceptible to MLs. Activity against adult filarial worms (including the canine heartworm) is limited, although the MLs do have potent activity against migrating heartworm larvae. Several are in widespread use as heartworm prophylactics (see Section 9.2.2).

Optimisation of ML potency against nematodes usually comes at the price of diminished efficacy against arthropods, and vice versa. Thus, ivermectin, which is highly effective against most nematodes, has little activity against fleas, whereas selamectin, widely used for flea control (Section 3.5.2), has useful but nevertheless limited activity against nematodes.

Table 7.4 General spectrum of activity of levamisole

Nematodes		Other parasites	
Adult worms	▼▼▼	Trematodes	0
Mucosal larvae	▼	Cestodes	0
Hypobiotic larvae	0	Arthropods	0

Note: activity may vary according to host, parasite species and formulation.

Table 7.5 General spectrum of activity of macrocyclic lactones.

Nematodes		Other parasites	
Adult worms	▼▼▼	Trematodes	0
Mucosal larvae	▼▼▼	Cestodes	0
Hypobiotic larvae	▼▼▼	Arthropods	▼▼ (blood-sucking and tissue dwelling only)

Note: activity may vary according to host, parasite species, compound and formulation.

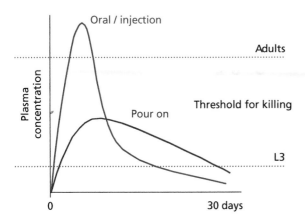

Figure 7.44 Macrocyclic lactone plasma concentrations following a single treatment at the therapeutic dose for injection/oral formulations: a comparison of administration by injection/oral and pour-on routes (notional diagram).

Pharmacokinetics

As with levamisole, MLs are absorbed more slowly as pour-on formulations and a higher dose-rate is required to achieve the same plasma peak for immediate anthelmintic effect (see Figure 7.44).

MLs are excreted only slowly from the body so the plasma concentration curve has a very long 'tail'. (Note that the horizontal time-scale in Figure 7.44 is measured in days whereas that for levamisole in Figure 7.43 was in hours.) This pharmacokinetic profile can be put to practical use as the ML plasma concentration required to kill strongyle infective larvae (L_3) is much lower than that needed for control of adult worms. Thus, the initial high plasma peak attained soon after dosing kills worms already in the animal at the time of treatment, while the 'tail' will ensure that any new infective larvae that are ingested for a period thereafter will be killed. Consequently, ML treatments provide a period of protection against reinfection. This is termed 'persistent activity' and is particularly useful for worm control programmes in cattle. The period of protection varies with the compound, formulation and host species, being much shorter in small ruminants than in cattle or horses.

The down-side of the long 'tail' of the plasma decay curve is that ML residues remain in the body for relatively long periods and statutory withdrawal periods (during which milk and meat may not be used for human consumption) are correspondingly long. Eprinomectin has been developed for use in dairy cattle as it is not excreted with milk.

In general, MLs are safe if used according to label recommendations. Some individual dogs, however, lack an efflux transporter protein to remove ML from the CNS allowing dangerous, sometimes fatal, concentrations to accumulate. This occurs mainly in rough coated collies but occasionally also in other breeds. The very low ML doses used for heartworm prophylaxis are fortunately too small to produce this effect. Some MLs (e.g. selamectin) have been selected for use in dogs as they are relatively safe in this respect.

MLs are excreted in faeces. Concentrations can be sufficient to disrupt the development of beetles and other beneficial insects that populate and help to disperse dung-pats. The ecological impact of this is often overstated but may be of significance in delicate ecosystems.

7.3.3 Benzimidazoles

The most widely used compounds in this large group are albendazole, fenbendazole and oxfendazole. Febantel and netobimin are examples of pro-benzimidazoles that are metabolised to active benzimidazoles (BZDs) by the liver. The BZDs have low water solubility and are therefore almost entirely restricted to oral administration.

Activity

BZDs exert their anthelmintic effect by binding to tubulin. This is the 'building brick' for constructing microtubules, which in turn support the internal structure of the cell. Microtubules are in a dynamic state and are constantly being reassembled. When a BZD-tubulin molecule becomes incorporated, it 'caps' the end of the microtubule and inhibits further polymerisation (see Figure 7.45). This leads to cellular disruption which particularly affects intestinal cells. Consequently, glucose uptake is reduced and glycogen stores become depleted. This condemns the nematode to a slow death.

Help box 7.7

Mode of action of the benzimidazoles

BZD binds to tubulin
- prevents self-association of tubulin molecules
- 'capping' of end of microtubule
- further polymerisation of microtubule inhibited
- disruption of microtubular structure of intestinal cells
- glucose uptake reduced
- glycogen depletion
- **slow death of parasite**

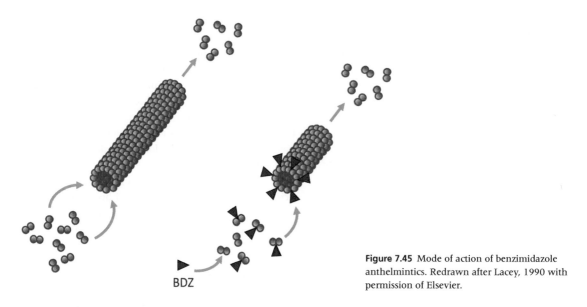

BDZ

Figure 7.45 Mode of action of benzimidazole anthelmintics. Redrawn after Lacey, 1990 with permission of Elsevier.

The BZDs have a broad spectrum of activity against adult and developing nematodes (see Table 7.6), but efficacy against hypobiotic forms at normal dose-rates varies from compound to compound. Some BZDs have limited but useful activity against tapeworms. Albendazole is also active against adult liver fluke. Albendazole and fenbendazole are effective against the protozoan parasite *Giardia*.

Triclabendazole is unique amongst the BZDs as it has no activity against nematodes but is highly effective against *Fasciola* (Section 5.7.1).

Pharmacokinetics

As BZDs kill worms slowly, potency is not determined by the peak plasma concentration (as was the case with levamisole and the MLs) but by the duration of exposure of the parasite to the compound (i.e. the area under the plasma concentration-time curve in Figure 7.46). This has several practical consequences:

a – Less soluble BZDs (such as Compound B in Figure 7.46) have greater potency than more soluble compounds.

b – Multiple low doses often give better results than a single large dose.

Table 7.6 General spectrum of activity of benzimidazoles (excluding triclabendazole)

Nematodes		Other parasites	More information in Section:
Adult worms	▼▼▼	Trematodes*	5.7.1
Mucosal larvae	▼▼▼	Cestodes*	5.5
Hypobiotic larvae	▼	Arthropods 0	
		Protozoa**	9.2.1

* Some have limited activity; ** some active against *Giardia*.
Note: activity may vary according to host, parasite species, compound and formulation.

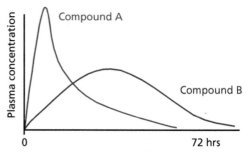

Figure 7.46 Benzimidazole plasma concentrations following a single oral administration with a more soluble BZD (Compound A) and a less soluble BZD (Compound B).

c – BZDs are more potent in ruminants and horses than they are in pigs or dogs. This is because the latter lack a rumen or enlarged caecum to act as a reservoir. Consequently, much of the dose passes through the gastrointestinal tract without dissolving and is excreted in the faeces. In dogs, potency is enhanced if the BZD is given with food as this extends the transit time through the alimentary tract.

The BDZs are generally safe to use at recommended dose-rates but some members of the group are teratogenic and should not be used in early pregnancy.

7.3.4 Newer chemical groups

Amino-acetonitrile derivatives

The amino-acetonitrile derivatives (AADs) act as nicotinic agonists, binding to a subfamily of nAChR-receptors unique to the nematodes. This novel mode of action makes them valuable for worm control as they can be used to control nematode strains resistant to the longer-established anthelmintic groups. They are particularly useful for quarantine treatments when new animals are introduced onto a farm. It is important that the AADs are used responsibly so that the onset of resistance to this new chemical class can be delayed as long as possible.

At the time of writing, the only commercially available AAD is a monepantel preparation for use in sheep. It is active against adult and immature stages, including hypobiotic larvae of a wide range of gastrointestinal nematodes.

Spiroindoles

Derquantel is a very recently introduced anthelmintic. It blocks neuromuscular transmission causing flaccid paralysis of the worms and is active against populations resistant to the major anthelmintic classes. To preserve this valuable property, it is currently presented as a multiple active product with an ML (abamectin) for use in sheep. It is active against a wide range of gastrointestinal nematodes, including hypobiotic larvae, and the sheep lungworm, *Dictyocaulus filaria*.

Practical tip box 7.2

Combination and multiple active parasiticides

Commercial parasiticidal products sometimes contain a mixture of active ingredients. These should be used only if there is a valid reason to do so. Otherwise, the patient is being unnecessarily exposed to pharmacologically active substances that might enhance the risk of side-effects, meat or milk residues, or the development of resistant strains of nontarget parasites.

The additional ingredient could be a synergist (e.g. the use of piperonyl butoxide to enhance the insecticidal properties of synthetic pyrethroids – see Section 3.5.2). More often, it is included to broaden the spectrum of activity. Sometimes the intention is to decrease the risk of resistance developing to the principle ingredient. It is important in veterinary practice to be able to distinguish these functions:

- Combination product: ingredients complement each other's spectrum of activity. Examples include the 'fluke and worm' products such as those containing triclabendazole and levamisole. Note that there are only a few occasions during the year when both treatments might be needed simultaneously (Section 8.2.1).
- Multiple active product: the purpose of the second ingredient in this case is to kill or render infertile any individuals in the target population that might otherwise have survived the primary treatment, thereby reducing selection pressure for resistance (e.g. derquantel with abamectin for worm control in sheep; fipronil with lufenuron for flea control).

Depsipeptides

The depsipeptides are a recently discovered group of semi-synthetic compounds. They are based on fermentation products produced by a fungus originally recovered from the leaves of a flowering *Camellia* species. They have a complex molecular ring structure and a novel mode of action affecting the nervous system. A cascade of presynaptic events culminates in the release of inhibitory neuropeptides producing flaccid paralysis and death of the nematode.

Emodepside is the only representative of the group commercially available at the time of writing. It is used as a 'spot-on' formulation to treat ascarid and hookworm infections in cats.

CHAPTER 8

Clinical parasitology: farm animals

8.1 Introduction

So far, this book has considered Veterinary Parasitology as a scientific discipline, albeit from a clinically-orientated viewpoint. Chapter 1 explored the nature of parasitism while Chapters 2–7 examined interactions between different types of parasite, their hosts and the environment. An understanding of these fundamental processes enables clinical judgements concerning parasitic disease to be made on a sound rational basis.

In practice, the veterinarian or animal health expert is usually concerned with an animal, flock or herd exhibiting, or at risk from, some alimentary, pulmonary, dermatological or other dysfunction which may, or may not, have a parasitological origin. The concluding chapters of this book therefore adopt a different perspective with emphasis placed on the diseased animal. The major parasites affecting each organ system are considered in a general context embracing clinical impact, diagnosis and strategies for treatment and control. To avoid unnecessary repetition, cross-references are made (e.g. 'see Section 1.1.1') to pertinent information in earlier chapters.

8.2 Ruminants

Parasite control is an integral component of livestock husbandry. This is especially true for herbivores. The higher the stocking density, the more opportunity there is for parasite transmission since greater numbers of host-seeking parasite life-cycle stages can accumulate per unit area. Traditional and organic farming systems show that much can be achieved by careful management, but intensive production often requires judicious use of pharmaceutical or other interventions. The experience of recent decades, however, has taught us that overdependence on chemotherapy is unsustainable because of resistance problems and concern over chemical residues in food products and the environment.

Principles of Veterinary Parasitology, First Edition. By Dennis Jacobs, Mark Fox, Lynda Gibbons and Carlos Hermosilla.
© 2016 John Wiley & Sons, Ltd. Published 2016 by John Wiley & Sons, Ltd.
Companion website: www.wiley.com/go/jacobs/principles-veterinary-parasitology

Table 8.1 Parasitic genera most likely to be encountered in the gastrointestinal tract and liver of cattle and sheep

	Cestodes	Trematodes	Nematodes	Protozoa
Host: CATTLE and SHEEP				
Rumen		*Paramphistomum* 5.6.3		
Abomasum		*Paramphistomum* (migrating) 5.6.3	*Ostertagia* [C] 6.3.2 *Teladorsagia* [S] 6.3.2 *Haemonchus* 6.3.2 *Trichostrongylus* 6.3.2	*Cryptosporidium* 4.9.1
Small intestine	*Moniezia* 5.3.5	*Paramphistomum* (migrating) 5.6.3	*Trichostrongylus* 6.3.2 *Cooperia* 6.3.2 *Nematodirus* 6.3.2 *Bunostomum* 6.3.4 *Toxocara* [C] 7.1.3 *Strongyloides* 7.1.2	*Cryptosporidium* 4.9.1 *Eimeria* 4.6.2 *Giardia* 4.5.2
Caecum/ large intestine			*Trichuris* 7.1.6 *Oesophagostomum* 6.3.3 *Chabertia* 6.3.3	*Eimeria* 4.6.2 *Buxtonella*[C] 4.3
Liver	*Echinococcus* (cyst) 5.3.4 *Taenia* (migrating cyst)[1] 5.3.3	*Fasciola* 5.6.2 *Dicrocoelium* 5.6.3		

Note: these lists are not comprehensive; other parasites do occur but less frequently or are of more restricted distribution or importance; numbers in red cross-reference to section of book with more detailed information. C – cattle; S – sheep; [1] – *T. hydatigena*.

8.2.1 Digestive system

The ruminant digestive system harbours a great variety of parasites (see Table 8.1). Protozoan diseases are particularly problematic in neonates and very young animals, as is the nematode *Toxocara vitulorum*. Other gastrointestinal nematodes, mostly trichostrongyloids, commonly cause diarrhoea and production losses in young grazing stock. The pathogenicity of different species varies markedly but their additive effect determines clinical outcome. Trematodes such as *Paramphistomum* and *Fasciola* can cause severe disease in wet climates, while heavy *Dicrocoelium* infections can be debilitating in drier habitats. Adult *Moniezia* in the small intestine (and related tapeworms in the bile ducts in some tropical countries) are usually relatively harmless, as are hydatid cysts in the liver.

Cattle

Ostertagia is the nematode most often associated with digestive problems in cattle. Other genera such as *Trichostrongylus*, *Cooperia* and *Nematodirus* may also contribute, while *Oesophagostomum* can be a primary pathogen in warmer climates. The blood-suckers *Haemonchus placei* and, less often, *Bunostomum* cause anaemia if present

in large numbers and can be responsible for serious disease, particularly in the wet tropics.

Bovine parasitic gastroenteritis

Bovine parasitic gastroenteritis (PGE) caused by *Ostertagia* is most commonly seen in calves during the second half of their first grazing season. Affected animals pass watery faeces, lose condition and become thin. Dehydration is evident in advanced cases. Smaller (subclinical) infections may significantly slow growth-rates without other overt sign of disease. This is associated with a reduced feed intake.

Type I disease (i.e. disease occurring shortly after ingestion of large numbers of infective larvae) is associated with high morbidity but mortality is generally relatively low. Type II disease, caused by the reactivation of arrested larvae in the abomasal wall (see Section 6.3.2), occurs mainly in yearlings in the late winter or early spring. Morbidity is generally low but affected animals, which often show submandibular oedema, are likely to die if untreated.

Clinical signs and grazing history are usually sufficient for a presumptive diagnosis to be made. The number of 'strongyle' eggs per gram of faeces (e.p.g.)

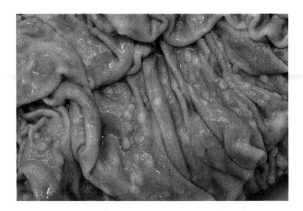

Figure 8.1 Ostertagiosis: nodules on abomasal mucosa. Reproduced with permission of J. McGoldrick.

in Type I PGE will be close to or greater than 1000 in at least some members of the group, but low or zero values are common in Type II disease (as many worms are still immature when clinical signs first appear). Blood biochemistry shows reduced serum albumin and raised pepsinogen concentrations (see Figure 6.22). At autopsy, abomasal contents have an unpleasant smell (because pH values approaching neutrality allow bacteria and moulds to flourish). Closer inspection of the mucosa reveals typical small nodules (see Figure 8.1) and the presence of brownish threadlike worms. These may number 40 000 or more.

Practical tip box 8.1

> **Recognition of abomasal worms**
>
> The three major nematode parasites of the abomasum are, in order of size: *Haemonchus* (2–3 cm); *Ostertagia* in cattle or *Teladorsagia* in sheep (1 cm); and *Trichostrongylus axei* (0.5 cm). The red and white 'Barber's Pole' appearance of *Haemonchus* (see Figure 6.25) is obvious in fresh specimens but the red colour tends to fade with storage.

PGE is most likely to occur on dairy farms as calves are weaned early in life and often grazed on permanent pastures at high stocking rates. In contrast, calves in beef suckler systems are grazed with their mothers. As most of the grass is utilised by the cows, there are relatively few calves per unit area. Cows produce large volumes of faeces with few *Ostertagia* eggs per gram. This has the effect of diluting the high e.p.g. faecal output of the calves and so correspondingly few infective larvae accumulate per kg grass.

Adult cattle are not usually clinically affected by PGE as they will have developed a substantial level of immunity. Nevertheless, abomasal damage can accrue if they graze heavily contaminated pasture and milk-yields may be affected to a small, but economically significant degree. An estimate of the level of herd exposure can be obtained by measuring specific antibody titres in bulk milk samples, but serum pepsinogen concentrations do not provide a reliable indicator as normal values tend to increase with age.

At the time of writing, resistance to anthelmintics has not become a serious problem in cattle nematode populations (although this is no reason for complacency, as will become evident in the ovine PGE section below). Compounds active against adult and immature worms include macrocyclic lactones (MLs – see Section 7.3.2), benzimidazoles (BZDs – see Section 7.3.3) and levamisole (see Section 7.3.1). Ideally calves should be moved to clean pasture after treatment but, if this is not an option, the persistent activity of MLs against incoming L_3 will protect against reinfection for three or more weeks (depending on the compound, formulation and method of administration).

The persistent activity of the MLs can also be utilised to prevent PGE from happening. This approach is based on the knowledge that, in temperate climates, the epidemiology of PGE in set-stocked calves (i.e. those kept on the same pasture all season) follows a stereotyped seasonal pattern (see Figure 6.18). Disease can be avoided in two ways:

a – Metaphylaxis: nature is allowed to take its course but the calves are dosed with an ML shortly before the density of L_3 on the pasture rises to potentially pathogenic levels (see Figure 8.2). The persistent activity of the chosen ML kills ingested larvae before they can cause disease. Some mucosal damage will occur, however, and this may influence growth-rates. On the other hand, the calves are given adequate opportunity to develop an immunity that will protect them in their second grazing season.

b – Prophylaxis: calves are treated with an ML early in the grazing season to ensure that worms derived from the ingestion of overwintered larvae are killed before they start to lay eggs. This is beneficial as, because no new eggs are dropped onto the pasture at this time, the subsequent disease-producing wave of infective larvae (the 'autoinfection peak') fails to

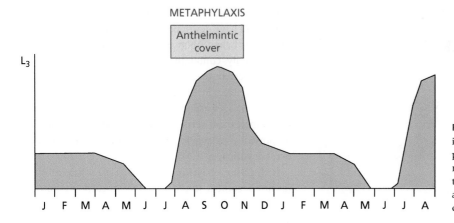

Figure 8.2 Prevention of PGE in calves on a set-stocked pasture by metaphylaxis: the numbers of infective larvae on the grass are shown in green and the period of anthelmintic cover in red.

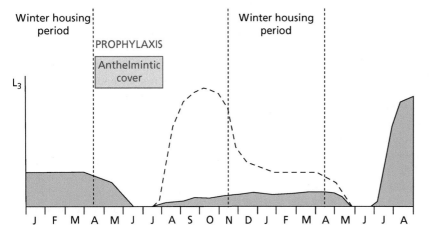

Figure 8.3 Prevention of PGE in calves on a set-stocked pasture by prophylaxis: the numbers of infective larvae on the grass are shown in green and the period of anthelmintic cover in red. The dotted line depicts expected pasture larval counts if the prophylactic treatment had not been given.

develop (see Figure 8.3). The pasture thereby remains 'safe' for the remainder of the year. This system works well if early season treatments are timed correctly and provided no untreated animals are introduced onto the pasture. As with all routine parasite control strategies dependent on a single chemical class, careful management is required to avoid resistance developing in the longer term.

For early season prophylaxis, the first dose of ML is usually given three weeks after spring turnout as this corresponds to the prepatent period (PPP) of *Ostertagia*. One or two further doses will be needed, depending on the period of persistency (PP) of the chosen ML. The dosing interval is calculated by adding together the PPP and PP as this determines the length of time over which no eggs will be dropped onto the pasture. Conservative values are used to

allow for possible biological variation. Thus, one such programme uses three doses of ivermectin administered at 3, 8 and 13 weeks after turnout. To reduce the number of times that calves need to be rounded up for treatment, the first dose of ML can be given at turnout (as, for example, in the doramectin 0, 8 week programme).

To eliminate the need for repeated dosing, intraruminal devices have been developed that continuously or intermittently release an appropriate amount of ML or BZD over a sufficient time-period to ensure prophylactic or metaphylactic protection. Although highly successful, most are no longer sold, partly because of the high cost of manufacture and partly because of a concern that, in some circumstances, recipient calves may not receive adequate antigenic stimulation to ensure immunity by the end of their first grazing season.

With ingenuity, other strategies can be devised for preventing PGE. For example, it is known that overwintered larvae die in the early part of the grazing season (see Figure 6.18). Pastures are therefore safe to use ('clean') after hay or silage has been harvested in the spring. Thus, calves that graze initially on contaminated permanent pasture can be treated to remove the worms that have established and then moved onto a harvested field (i.e. onto 'aftermath'). A potential disadvantage, however, of such 'dose-and-move' systems is that any eggs subsequently dropped onto the new pasture will have been derived from worms that survived treatment. This may enhance the prevalence of resistance genes in the parasite population.

Extra information box 8.1

'Clean' and 'safe' grazing

Recommendations for grazing programmes often differentiate between 'clean' and 'safe' pastures:

Clean grazing: pastures that are unlikely to carry infective larvae, e.g.

i) new recently sown grass;

ii) grass previously grazed but where:
  - a spring hay or silage cut has been taken (by which time overwintered L_3 will have died out);
  - pasture that has been grazed exclusively by another host species.

Safe grazing: pastures that have been grazed by the same host species but where contamination is likely to be at a very low level (e.g. if grazed only by immune animals).

Bovine toxocarosis

Somatic larvae of *Toxocara vitulorum* in the tissues of cattle and buffalo are activated towards the end of pregnancy. They migrate to the udder and are passed in colostrum for about a week. Adult worms establish in the small intestine of the calf and start to pass eggs at about three weeks of age. By five months, the worms have all been expelled. In the meantime, heavy infections cause enteritis, loss of condition and sometimes intestinal obstruction. Fatalities can occur, especially in buffalo. Losses can be avoided by treating vulnerable calves at 10–16 days of age using an anthelmintic with high efficacy against adult and immature stages.

Bovine fasciolosis

Cattle rarely suffer from acute fasciolosis but the chronic form of the disease does occur. Clinical signs are confined

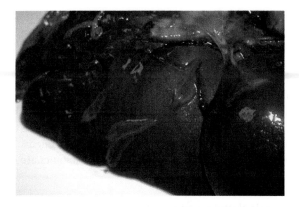

Figure 8.4 Adult *Fasciola hepatica* (released from bile duct). Reproduced with permission of T. de Waal.

mostly to younger grazing stock as a partial immunity follows initial infection. Affected animals show weight-loss accompanied by anaemia and sometimes submandibular oedema. Subclinical infection is responsible for reduced weight gains in growing animals or depressed milk production in dairy cows. The susceptibility of cattle to certain other diseases (e.g. salmonellosis) is increased and the sensitivity of the tuberculin test (an intradermal test to detect cattle infected with bovine tuberculosis) reduced. This is probably the result of powerful immunomodulatory factors released by *Fasciola* as part of its defence against host immune attack (see Section 5.6.1).

As bovine disease is associated with the presence of adult flukes (see Figure 8.4), faecal examination for parasite eggs is a useful diagnostic aid. Further evidence of infection is provided by elevated plasma enzyme concentrations indicating liver or bile duct damage, e.g. glutamate dehydrogenase and gamma-glutamyl transpeptidase. Specific antibodies can be assayed in serum or bulk milk samples. Almost all commercially available flukicidal drugs are active against the adult worm, although strict regulation controls their use in animals for milk production.

A recombinant vaccine is being developed for use in cattle but is not commercially available at the time of writing. It exerts its effect by stimulating a range of immune responses not normally occurring in chronically infected animals (including Th1-type responses).

Bovine paramphistomosis

Although paramphistomes are cosmopolitan, disease is associated mostly with warmer, wetter regions, especially those prone to flooding, as these are the conditions most favourable for the aquatic intermediate hosts. Large numbers of migrating immature flukes in the duodenum provoke persistent afebrile foetid diarrhoea. This leads to depression, dehydration, weakness and often death. Grazing history and local knowledge are important factors in reaching a presumptive diagnosis. Faecal egg-counts are not dependable since the causal organisms are immature. Small plump flukes may, however, sometimes be seen in faeces. Treatments have to be selected with care as few anthelmintics are effective against this trematode.

Intestinal protozoan infections

Intestinal protozoa are mainly problematic in young stock. Asymptomatic infections are common. Cryptosporidiosis and coccidiosis are the most frequent clinical conditions, although *Giardia* can also provoke diarrhoea on occasion.

Cattle harbour numerous *Eimeria* species. Two, *E. bovis* and *E. zuernii*, are recognised as serious pathogens in young calves. A third species, *E. alabamensis*, sometimes affects older calves at pasture producing a milder diarrhoea and weight loss.

E. bovis and *E. zuernii* sporozoites invade villi along the ileum. They enter endothelial cells lining the lacteals and develop into giant macroschizonts. The consequent tissue damage provokes blood-stained diarrhoea, which often contains strands of sloughed mucosa. The disease occurs mostly in calves kept in poor conditions but can strike when young stock are newly introduced into a herd or when they are turned out to grass. A high faecal oocyst count (>5000 o.p.g.) is suggestive of a causal relationship, although diarrhoea can start shortly before patency becomes evident. Speciation of oocysts is necessary to determine the proportion attributable to pathogenic species. Control revolves around management of the immediate environment, e.g. by ensuring that susceptible animals are not overcrowded or exposed to stress, by keeping buildings dry and by changing bedding regularly, etc.

Cryptosporidiosis is one of the commonest infections detected in diarrhoeic calves, especially in those 1–2 weeks of age. It is more likely to occur if calves are colostrum-deprived, or if other potential enteropathogens (such as rotavirus, coronavirus or enterotoxigenic *Escherichia coli* bacteria) are also present on the farm. In faecal smears stained by the Ziehl-Neelsen method, oocysts measuring 4–5 μm appear red against a blue-green background (see Figure 8.5). Few drugs are completely effective against *Cryptosporidium*, so supportive therapy including

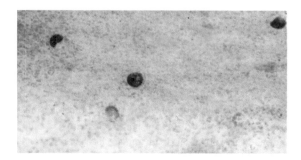

Figure 8.5 *Cryptosporidium* oocysts (red) in faecal smear. Reproduced with permission of F.M. Barakat.

fluids and electrolytes are particularly important. Control requires scrupulous hygiene in calf rearing facilities. Calves should receive adequate amounts of colostrum.

Sheep

Although most gastrointestinal nematodes of sheep and cattle belong to the same genera, each host has its own species and there is limited transmission between them. An exception to this rule is *Nematodirus battus* which, although primarily an ovine species, is nevertheless able to establish in calves. These can, therefore, act as an alternative source of pasture contamination for lambs.

Lambs can be adversely affected by intestinal protozoa. *Eimeria* spp. (which are strictly host specific) can be particularly damaging if infection occurs at the same time as *Nematodirus*.

Ovine PGE

Parasitic gastroenteritis in sheep is more complex than the corresponding condition in cattle. This is because a greater variety of abomasal and intestinal nematodes contribute to the disease process. Mixed infections are the norm, with *Teladorsagia* (the ovine equivalent of *Ostertagia*) and *Trichostrongylus* tending to dominate, although other genera can be primary pathogens. Two gastrointestinal nematodes, *Haemonchus* and *Nematodirus*, are so different from the others that they are discussed below under separate headings.

The epidemiology of the ovine condition is complicated by the occurrence of two separate sources of pasture contamination in the spring: larvae from the previous year that have overwintered on the grass and eggs dropped by the ewes as a result of their periparturient relaxation of immunity (see Figure 6.19). Development rates from egg to L$_3$ on pasture differ for each parasite so that the risk period tends to start earlier for *Teladorsagia* than for *Trichostrongylus*, for example.

PGE is a serious constraint on sheep farming world-wide. It mostly affects weaned lambs grazing in summer and autumn, although Type II disease can occur early in the following year. Older sheep are protected by an acquired immunity, although this is partially compromised during lactation.

Ovine PGE progresses from an initial retardation of growth-rate to more obvious general unthriftiness, often accompanied by soiled hindquarters indicating diarrhoea. In severe cases, weight-loss, depression and death can ensue. Not all members of the flock will be equally affected. Representative faecal sampling will reveal high strongyle egg-counts (>750 e.p.g.) in at least a proportion of the animals. This can be followed up by larval culture if there is a need to know the composition of the worm burden.

Extra information box 8.2

Interpretation of faecal egg-counts

Faecal egg-counts can be difficult to interpret as they do not always reflect the size of the gastrointestinal nematode population. This is because e.p.g. values can be influenced by a number of factors including:
i) Some genera produce many more eggs than others (e.g. *Haemonchus* > *Teladorsagia*).
ii) With some genera (e.g. *Teladorsagia*), egg production per female is inversely related to the size of the population within the host.
iii) Female worms produce fewer eggs once their host has developed acquired immunity.
iv) Inappetence increases the e.p.g. value (by reducing faecal volume); diarrhoea has the opposite effect.
v) Clinical signs may start while worms are still immature (e.g. *Haemonchus* and *Nematodirus*) or may continue after treatment if residual damage is slow to resolve. In either case, faecal egg-counts will be low despite worms being the direct cause of the clinical problem.

Until recently, recommendations to control ovine PGE included:

a – Dosing ewes around lambing time: to eliminate the periparturient egg-rise and thereby prevent ewes from contaminating the pastures.

b – Dosing lambs: with a view to:

i) expelling worms to minimise pathological damage and maximise growth-rates;
ii) minimising egg-deposition and future pasture contamination.

Experience has shown that the routine application of this approach exerts undue selection pressure on nematode populations leading eventually to anthelmintic resistance. This does not become clinically apparent until resistance genes have reached a high prevalence within the parasite population, by which time it is often too late to reverse the trend. Strains resistant to BZDs, levamisole or MLs are becoming ever more frequent worldwide and multiresistant worm populations are also appearing.

It is imperative therefore that sustainable worm control practices should be developed and implemented. Much research and education is currently underway to attain this goal. With so few classes of broad-spectrum anthelmintic available, it is essential that the remaining usefulness of older compounds is retained as long as possible and that the efficacy of newly introduced chemical groups (such as AADs and spiroindoles – see Section 7.3.4) is conserved.

Some countries are evolving protocols to assist veterinary advisers and farmers aspire to this ideal. In the UK, for example, guidelines issued by an organisation entitled 'SCOPS' ('Sustainable Control of Parasites in Sheep') provide detailed advice based on the following broad principles:

a – Work out a control strategy: which should be appropriate for the particular needs of the farm and designed to reduce selection pressure on parasite populations (remembering that some treatments impinge upon more than one type of parasite, e.g. MLs are used for sheep scab control as well as PGE).

b – Use a quarantine procedure: to ensure that resistant strains are not introduced onto the farm. New stock should undergo a rigorous treatment programme and be kept quarantined until they no longer pass parasite eggs.

c – Test for anthelmintic resistance on the farm: if this is not done, it is not known which chemical classes will give reliable control.

d – Administer drugs correctly: this may sound obvious, and maybe patronising, but experience has shown that many resistance problems originate because of simple mistakes, e.g. underdosing because body-weights are estimated inaccurately rather than measured, or because dosing equipment is poorly calibrated.

e – Use anthelmintics only when necessary: avoidable or inappropriate treatments are an unnecessary expense and likely to increase selection pressure on parasite populations. Faecal egg-counts performed on a representative sample of the flock can help to determine when treatment is necessary.

f – Select an appropriate anthelmintic for each task: as products vary with regard to both biological and physical characteristics. The chemical class being used should be changed ('rotated') at appropriate intervals (so parasite populations are not constantly exposed to the same mode of action), but only anthelmintics that are still fully active should be used (see point 'c' above).

g – Preserve susceptible worms on the farm: As it is impossible to eliminate all worms from a farm, it is essential to avoid or modify any control strategy that might exert undue selection pressure on the parasite population. This principle is best illustrated with an example: in the traditional dose-and-move system (as described in the last paragraph of the section on 'Bovine parasitic gastroenteritis' above), treated animals contaminate their new pasture with eggs from surviving worms, thereby encouraging resistance to develop. Two alternative adjustments can be made to counter this tendency. These 'dilute' eggs from dosed animals with those from worms not exposed to treatment, thereby maintaining the diversity of the gene-pool:

i) A proportion of the group (e.g. the strongest lambs) can be left undosed so they drop 'drug-susceptible' eggs onto the new pasture.

ii) The move to the clean pasture can be delayed for a short time after dosing so that all animals in the group acquire a light infestation of 'drug-susceptible' worms from the old pasture.

h – Reduce dependence on anthelmintics: disease risk can be reduced by means of carefully considered management and grazing plans. For example, the safest grassland should be reserved for the most vulnerable animals (e.g. twin-lambs and triplets), while contaminated sheep pastures are reserved for nonsusceptible stock (ewes, cattle etc.). Consideration should also be given to alternative technologies such as those discussed in Section 1.6.6 (e.g. the use of rams for breeding that have been selected for enhanced genetic resistance/resilience to worms).

Extra information box 8.3

Suppressing the periparturient egg-rise

When to dose ewes around parturition presents a particular problem. One dose soon after lambing is insufficient to eliminate the periparturient egg-rise (see Figure 6.19) but a second dose has been shown to apply significant selection pressure on the worm population. This is because ewes do not become reinfected once they regain their full immune status. As a consequence, worms that survived treatment are not 'diluted' with a new intake of susceptible genotypes. Selection pressure for anthelmintic resistance can be reduced by withholding the second treatment or by leaving a proportion of ewes untreated, but either way the ewes remain a potential source of pasture contamination for their lambs.

Haemonchosis

Both L_4 and adult *Haemonchus* suck blood and heavy infections cause a potentially fatal haemorrhagic anaemia. Diarrhoea is not usually a feature. Disease occurs during the wet season in the tropics and is most likely to happen during hot thundery summer periods in temperate regions. Different forms of disease occur depending on the rate of larval intake:

a – hyperacute: lasting 0–7 days. This is most commonly seen in the wet tropics. Apparently healthy sheep die with little or no prior warning. Autopsy reveals signs of severe anaemia and large numbers of immature *Haemonchus* in the abomasum.

b – acute: lasting 1–6 weeks. A loss of condition with pallor, oedema, lethargy and death is associated with haemorrhagic anaemia and hypoalbuminaemia.

c – chronic: lasting 2 months or more. Progressive weight-loss or reduced weight-gain is accompanied by a low level anaemia. This condition can be difficult to differentiate from malnutrition, especially in stock grazing marginal land.

Haemonchus produces many more eggs than most other trichostrongyloids, which complicates the interpretation of faecal egg-counts. For example, e.p.g. values in the upper hundreds are of little consequence if *Haemonchus* is predominant but, in its absence, could indicate a PGE problem. Traditionally, this problem has been overcome by culturing the faeces and identifying third-stage larvae to determine which genera are present, but quicker and more convenient tests are being developed, including a fluorescent staining technique and molecular probes.

Haemonchus populations develop anthelmintic resistance more quickly than do other gastrointestinal nematodes. This is because:

a – in the tropics: *Haemonchus* has a short generation time and a large biotic potential. L_3 develop quickly in the wet season, so several parasitic generations are possible each year. The severity of the disease encourages frequent dosing which applies extra selection pressure. Each surviving female produces up to 10 000 eggs per day, so the prevalence of resistance genes in subsequent generations can escalate quickly.

b – in temperate regions: winter temperatures can be cold enough to kill *Haemonchus* L_3 overwintering on grass, so in spring the entire surviving population is resident in the abomasum. Treatments given to ewes to eliminate the periparturient egg-rise therefore exert much greater selection pressure on *Haemonchus* than they do on other gastrointestinal nematodes, which have overwintering L_3 on the pasture *in refugia* (see Section 1.6.3).

Anthelmintic resistance has either become, or is becoming, a severe problem in many warmer regions. Sheep production has already been abandoned on some farms in South Africa and Australia because of an inability to control multiresistant strains of *Haemonchus*.

Novel and sustainable control methods are being developed for both advanced and low-input farming systems. Selection pressure can be reduced by dosing only the most vulnerable individuals within a flock (see Section 1.6.6). A simple but ingenious and effective method of determining which animals to treat is the FAMACHA© system. This measures the pinkness of the conjunctival mucosa against a calibrated colour chart to indicate the degree of anaemia being experienced by each individual animal (see Figure 8.6).

In addition to the mainstream anthelmintic groups, the flukicidal drug closantel (see Section 5.7.2) is used in some control programmes as it is effective against blood-sucking nematodes. It has residual activity and prevents reinfection with *Haemonchus* for a period of four weeks.

A hidden-antigen vaccine (see Section 1.6.5) is being developed but is not commercially available at the time of writing.

Nematodirosis

Nematodirosis is a seasonal disease, occurring in the spring, which affects lambs around 6–10 weeks of age. Sudden onset profuse diarrhoea follows a mass hatch of L_3 from eggs that have overwintered on the pasture (see Figure 6.29). The mortality rate can be high, especially if there is concurrent coccidial infection.

Diagnosis is based primarily on clinical history as death can occur before eggs start to appear in the faeces (i.e. within two weeks of infection). *Nematodirus* eggs are larger than the usual strongyle ova. Those of the most pathogenic species, *N. battus*, are characteristically brown-coloured with parallel sides (see Figure 6.28).

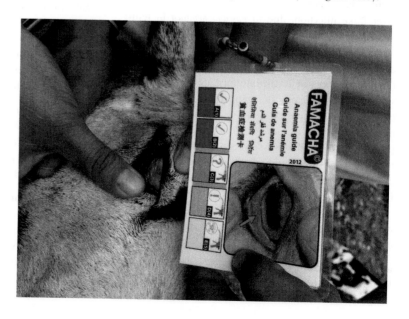

Figure 8.6 The FAMACHA© system in use to identify anaemic sheep needing treatment. Reproduced with permission of J.F.J. Torres Acosta.

As infections are passed from one batch of young lambs via overwintering eggs to the following year's lamb crop, trouble can be avoided by withholding vulnerable lambs from potentially contaminated pastures during the danger period. If this is not possible, treatments with an anthelmintic active against immature *Nematodirus* can be given in anticipation of the onset of disease. The precise timing of such interventions is critical and is aided in some countries by disease forecasts based on local meteorological data.

Practical tip box 8.2

Recognition of small intestinal worms

With care, the composition of small intestinal worm populations from cattle and sheep can be deduced at autopsy by visual inspection. When washed off the small intestinal mucosa, *Nematodirus* worms, if present in large numbers, tangle together resembling cotton-wool. *Trichostrongylus* do not do this and are much smaller (< 1 cm), like short lengths of thread. *Cooperia* is about the same size as *Trichostrongylus* but the ovine species is always comma-shaped or coiled, while males of the bovine species have a bursa so big that it looks like a knot tied at the end of the worm. Iodine staining with partial decolourisation can make the worms stand out better against background debris. Microscopic examination of a few representative specimens is advisable to confirm diagnosis.

Ovine fasciolosis

Liver fluke infection, due to *Fasciola hepatica* in temperate and *F. gigantica* in warmer regions, is a common cause of disease and suboptimum productivity wherever there is a wet climate and poorly drained pastures that are not too acid for the intermediate host, the mud snail, *Galba* (*Lymnaea*). In contrast to the equivalent bovine disease (discussed earlier in this section), ovine immune responses to *Fasciola* do not provide any useful protection against disease, so sheep remain susceptible to fasciolosis throughout their lives. Unlike cattle, they can succumb during the migratory phase of the liver fluke life-cycle.

Ovine fasciolosis exhibits as a spectrum of disease manifestations with no clear demarcation between each:

a – acute fasciolosis: a few animals in the flock are found dead each day with few if any warning signs. In temperate zones, most outbreaks occur in the autumn.

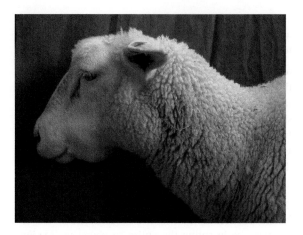

Figure 8.7   Sheep with mandibular oedema ('bottlejaw'). Reproduced with permission of W.E. Pomroy.

b – subacute fasciolosis: rapid weight-loss becomes evident over 1–2 weeks, usually during the autumn or early winter. Affected animals have pale mucous membranes and may die. Fluke infection can predispose to Black Disease caused by *Clostridium novyi* type B.

c – chronic fasciolosis: progressive weight-loss extends over weeks or months becoming obvious during the winter or early the following spring. Lethargy and submandibular oedema are other frequent signs (see Figure 8.7).

d – subclinical effects: fleece weight and wool-fibre quality are affected even by small fluke burdens. Reproductive performance (as measured by number of lambs born and the growth-rate of unweaned lambs) may be adversely influenced (although this is less well documented). Poor carcase quality and liver condemnations reduce value to the meat industry.

The presence of snail habitats on a farm, together with time of year and prevailing weather patterns, will alert the clinician to the possibility of fasciolosis as an explanation for deaths or poor performance. Other indications include:

a – acute fasciolosis: there is seldom opportunity to examine animals prior to death but at autopsy the liver is enlarged, pale, friable and haemorrhagic (see Figure 5.40). Squeezing slices of liver will reveal large numbers of immature flukes in the parenchyma. These are leaf shaped, pale coloured and lack the 'shoulders' typical of adult *Fasciola*.

b – subacute fasciolosis: haematology reveals normochromic anaemia. The liver is enlarged and subcapsular haemorrhages are often present (see Figure 5.41). There will be more than 500 flukes of which about half will be adult.

c – chronic fasciolosis: diagnosis is usually confirmed by demonstrating characteristic eggs in faeces (see Figure 5.38), although egg-output can be erratic. A recently introduced coproantigen test promises to provide greater sensitivity and is able to detect the presence of flukes in bile ducts before they start to produce eggs. The anaemia is initially normochromic but later becomes hypochromic; afflicted animals are also hypoalbuminaemic and hyperglobulinaemic. Liver enzyme concentrations in the blood are raised. At autopsy, the liver is small, cirrhotic and distorted, with gross enlargement of bile ducts (see Figure 5.42). Opening these and the gall bladder will reveal more than 250 adult flukes. Their size (2–5 cm) and 'shoulders' (see Figure 8.4) differentiate them from *Dicrocoelium* which may be also found in bile ducts, although usually in animals grazing drier environments.

Practical tip box 8.3

Diagnosis of liver fluke

Fluke eggs are relatively dense structures that do not float readily in the saturated salt solution often used for routine faecal egg-counts. A flotation fluid with a higher specific gravity (e.g. $ZnSO_4$) is therefore required for diagnostic purposes. Better still are techniques that rely on sedimentation rather than flotation. Even so, infections can be missed as egg-output can be irregular.

The eggs of *Fasciola* and *Dicrocoelium* are easily differentiated as the latter are much smaller and darker in colour (see Figure 8.8).

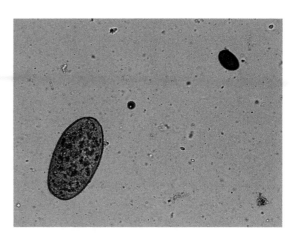

Figure 8.8 Eggs of *Fasciola* (below left) and *Dicrocoelium* (above right).

Few flukicides kill all parasitic developmental stages (see Table 8.2). Not all products, therefore, are suitable for controlling outbreaks of acute disease. The anthelmintic with the broadest spectrum of activity against immature and adult *F. hepatica* is triclabendazole, but resistant strains are beginning to emerge and so alternatives should be used when possible in order to preserve the activity of this clinically valuable product.

The prevention of fasciolosis requires an understanding of the epidemiology of the disease. This is determined by the breeding cycle of the intermediate host and the influence of ambient temperature on the rate of fluke development within both the egg and the snail (see Section 5.6.2). The precise timing of the resulting sequence of events varies with local circumstances and so an example (from Great Britain) is used to illustrate the principles underlying control strategies (see Figure 8.9).

Table 8.2 Relative efficacy of some flukicides in sheep (adapted from Abbott *et al.*, 2012)

	Age of fluke in sheep (weeks)													
	1	2	3	4	5	6	7	8	9	10	11	12	13	14
Albendazole							–	.		+		+++		
Oxyclozanide	–													
Nitroxynil							++			+++				
Closantel														
Triclabendazole	+++			++++										

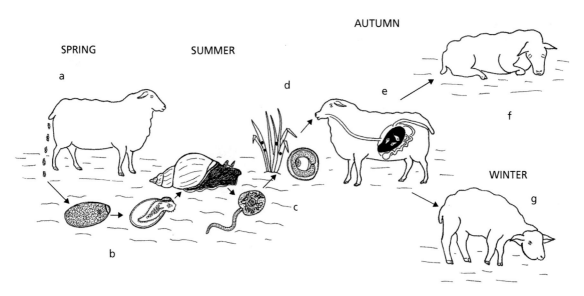

Figure 8.9 Epidemiology of fasciolosis in Great Britain: a – eggs dropped in spring; b – eggs hatch and snails infected in June; c – flukes develop in snail during summer; d – metacercariae on herbage from late-August; e – flukes migrating in sheep; f – acute disease from late-September; g – chronic disease from January. Sheep images f and g redrawn after Taylor, 1964 with permission of FAO; immature stages after J.N. Oldham's drawings in RVC collection.

There are two main control objectives:

a – to prevent fluke eggs dropping onto pasture: Most fluke eggs die during the winter. Treating sheep in the late winter or early spring to remove adult flukes will ensure that no new eggs are dropped onto the pasture during the spring and early summer ('a' in Figure 8.9). As a result, there will be few miracidia hatching to infect the new generation of snails ('b' in Figure 8.9) and this will substantially reduce the numbers of metacercariae appearing on the pasture later in the year ('d' in Figure 8.9).

b – to protect grazing animals during times of high risk: this applies especially to sheep grazing a snail habitat during the autumn of a year when a 'bad' fluke season is forecast ('d' in Figure 8.9). In the knowledge that such animals are likely to ingest considerable numbers of metacercariae, treatment with a compound active against immature flukes can be given during the incubation period, i.e. while the flukes are in the liver but before they have grown large enough to cause substantial damage ('e' in Figure 8.9). A second treatment may be necessary if stock cannot be moved to safer pasture, the dosing interval depending on the persistency of the drug used.

Historically, molluscicides have been employed to control fasciolosis by eliminating snail populations. Although technically successful, they were not commercially viable. This was due partly to environmental concerns and partly because any snails surviving (e.g. if protected from the spray by thick vegetation) could quickly recolonise available habitat.

An ability to recognise and define the extent of snail habitat on an affected farm allows alternative cost-effective control options to be practised, such as fencing, drainage and the removal of vulnerable stock to safer pastures at times of high risk.

Ovine coccidiosis

Sheep harbour many *Eimeria* species, some producing macroschizonts visible as white spots in the intestinal mucosa. One nonpathogenic species induces papillomatous growths. Two species, *E. ovinoidalis* and *E. crandalis*, are commonly responsible for diarrhoea in lambs of about 6 weeks old.

Ewes act as immune carriers passing small numbers of oocysts which accumulate indoors in poorly managed litter or, outdoors, around feed and water troughs. Early lambs amplify the parasite population exposing later lambs to heavier infection pressure. Twins and triplets are particularly vulnerable. Disease is usually associated with high faecal oocyst counts although death can occur within the two week prepatent period. Outbreaks may be coincident with *Nematodirus* or *Cryptosporidium* infections, which can complicate diagnosis and control.

Goats

Goats share many nematode species with sheep, but in extensive husbandry systems they are not necessarily equally exposed to infection. This is because goats are browsers rather than grazers. Heavy worm burdens can cause disease but goats are generally more resilient than sheep. On the other hand, they mount a weaker immune response to gastrointestinal nematodes and continue to void eggs throughout their lives.

Anthelmintic resistance tends to develop more rapidly in goats than in sheep. Consequently, sheep should not be grazed on pastures previously used by goats. To overcome potential resistance problems, zero grazing systems are commonly employed in goat husbandry (i.e. forage cut in the field is brought to animals kept in pens or yards). Otherwise, the general principles described for ovine PGE are applied to goats with a view to keeping the number of anthelmintic treatments to an absolute minimum. Some anthelmintics are metabolised more quickly by goats than sheep and may therefore require a higher dose-rate. Inadvertent underdosing is one of the factors that accelerates the development of anthelmintic resistance in goats.

Goats have their own *Eimeria* species. Of these, two (*E. ninakohlyakimovae* and *E. arloingi*) are common pathogens causing diarrhoea in kids and a check in growth-rate.

8.2.2 Respiratory system

The sheep nasal fly, *Oestrus ovis*, is widely distributed, but is mostly troublesome in some regions with warmer climates such as the Mediterranean region and South Africa. Further down the respiratory tree (see Table 8.3), the cattle lungworm, *Dictyocaulus viviparus*, is responsible for sporadic and potentially lethal disease in some temperate regions, while in small ruminants *D. filaria* and *Protostrongylus* are seen more commonly in warmer, drier terrains. Hydatid cysts (the metacestodes of *Echinococcus granulosus*) and the tiny greenish lesions associated with the sheep metastrongyloid, *Muellerius*, rarely cause inconvenience to their host even though they are commonly present in the lungs.

Table 8.3 Parasitic genera most likely to be encountered in the respiratory tract of cattle and sheep

	Nasal passages	Trachea/ bronchi	Lung
Host: **CATTLE and SHEEP**			
Nematodes		*Dictyocaulus* 6.3.5 *Protostrongylus*[S] 6.3.5	*Echinococcus* (cyst) 5.3.4 *Muellerius*[S] 6.3.5
Insects	*Oestrus*[S] 2.2.6		

Note: these lists are not comprehensive; other parasites do occur but less frequently or are of more restricted distribution or importance; numbers in red cross-reference to section of book with more detailed information. S – sheep only.

Nasal myiasis

When the adult nasal fly, *Oestrus ovis*, is on the wing and attempting to deposit larvae, sheep become restless, either shaking their heads or pressing their nostrils into each others' fleeces or against the ground. This interrupts feeding which can result in poor weight gain if they are constantly troubled. Larvae in the nasal cavities and sinuses provoke the formation of thick mucus that can block the nostrils forcing mouth breathing which interferes still further with food intake. Bone erosion with perforation into the cranial cavity sometimes follows. This induces neurological signs such as a high-stepping gait and incoordination.

Little can be done to protect grazing sheep from the adult flies but after an attack systemic treatment (e.g. with some ML endectocides) can be used to kill the parasitic larvae before they are large enough to produce significant damage.

Bovine parasitic bronchitis

Lungworm disease of cattle is a complex condition. It is sporadic in nature as calves in endemic areas generally acquire immunity quickly enough to protect themselves against rising numbers of L_3 on pasture. This natural epidemiological balance can be easily upset by weather conditions favouring a faster accumulation of L_3 on grassland, or by inappropriate husbandry practices (such as putting susceptible calves onto pastures contaminated by older stock). Disease occurs when the daily intake of infective L_3 reaches a level that overwhelms the developing immunity of the calves.

Table 8.4 Summary of the main disease processes occurring in parasitic bronchitis

Phase of disease	Timing (pi)	Main lesion	Prognosis
Prepatent (migrating larvae)	1–3	Bronchioles blocked; alveolae collapsed	Rapid and complete recovery
Patent (adult worms in trachea and bronchi)	4–8	Aspiration pneumonia	Guarded; slow recovery
Postpatent (worms expelled by treatment or immunity)	8–12	Epithelialisation of alveolar lining	Very poor

pi = weeks postinfection.

Clinical signs, diagnostic procedures, responses to treatment and prognosis all vary according to the stage of parasitic development. The earlier that diagnosis is made and treatment started, the more satisfactory the outcome. The underlying pathogenic processes were described in Section 6.3.5 and are summarised in Table 8.4. The spectrum of disease encompasses:

a – Acute (prepatent) disease: eosinophilic exudates block the bronchioles bringing air to the alveolae, which collapse. If a large volume of lung tissue is affected, breathing becomes rapid and shallow with a frequent bronchial cough. Initially the calves are bright and attempt to graze, but later stand with necks outstretched, breathing heavily through their mouths assisted by exaggerated flank movements. Recumbency and death can follow if treatment is not given. As there is no physical damage to the lung at this stage, response to treatment is rapid and the prognosis favourable.

b – Subacute (patent) disease: an increased respiratory rate is accompanied by a greater depth of breathing and fits of coughing. Foaming at the mouth is indicative of pulmonary oedema (see Figure 8.10). Dyspnoeic calves lose weight and are prone to secondary pulmonary infection. As the dominant pathology at this stage is aspiration pneumonia, and as consolidated lung tissue takes a long time to resolve even after removal of the worms, recovery is slow. Prognosis has to be guarded because of the possibility of postpatent disease occurring subsequently.

c – Postpatent disease: a small proportion of cases may relapse some two months after the initial onset of clinical signs. Anthelmintic therapy at this stage is inappropriate as the lungworm population will already have been expelled by immune responses. As the pathology at this stage is

likely to include an irreversible thickening of alveolar walls (see Figure 6.58), the prognosis is grave.

Animals suffering from parasitic bronchitis should be removed from contaminated pasture. If this is impossible, reinfection can be blocked by use of ML anthelmintics as these provide good persistent activity against *D. viviparus* larvae.

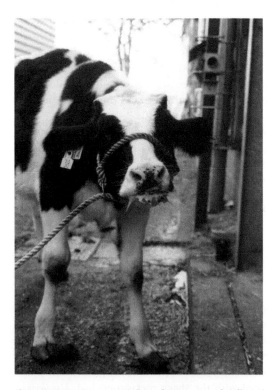

Figure 8.10 Bovine parasitic bronchitis: a severely affected calf: note the outstretched neck and foam around the mouth. Reproduced with permission of D. Brown.

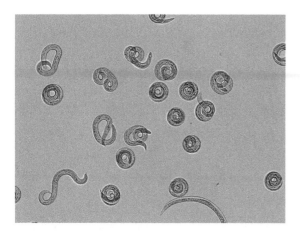

Figure 8.11 Typical appearance of *Dictyocaulus viviparus* larvae harvested from faeces (the sheath just visible on some larvae indicates that larval development has commenced).

Immune animals exposed to a high level of pasture contamination may cough and their respiratory rate may be raised slightly (mild tachypnoea), but these signs are usually transitory and of little consequence, although there can be a sudden and expensive drop in milk yield in dairy cows.

Diagnosis is largely dependent upon a consideration of clinical signs, seasonal incidence and grazing history. During the patent phase of the disease, confirmation is provided by recovering L_1 from faeces using the Baermann apparatus (see Section 1.5.1). The L_1 (see Figure 8.11) does not have the 'S'-shaped tail typical of other lungworms but can be recognised microscopically by the greenish refractile granules present in its intestinal cells.

Immunoassays and the presence of an eosinophilia can provide further evidence of infection in adult cows but these have to be interpreted with caution. Currently, eprinomectin is the only ML licensed for use in cows producing milk for human consumption.

Control strategies are designed to ensure that calves do not graze contaminated pastures before they have developed adequate immunity. Such measures have to be integrated with PGE prevention as *Ostertagia* is a concurrent consideration in herd health schemes. Early season prophylactic schemes for PGE (described earlier in this section) are generally effective against lungworm but can break down as relatively few *D. viviparus* larvae need to be ingested by susceptible calves to cause disease. Also, the speed of development from L_1 to L_3 is much

faster for *D. viviparus* than for most gastrointestinal trichostrongyloids, so pathogenic numbers can accumulate very quickly. Furthermore, by suppressing early-season infection, the onset of protective immunity may be delayed leaving calves more vulnerable later in the year.

It is more satisfactory, therefore, to employ a method that ensures adequate immunity early in the season and this can be achieved by vaccination. Currently, the only commercially available vaccine utilises attenuated larvae (see Section 1.6.5). This provides effective protection against overt disease but vaccinated calves, in common with all immune cattle, may still cough if exposed to infection and can even harbour small numbers of adult worms. They can therefore act as carriers and for this reason should never be grazed on pastures used by susceptible unvaccinated stock. Immunity can wane if not naturally boosted by grazing contaminated grassland.

Sheep lungworm infection

Dictyocaulus filaria like *D. viviparus*, has a direct life-cycle. It is a sporadic cause of bronchitis. Coughing and loss of condition can occur in sheep and goats of any age but is seen most commonly in the 4–6 month age-group. Infection with *Protostrongylus* arises when the snail intermediate host is accidentally eaten, so heavy infections are infrequent.

Lungworm infections in small ruminants can be differentiated by the appearance of the larvae recovered from faeces. *D. filaria* L_1 are similar to those of *D. viviparus* from cattle, except that there is a small protrusion at the head end (the 'protoplasmic knob'). This is lacking on the L_1 of other ovine lungworm genera, which all have a typical 'S'-shaped tail. The tail of the non-pathogenic *Muellerius* has an additional small spine (see Figure 8.12) not seen in *Protostrongylus*.

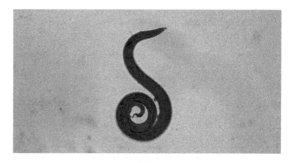

Figure 8.12 *Muellerius*: first stage larva. Reproduced with permission of J.A. Figueroa-Castillo.

8.2.3 Cardiovascular system

Blood-borne protozoan infections of major significance include: *Babesia* in erythrocytes, *Theileria* which also infects leukocytes, and *Trypanosoma* that swims freely in blood plasma (see Table 8.5). Schistosomes inhabiting blood vessels cause animal welfare problems throughout the wet tropics.

Babesiosis

Babesiosis is an acute disease that strikes either:

a – after a nonimmune animal has been bitten by an infected tick; or

b – if a chronically infected animal becomes stressed.

After an incubation period of up to two weeks, animals develop fever followed by inappetence, depression and weakness. Signs of anaemia and jaundice become increasingly apparent. The heartbeat may be audible and the respiratory rate increased. The urine turns reddish-brown (haemoglobinuria) and there may be diarrhoea. In *B. divergens* infections, spasm of the anal sphincter results in the production of 'pipe stem faeces'. Severely affected animals lose weight rapidly and may become comatose and die. Pregnant cattle may abort. Infection with *B. bovis* may be further complicated by neurological signs such as aggression or convulsions. In animals surviving the acute haemolytic crisis, the disease lasts about three weeks followed by a slow recovery. Milder forms of the disease may occur in younger or partly immune stock.

For diagnosis, parasitized cells are most easily found in capillary blood (obtained by pricking the skin of the inner side of the tail or ear). Thick smears on glass slides are examined microscopically after staining with Giemsa (see Figure 8.13). The degree of parasitaemia correlates

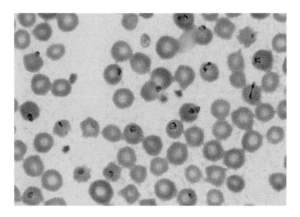

Figure 8.13 *Babesia divergens* (a 'small' *Babesia* species) within RBCs in a blood smear.

only poorly with the level of anaemia as measured by haematology. Parasites can be difficult to find after the haemolytic crisis, but this problem can be resolved by application of DNA or serological tests.

In view of the rapid rate of haemolysis in the acute phase of the disease, treatment must be started as quickly as possible. Treatment options are limited and in some countries restricted to just one compound: imidocarb. This can be used therapeutically and, at a higher dose, prophylactically to protect animals at high risk. There are, however, strict regulations governing its use in meat- or milk-producing animals as it has a very protracted half-life in the body.

The incidence of disease is generally low where a high transmission rate maintains herd immunity (see Section 4.8.1). Set against this background, there are a number of predisposing factors that can trigger disease:

i) introducing susceptible (nonimmune) animals onto a pasture with infected ticks;
ii) introducing infected ticks onto a previously clean pasture (e.g. attached to newly acquired stock);
iii) introducing infected cattle onto a pasture with clean ticks;
iv) a decrease in tick population leading to a reduced transmission rate (e.g. as a result of drought conditions, pasture improvement schemes or tick control measures);
v) stress (e.g. calving or transportation).

The incidence of babesiosis can be minimised by avoiding or appropriately managing these potentially hazardous situations.

Table 8.5 Parasitic genera most likely to be encountered in the cardiovascular system or blood of cattle and sheep

	Host: CATTLE and SHEEP
Protozoa	*Babesia* 4.8.1
	Trypanosoma 4.5.1
	Theileria 4.8.2
Trematodes	*Schistosoma* 5.6.3

Note: these lists are not comprehensive; other parasites do occur but less frequently or are of more restricted distribution or importance; numbers in red cross-refer to sections with more detailed information.

Attenuated vaccines have been used successfully in some regions where babesiosis is a severe constraint on cattle production, including parts of Australia, South America and Africa. As the attenuated organisms are intra-erythrocytic, vaccination programmes have to be managed carefully to reduce the risk of blood-group sensitisation problems (e.g. haemolytic disease in calves born to vaccinated dams). Vaccines utilising recombinant antigens are under development.

Trypanosomosis

Livestock production is severely impacted by several species of tsetse-transmitted *Trypanosoma* species in sub-Saharan Africa and by *T. evansi* in parts of Africa, Asia and Latin America. The latter is spread mechanically by blood-feeding flies and vampire bats.

The pathogenicity of trypanosomosis varies with parasite species and between host breeds. The disease may pass through an acute stage but often becomes chronic. The clinical presentation is inconsistent and is without any unambiguously characteristic (pathognomonic) signs, although most cases develop an intermittent fever and anorexia. Afflicted animals are dull and rough-coated with enlarged lymph-nodes and pale mucous membranes. They become emaciated and may die after a period of weeks or months.

Motile trypanosomes can be demonstrated in fresh blood films (see Figure 8.14), but numbers vary due to the remission cycle (see Figure 4.12). Increased sensitivity can be obtained by centrifuging blood in a haematocrit tube and examining the plasma/ buffy coat interface. Thick and thin blood smears can be prepared in the field for later processing in the laboratory. Trypanosome

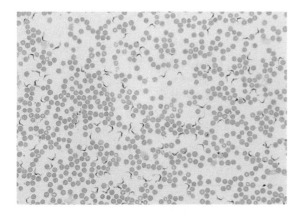

Figure 8.14 Trypanosomes in a blood smear.

species can be differentiated by subtle morphological differences. Some species are 'pleomorphic', meaning there may be more than one morphological form in a single blood sample. Mixed infections (i.e. with more than one species) are common in Africa.

Not all trypanosome species or strains are dangerous. In the British Isles, for example, nonpathogenic trypanosomes are transmitted between cattle by tabanid flies and between sheep by keds. Finding trypanosomes in a blood sample, therefore, does not necessarily pinpoint the cause of a health problem.

The range of drugs available for the treatment and prophylaxis of *Trypanosoma* infections is limited and their cost restrictive for poorer communities. Most have been in use for many years and resistance problems are emerging. In Africa, the main control strategy is regulation of the tsetse fly population with baited traps. Local trypanotolerant cattle thrive better than more vulnerable imported breeds. Vaccine development is hindered by the ability of the parasite to change its surface antigens at regular intervals.

Theileriosis

There are different forms of theileriosis in the Mediterranean region, Asia and Africa. The disease in Africa is known as East Coast Fever. Clinical cases are infrequent while herd immunity levels are high but any disturbance in epidemiological stability can lead to an outbreak. Morbidity is greatest in nonnative breeds. Signs include enlarged local lymph nodes (especially the parotid as the tick vector feeds in the ear), followed by pyrexia and loss of condition. This can progress to anorexia, emaciation, recumbency and death within three weeks.

Biopsy smears from enlarged lymph nodes, stained with Giemsa, will reveal parasites within the cytoplasm of lymphoid cells. Parasitised erythrocytes appear in peripheral blood during the later stages of infection. Treatment is difficult and prognosis poor. An integrated approach to control is advised which places emphasis on the management of risk factors rather than attempting to eradicate the tick vector. Attempts have been made to induce immunity by infecting animals with a low virulence strain and terminating subsequent parasitic development by chemotherapy.

Schistosomosis

Schistosomosis is widespread in tropical regions where animals have access to water courses that provide a habitat for aquatic snail intermediate hosts. As treatment is often uneconomic, control is focussed on reducing the number of snails or restricting grazing to safer pastures.

Clinical signs are mostly attributable to the entrapment of schistosome eggs within capillary beds in the intestine, liver, urinary bladder or nasal passages (depending upon the *Schistosoma* species). A massive invasion of cercariae may provoke acute disease but schistosomosis is primarily a chronic condition with diarrhoea, anorexia, emaciation and anaemia as the main signs.

As these signs are nonpathognomonic, diagnosis is based on grazing history and demonstration of characteristic eggs (see Figure 5.49) in faeces or other appropriate excretion. Autopsy will reveal adult worms within blood vessels, e.g. the mesenteric veins in the case of *S. bovis* (see Figure 8.15).

8.2.4 Integument

The skin is prone to attack by many different types of arthropod (see Table 8.6). Some visit temporarily to feed (e.g. nuisance and biting flies, ticks etc.), or fleetingly, like the myiasis flies, to lay their eggs. Control may be necessary to ameliorate the irritation and annoy-

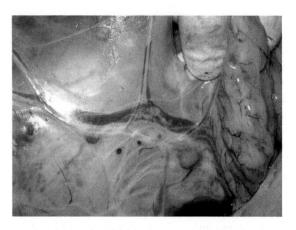

Figure 8.15 Several schistosome pairs in a mesenteric blood vessel. Reproduced with permission of J. Vercruysse.

ance they all provoke, or to prevent more serious welfare issues such as blowfly strike, screwworm infestation, tick-paralysis or the transmission of a multitude of vector-borne diseases. Other parasites have a more intimate relationship with their host and are often associated with dermatological problems. Lice, mites, keds and warbles come into this category. Each ectoparasite

Table 8.6 Parasitic genera most likely to be encountered on, in or under the skin of cattle and sheep

	Host	
	CATTLE	**SHEEP**
Ticks / nuisance and biting flies	Many	Many
Myiasis flies	*Hypoderma* 2.2.6	*Lucilia* etc. 2.2.6
	Lucilia etc. 2.2.6	Screwworms etc. 2.2.6
	Screwworms etc. 2.2.6	
Lice	*Bovicola*[1] 2.2.3	*Bovicola*[1] 2.2.3
	Linognathus 2.2.3	*Linognathus* 2.2.3
	Haematopinus etc. 2.2.3	
Keds		*Melophagus* 2.2.5
Surface mites	*Chorioptes* 3.3.3	*Psoroptes* 3.3.3
		Chorioptes 3.3.3
		Psorergates 3.3.3
Subsurface mites	*Sarcoptes* 3.3.2	*Sarcoptes* 3.3.2
	Demodex 3.3.2	*Demodex* 3.3.2
Protozoa	*Besnoitia* 4.7.2	
Helminths	*Parafilaria* 7.1.5	
	Stephanofilaria 7.1.5	

Note: these lists are not comprehensive; other parasites do occur but less frequently or are of more restricted distribution or importance; numbers in red cross-reference to section with more detailed information.
[1] Also called *Damalinia*.

has its own biological and ecological characteristics and there is no magic spray that will stop them all. Examples will be used to illustrate some common approaches to controlling these difficult infestations.

Not all integumentary parasites are arthropods. A protozoan infection, besnoitiosis, is an emerging disease spreading across southern Europe. The filarial worms *Parafilaria* and *Stephanofilaria*, are both spread by muscid flies. The former causes small bleeding lesions on the flanks of its host in the summer, while the latter produces nodules and ulcers on the udder and underside of the body.

Cattle tick control

Cattle production would be severely curtailed in many tropical and subtropical areas if ticks could not be controlled. The task is, however, becoming more difficult as tick populations increasingly develop resistance to acaricides. While some infestations may be amenable to systemic MLs or acaricide-impregnated ear-tags and tail-bands, control is mostly dependent on dipping or spraying which may be practised on a large or small scale depending on circumstances (see Figure 8.16 and Figure 8.17).

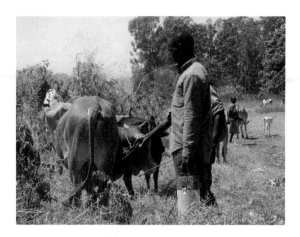

Figure 8.17 Tick control: cattle being sprayed with acaricide. Reproduced with permission of V. Lorusso.

Careful management of these procedures is essential when acaricidal wash draining off animals, after passing through a dip-tank or spray-race, is recycled. The concentration must be kept within strict limits. If too high, there is a danger of toxicity and if too low, underdosing will give unsatisfactory results and will encourage acaricide-resistance. Some compounds bind to skin or hair and so their concentration in recycled wash becomes progressively weaker (known as 'stripping'). In such cases, concentrated acaricide is added at intervals to restore the balance ('replenishment'). Thorough mixing is needed to ensure an even distribution of the acaricide through the wash. Strict precautions should be taken to ensure that people involved in these operations are not exposed to acaricide by skin contact, ingestion or by aerosol.

The treatment interval is determined by the residual activity of the acaricide on the skin, hair or wool (usually a few days on cattle, longer on sheep), the tick pressure (i.e. the number of host-seeking ticks in the environment) and the time spent on the host (which varies from 5 days for some three-host ticks to 21 days for one-host species). To discourage acaricide-resistance, the number of treatments should be kept to the minimum required to attain defined control objectives (see 'Integrated Parasite Management' in Section 1.6.4). Use should be made, wherever practicable, of management strategies that eliminate or substantially reduce the numbers of off-host life-cycle stages, such as:

a – pasture improvement: to make the microhabitat less favourable for tick survival;

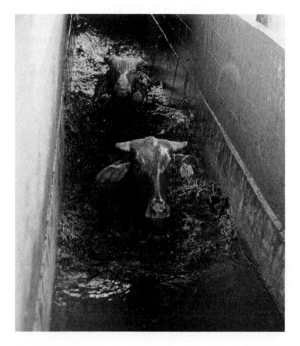

Figure 8.16 Tick control: cattle passing through an acaricidal plunge dip. Reproduced with permission of the Queensland Department of Agriculture, Fisheries and Forestry.

b – periodic burning of pastures: to destroy the off-host ticks;

c – removal of stock from pasture: for an adequate period to starve the off-host ticks: this is known as 'spelling' and only works in the case of species with a very narrow host range, e.g. *Boophilus microplus* which feeds solely on cattle.

Stock hybridisation programmes are used in some regions to reduce dependence on chemical control. These exploit the natural resistance of zebu-type cattle to tick infestation. In Queensland, for example, European cross-bred cattle with three- to five-eighths of their genetic material originating from *Bos indicus* can provide an acceptable compromise between productivity and tick resistance (see Figure 8.18).

A hidden antigen vaccine (see Section 1.6.5) has been developed for use against *Boophilus*. It does not protect the vaccinated animal *per se* from biting ticks but greatly reduces the reproductive potential of the ticks that attach and feed on the vaccinated animal. In this way, vaccination reduces future numbers of host-seeking larvae on the paddock, thereby decreasing the number of acaricidal treatments needed during the year.

Mange and sheep scab

Although sarcoptic and psoroptic mange do occur in cattle and can produce extensive lesions, the commonest bovine infestation is caused by *Chorioptes*. It is found on the lower leg and is usually asymptomatic. Clinical signs are mostly seen in housed dairy cattle during the winter. Heavy infections spread up to the udder and tail-base, causing papules, crusty lesions and hair-loss.

In sheep, psoroptic mange ('sheep scab') is the main problem and is economically important in Europe, Asia and South America. The condition is intensely pruritic making sheep rub, scratch and nibble. This exacerbates the damage caused by the parasites and wool can be lost from large areas of the body. Distress can, in some cases, be severe enough to trigger epileptiform fits. The mites are active only at the moist circumference of the expanding lesion, which can become very extensive (see Figure 8.19). The recovering skin in the centre of the lesion is often covered with a dry, yellowish crust.

Sheep scab is primarily a disease of late autumn and winter when the fleece provides optimal conditions for the mites. Population numbers decline markedly in summer, particularly after shearing. The lesions heal but nevertheless small numbers of mites survive under scabs or in skin folds. Infection can be passed from these apparently healthy animals to in-contact sheep, for example at market. Indirect spread between batches of sheep is also possible as mites can survive off the host for a few days in trucks, handling pens etc. An adult female lays up to 100 eggs during her month-long life-span and the life-cycle is completed in about 10 days, so parasite numbers can build up rapidly when the winter fleece starts to grow.

Diagnosis is confirmed by the presence of mites in scrapings taken from the edge of active lesions. Collected material should be cleared in a drop of potassium hydroxide solution so that the mites can be closely examined. (Caution – KOH is corrosive to living animal and human skin). If the mite is *Psoroptes*, the stalks joining the end of each leg to the sucker will be segmented (see Figure 3.20).

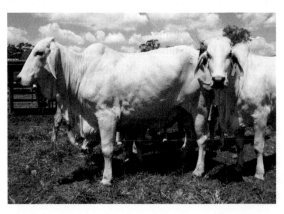

Figure 8.18 Tick resistant hybrid cattle in Queensland, Australia. Reproduced with permission of C. Gardiner.

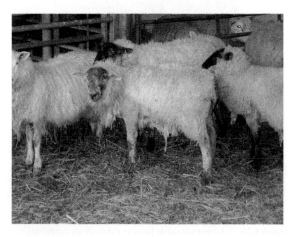

Figure 8.19 Sheep scab infestation. Reproduced with permission of P. Bates.

The choice of acaricide for treatment and prophylaxis is limited by the necessity for all mites on the animal to be killed. Sheep will remain infectious for others if there are any survivors. For the same reason, infected sheep have to be plunged through a dip bath – spraying is not adequate. They have to remain in the acaricidal wash long enough for the fleece to be thoroughly wetted. Alternatively, injectable MLs can be used for systemic treatment, but strict compliance with label instructions is essential to achieve satisfactory results. Only one ML (moxidectin) is currently licensed for prophylactic use.

Calliphorine myiasis

Calliphorine myiasis (blowfly strike) is caused by the greenbottle *Lucilia sericata* in cooler climates and by *L. cuprina* in warmer regions. Strike is a serious animal welfare problem, particularly in sheep. In England and Wales, for example, up to 80% of sheep farms and 2% of the national flock may be affected in an average season.

Female *Lucilia* are most active on warm, still days with high relative humidity. They are attracted by open wounds or the odour of wool soiled with urine or faeces. They lay clusters of yellow-cream eggs which hatch within 24 hours. The larvae lacerate skin and liquefy underlying tissues to produce large wounds. The growing maggots (see Figure 8.20) reach a length of 1 cm within two weeks.

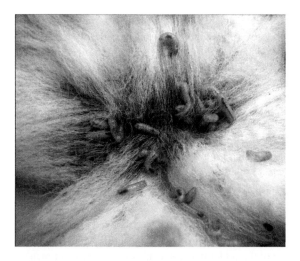

Figure 8.20 Calliphorine myiasis: sheep infested with blowfly maggots. Reproduced with permission of M. Walters and R.L. Wall.

Affected sheep are anorexic, dull and often stand apart from the rest of the flock. The full extent of the damage may not be immediately apparent as the infestation may be hidden by overlying wool. In severe cases, the fleece is discoloured, damp and has a foul smell.

Extra information box 8.4

Epidemiology of blowfly strike in northern temperate regions

The seasonal incidence of strike depends on the activity of the fly (June to September) and the suitability of the microclimate within the fleece of individual animals. Strike tends to occur in two waves in British hill flocks:

First phase (early summer): Adult sheep tend to be affected most because they have a long fleece; lambs are less likely to be struck as their fleece is too short.

Interim phase (mid-summer): Few new strikes occur after shearing.

Second phase (late summer): Lambs become increasingly vulnerable as their wool grows.

Insecticides or insect growth regulators (see Section 3.5.3) with a long period of persistence in the fleece (weeks or months) can be used to protect sheep against blowfly strike. They are applied by dipping, spraying or as a pour-on formulation. Insecticide-resistance is becoming a problem in some *L. cuprina* populations.

Management practices that reduce the risk of blowfly strike include:

a – effective worm control: to minimise diarrhoea and fouling of the fleece;

b – removal of excess wool: from around the tail, hind legs and other areas likely to become soiled with faeces or other excretions;

c – tail docking: welfare investigations have confirmed the traditional belief that shortening the tail of lambs soon after birth reduces the incidence of blowfly strike substantially later in life;

d – carcase disposal: removal of dead stock and wild-life carrion limits blowfly numbers by depriving *L. sericata* of additional breeding sites.

Some breeds of sheep, like the Merino, tend to accumulate malodorous deposits under deep folds of skin. The risk of strike can be substantially reduced by surgical removal of the folds situated at the back of the thighs (Mule's operation). This is done at a time of year when the flies are inactive.

Warble fly

Warble flies are damaging in a number of ways. Adults on the wing cause distress to cattle ('gadding') which can reduce milk-yield. Migrating larvae leave trails marked by greenish exudate ('butcher's jelly') which must be removed during meat processing. Host reaction to the presence of overwintering *H. lineatum* larvae in the oesophageal wall may induce bloat by impairing regurgitation, while that provoked by the death of *H. bovis* larvae (e.g. following the injudicious use of some insecticides) in the spinal canal may result in paraplegia (see Figure 8.21). Finally, and most commonly, warble cysts and breathing holes reduce the value of affected hides for the leather industry (see Figure 8.22).

As there is only one warble fly generation per year, the entire population is within the bovine host throughout the winter and therefore vulnerable to attack with systemic insecticides. These should, however, be applied in the autumn before larvae have reached their winter resting sites or in the spring after they have left them, although in the latter case some hide damage may already have occurred. Warble flies have been eradicated in some countries and the prevalence of infection in cattle has declined dramatically in recent years in others. This is thought to be due to the widespread use of endectocides for worm control.

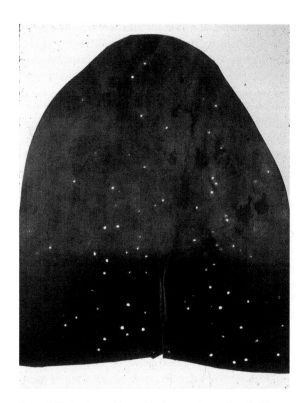

Figure 8.22 Leather with warble damage. Reproduced with permission of Agriculture and Agri-Food Canada Lethbridge Research Centre.

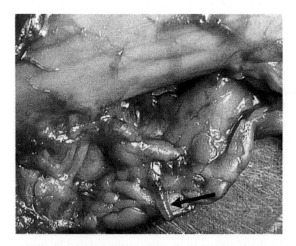

Figure 8.21 Dissected spinal cord showing a warble larva (*Hypoderma bovis*) on epidural fat. Reproduced with permission of Agriculture and Agri-Food Canada Lethbridge Research Centre.

Bovine besnoitiosis

The life-cycle and routes of transmission of *Besnoitia* are still only poorly understood, so the reason for its sudden increase in prevalence in Europe is currently unknown. Affected farms can suffer severe losses in terms of mortality, weight-loss, depressed milk-production, abortion and male sterility. Disease severity varies widely between infected individuals.

There are three clinical phases:

a – Febrile: lasting up to 10 days with ocular and nasal discharges, photophobia, ruminal atony and anorexia;

b – Intermediate: body temperature returns towards normal but lymph nodes start to enlarge and oedematous swellings appear on the head and lower parts of body. The skin becomes thickened and painful. There is congestion of the udder in cows, while orchitis occurs in males.

c – Chronic: The skin is now markedly thickened and hair is lost (see Figure 8.23). Body condition deteriorates

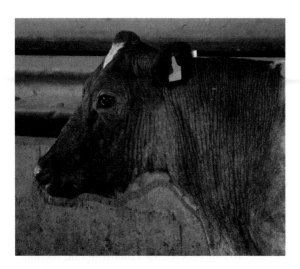

Figure 8.23 Chronic besnoitiosis: showing thickened skin. Reproduced with permission of A. Gentile.

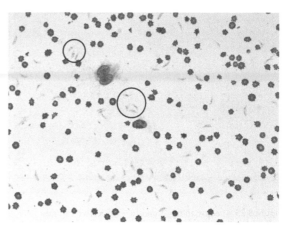

Figure 8.24 Chronic besnoitiosis: fine needle aspiration skin biopsy from cow showing numerous banana-shaped bradyzoites (pale blue structures among RBCs and monocytes). Reproduced with permission of G. Militerno.

despite a restored appetite. If recovery occurs, it is very slow and it is often uneconomic to keep convalescent animals.

In the chronic phase, the clinical appearance is characteristic and diagnosis can be confirmed with a skin biopsy smear revealing evidence of parasitism (see Figure 8.24). *Besnoitia* cysts can sometimes be seen on examination of the eye (see Figure 4.33). Diagnosis is more difficult in the earlier phases of the disease process as the signs are nonspecific and antibodies are not easily detected in the first two weeks.

More knowledge is required before control measures can be formulated. In the meantime, care should be taken to exclude seropositive carrier animals from the herd. Exposure to biting flies (suspected mechanical vectors) should be reduced as far as it is possible to do so.

8.2.5 Other body systems

The most important conditions listed in Table 8.7 are toxoplasmosis in ewes and neosporosis in cows, both common causes of abortion. As far as the other parasites are concerned, eye-worms in cattle generally cause little

Table 8.7 Parasitic genera most likely to be encountered in other body systems of cattle and sheep

	CNS	Eyes	Urogenital	Musculature
Host: **CATTLE**				
Nematodes		*Thelazia* 7.1.5		
Cestodes				*Taenia*[1] 5.3.3
Protozoa			*Neospora* 4.7.4	*Sarcocystis* 4.7.1
			Tritrichomonas 4.5.2	
Insect	*Hypoderma* 2.2.6			
Host: **SHEEP**				
Cestodes	*Taenia*[2] 5.3.3			
Protozoa			*Toxoplasma* 4.7.3	*Taenia*[1] 5.3.3
				Sarcocystis 4.7.1

Note: these lists are not comprehensive; other parasites do occur but less frequently or are of more restricted distribution or importance; numbers in red cross-reference to section with more detailed information.
[1]Cysticerci; [2] Coenurus.

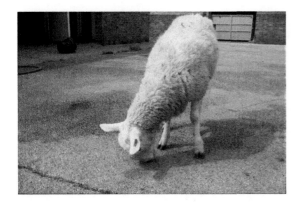

Figure 8.25 Sheep standing in posture indicative of brain damage due to the presence of a *Taenia multiceps* metacestode (coenurus). Reproduced with permission of M. Stallbaumer.

more harm than increased lacrimation and occasional conjunctivitis, although they can predispose to a bacterial condition (infectious keratoconjunctivitis). Tapeworm cysticerci and larger sarcocysts in muscle cause economic losses at meat inspection. *Tritrichomonas* is a venereally transmitted protozoan that causes infertility in cows, although it has been eradicated in many countries. The warble-fly, *Hypoderma bovis*, can cause spinal injury in cattle if its larval stage dies while at the winter resting site (as noted in the previous section). A *Taenia multiceps* coenurus growing within the cranium of a sheep can cause atrophy of brain tissue, thereby affecting head posture and gait (see Figure 8.25).

Toxoplasmosis

Toxoplasma gondii is one of the commonest causes of abortion in all major sheep-rearing regions. Infection derives from the ingestion of oocysts that have originated from cats (see Figure 4.39). In many localities between 30% and 80% of cats are seropositive for *T. gondii*, although each infected cat sheds oocysts for no more than 1–2 weeks over its total lifespan. Nevertheless,

massive numbers are produced during this brief period. The oocysts are long-lived and easily dispersed. Opportunities therefore arise for the contamination of pastures and feed stores by feral, stray and farm cats.

Infection of nonpregnant sheep causes no clinically discernible effect and results in solid immunity. When this happens early in life or prior to tupping, ewes will be refractory to the potentially detrimental effects of infection during pregnancy. Ovine toxoplasmosis therefore tends to be a sporadic disease dependent on the coincidence of two independent events:

a – individuals within a flock failing to acquire immunity before they are bred; and

b – the presence of sporulated oocysts on feedstuffs (pasture, hay or concentrate rations) during the time that susceptible animals are pregnant.

The absence of clinical disease in a breeding flock signifies either:

a – that all the animals are immune, and therefore not at risk; or

b – that there has been no recent exposure to sporulated oocysts; in which case, some or all of the ewes will be highly vulnerable.

Depending on the stage of pregnancy at the time of infection, *T. gondii* infection can provoke foetal absorption, abortion, still-birth or the birth of a congenitally infected lamb (see Figure 8.26). Diagnosis is based on the presence of 2 mm white focal necrotic lesions on the cotyledons of the placenta or in the aborted foetus (see Figure 8.27). Immunohistochemistry may confirm the presence of *T. gondii* in cotyledons or foetal brain. A rising IgM antibody titre differentiates recent infection from past exposure (as might be indicated, for example, by high IgG levels).

It is impossible to maintain an oocyst-free grazing environment and this would, in any case, hinder the natural acquisition of immunity. Risk during

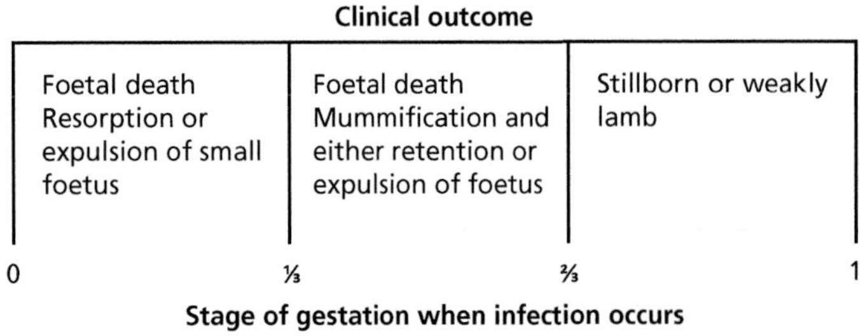

Clinical outcome

Foetal death Resorption or expulsion of small foetus	Foetal death Mummification and either retention or expulsion of foetus	Stillborn or weakly lamb

0   ⅓   ⅔   1

Stage of gestation when infection occurs

Figure 8.26 Effect of a primary *Toxoplasma gondii* infection at different stages of pregnancy in the ewe.

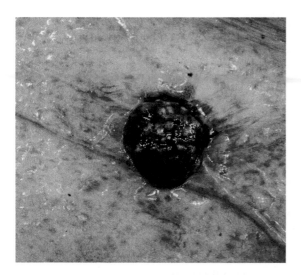

Figure 8.27 Placenta from aborted ewe showing white *Toxoplasma* lesions on cotyledon. Reproduced with permission of AHLVA, RVC Surveillance Centre © Crown copyright 2013.

pregnancy can be reduced by ensuring that cats cannot foul stored hay or concentrate rations. Medicated feed containing a suitable antiprotozoal drug (e.g. decoquinate) can be given daily, if practicable, to prevent infection during the main risk period (i.e. the 14 weeks before lambing).

An attenuated vaccine (see Section 1.6.5) given prior to tupping is used with success in some countries. The first time it is used, all ewes should be vaccinated as it is usually uneconomic to screen all of them to determine which are vulnerable, but in subsequent years only new additions to the breeding flock need be done. The vaccine strain of *T. gondii* can infect humans and so veterinarians administering this vaccine must take appropriate precautions.

Neosporosis

While only recognised in recent years, *Neospora caninum* is nevertheless one of the commonest causes of abortion in cattle. Although susceptible cows can be infected by ingesting oocysts from dogs (the exogenous route in Figure 4.41), most abortions are triggered by the recrudescence of a congenitally-derived infection (the endogenous route in Figure 4.41).

The clinical outcome depends on the stage of pregnancy when actively proliferating tachyzoites invade the placenta. Foetuses are lost mostly around the 5th or 6th months of gestation. Infections occurring in the last trimester can give rise to live calves with encephalomyelitis and paresis (weakness of the limbs). Many full-term calves born to infected dams appear healthy but are likely to be harbouring tissue cysts that will persist into later life.

Serological tests for *Neospora* infection need to be interpreted with care as:

a – specific antibodies in chronically infected cows have fluctuating titres which are periodically difficult to detect;

b – a positive result in an aborted cow does not necessarily establish a causal relationship as the death of the foetus could have been due to another, concurrent aetiological factor.

As *N. caninum* is passed to successive generations endogenously and chronic infections can remain unrecognised, bovine neosporosis is very difficult to eradicate from a herd. Much work is currently underway to find practical solutions for this problem. Culling all seropositive cows from a herd would have a drastic short-term effect on milk production and could lose valuable genetic blood-lines. Embryo transfer from infected cows to uninfected surrogate dams can overcome the latter concern. Otherwise, replacement stock has to be selected from uninfected dams. Dogs should not be fed raw meat or offal. As far as is practicable, they should not be allowed to defecate near pregnant cows or their fodder. No vaccine is widely available at the time of writing.

8.3 Pigs (swine)

Where pigs are reared intensively, the profitability of pig production is cyclical and economic returns are periodically squeezed, so any small differences that parasitism may make to the food conversion ratio or to the number of days needed to reach slaughter weight can be critical.

In some nonintensive systems, pigs are used to convert human food-waste to meat (swill feeding) or are allowed to roam free to scavenge. These practices expose pigs to other parasitic hazards, particularly *Trichinella* and *Taenia solium*. These are relatively innocuous infections in pigs but they can be transmitted to humans with catastrophic consequences and so discussion is deferred to the 'Zoonoses' section of Chapter 9 (see Section 9.3.1).

8.3.1 Internal organs

In general, the effect of helminth parasites on growing pigs in well-run intensive systems is considerably less than is the case with young grazing ruminants. This difference relates at least in part to the environmental influences listed in Table 8.8.

If there are any deficiencies in pig husbandry standards, however, then even low worm burdens can exert an economically significant effect on days to slaughter or food conversion ratio. Free-range pigs are exposed to greater variation in environmental conditions and to challenge from a greater range of parasites (see Table 8.9), especially from those utilising intermediate hosts (the gastric spiruroids, the thorny-headed worm and *Metastrongylus*) or paratenic hosts (*Stephanurus*).

Helminth infections

Strongyle worms

The strongyle worms (*Hyostrongylus* and *Oesophagostomum*) do not invoke a strong immune response and so large worm burdens can accumulate in adults yarded on deep-litter or kept outdoors. Infected in-pig sows can become very thin if also on a restricted diet. Although sows can have very high strongyle eggs-counts (thousands of eggs per gram faeces), little transmission to piglets occurs provided the farrowing house is kept clean and dry. Milk production, and therefore weaning weights, may be affected, however.

Faecal egg-counts cannot be used to confirm suspected gastritis due to *Hyostrongylus* as this worm produces few

Table 8.8 Intensively reared pigs and grazing ruminants: comparison of environmental influences

	Indoor growing pigs	Calves/lambs at grass
Ambient temperatures	Constant	Variable: day/night
Amount of food and nutrient value	Controlled/ optimal	Variable: seasonal / weather dependent
Faeces	Removed daily or passes through slatted floors	Accumulates on pasture
Parasitic challenge	Usually low	Can be seasonally high
Stress	Minimal (if not overcrowded)	Bad weather / predators / biting and myiasis flies etc.

Table 8.9 Parasitic genera most likely to be encountered in the gastrointestinal tract, internal organs and tissues of pigs

	Cestodes	Helminths	Protozoa
Host: PIG			
Stomach		*Hyostrongylus* 6.3.2 Spiruroids 7.1.5	*Cryptosporidium* 4.9.1
Small intestine		*Ascaris* 7.1.3 *Strongyloides* 7.1.2 Thorny-headed worm 7.2.1	*Isospora* 4.6.1 *Eimeria* 4.6.2 *Cryptosporidium* 4.9.1 *Giardia* 4.5.2
Caecum/ large intestine		*Trichuris* 7.1.6 *Oesophagostomum* 6.3.3	*Balantidium* 4.3 *Entamoeba* 4.4
Liver	*Echinococcus* (cyst) 5.3.4 *Taenia*[1] (cyst) 5.3.3	*Ascaris* (migrating) 7.1.3 *Stephanurus* (migrating) 6.3.3	
Lungs	*Echinococcus* (cyst) 5.3.4	*Metastrongylus* 6.3.5 *Ascaris* (migrating) 7.1.3	
Kidney		*Stephanurus* 6.3.3	
Musculature	*Taenia*[2] (cyst) 5.3.3	*Trichinella* 7.1.6; 9.3.1	*Sarcocystis* 4.7.1

Note: these lists are not comprehensive; other parasites do occur but less frequently or are of more restricted distribution or importance; numbers in red cross-reference to section of book with more detailed information.
[1] *T. hydatigena*; [2] *T. solium*.

eggs (in contrast to *Oesophagostomum* which is very pro-lific). It is, however, simple to differentiate living L_3 in a water-filled Petri dish as *Hyostrongylus* larvae are longer, thinner, and swim with a thrashing action, while *Oesophagostomum* L_3 squirm on the bottom.

Ascaris

If present in large numbers, larvae of the pig ascarid, *Ascaris suum*, can cause substantial tissue reaction as they migrate through liver and lungs, while the dele-terious effects of adult worms are attributable to their impressive bulk.

The effect on health and productivity depends on the level of exposure to embryonated eggs, which in turn depends on the husbandry system and standard of hygiene:

a – Light infection: which is common, even in inten-sive units:

i) Migratory phase: hepatic damage leads to con-demnation of liver tissue at the abattoir (e.g. 4.2% of pig livers were affected in a recent British abattoir survey).

ii) Intestinal phase: little, if any, discernible effect.

b – Heavy infection: usually associated with unhy-gienic buildings or contaminated yards:

i) Migratory phase: lung damage increases suscepti-bility to respiratory disease and provides a portal of entry for pyogenic organisms. Abattoir condemna-tions result from internal abscesses as well as para-sitic liver lesions.

ii) Intestinal phase: reduced growth-rate and/or increased food conversion ratio.

c – Massive infection: usually seen only in scavenging or back-yard pigs. Diarrhoea, jaundice, severe weight-loss, stunting and death result from:

i) Migratory phase: respiratory distress and liver damage.

ii) Enteric phase: obstruction of the small intestine by masses of large worms and of the main bile duct (by aberrant adult worms).

Ascarids are prolific egg-producers and patent infec-tions are easily diagnosed by finding characteristic rough-walled brown eggs at faecal examination (see Figure 8.28).

Pigs with 'milk-spot' liver lesions (see Figure 7.11) often have zero egg-counts. This is because larvae migrat-ing in partially immune pigs manage to pass through the liver before succumbing to host adaptive responses.

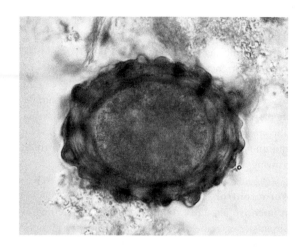

Figure 8.28 *Ascaris suum* egg. Reproduced with permission of Merial GmbH.

Consequently, control of milk-spot in problem herds depends on meticulous elimination of ascarid eggs from pig houses. The longevity and adhesiveness of these eggs enables transmission to continue at a low level in mod-ern intensive units unless all patent infections are con-trolled and hygiene is maintained at a very high level.

Fibrous liver lesions in pigs can also be provoked by the migrating larvae of *Stephanurus* (the swine kidney worm), the dog ascarid, *Toxocara*, and immature *Fasciola* (liver fluke).

Other gastrointestinal worms

The whipworm, *Trichuris suis*, like *Ascaris*, induces a strong immune response and is seen in greatest numbers in younger pigs. *Trichuris* can provoke intermittent diar-rhoea or dysentery. Disease mostly occurs in outdoor pigs or those kept in unhygienic conditions. The eggs have a characteristically double-plugged barrel-shaped appear-ance (see Figure 7.31) but fluctuate in number and do not always float well in routine faecal examinations. Not all anthelmintics are fully effective against whipworms.

Strongyloides affects unweaned piglets as infection is transmitted via colostrum and milk. The sow acquires infection through lying on damp straw or other materi-als that provide ideal conditions for the free-living phase of the life-cycle (see Figure 7.3).

Lungworm

Metastrongylus is found only in pigs that have access to earthworm intermediate hosts. As pig lungworms are found mostly in the smaller bronchi of the distal diaphragmatic lobe of the lung, damage is less extensive than the equivalent condition in calves (dictyocaulosis). Infection can, nevertheless, produce a marked check in the growth-rate which may be accompanied by coughing or dyspnoea. Larvated eggs with a wrinkled surface are passed in faeces but a flotation fluid with a high specific gravity is needed for their demonstration. A solid immunity develops quickly so disease occurs mostly in growing pigs.

Worm control

In intensive pig units, the most convenient method of administering anthelmintic treatment is to dose all stock simultaneously by filling food hoppers with a medicated ration. Cost and concerns about the possible induction of anthelmintic resistance dictate that the number of doses is kept to a minimum and determined by the results of routine faecal examination. In other circumstances, treatments can be strategically targeted: for example, sows as they enter the farrowing house (to eliminate egg-output and to redress any adverse effect on lactation) and growing pigs before they enter new premises (e.g. when weaners are moved into fattening pens).

Porcine coccidiosis

Isospora suis is considered to be one of the main causative agents of 'scours' (diarrhoea) in piglets 1–3 weeks old (the others being a variety of bacterial and viral conditions). *I. suis* has been found on a majority of pig farms in all regions surveyed. Piglets become infected within the first few days of life.

Scours is a very common condition in pig breeding units and is characterised by pasty cream-white faeces (see Figure 8.29) or profuse watery diarrhoea. Mortality is generally low in *I. suis* infections but weight-gains may be affected even in the absence of obvious disease. *Eimeria* infections tend to occur when the pigs are a little older.

Laboratory confirmation of *I. suis* infection can be challenging as diarrhoea starts during the prepatent period of the parasite (i.e. before oocysts start to be shed in faeces) and affected piglets often do not die until after the coccidia have completed their developmental cycle and left the host. If oocysts are found, they have to be sporulated to differentiate them from those of *Eimeria*, which are of similar size. Sporulated *Isospora* oocysts contain two sporocysts while *Eimeria* have four (see Figure 4.6).

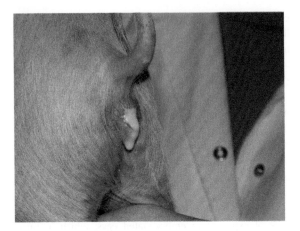

Figure 8.29 Piglet with 'scours' due to *Isospora suis*. Reproduced with permission of A. Joachim.

At least one effective treatment is available for piglets affected with *I. suis*. In the longer term, however, control depends on reducing infection pressure by providing a dry, hygienic environment for farrowing sows. Farrowing pens should be cleaned scrupulously after each occupation using detergent, a disinfectant known to kill oocysts, or steam sterilisation.

8.3.2 Integument

In intensive systems, lice and sarcoptic mange are the commonest parasitic skin infestations (see Table 8.10). The adult pig louse, *Haematopinus suis*, is large (5 mm long) and dark coloured (see Figure 8.30), so it is easily spotted (unless hidden in a skin fold). It sucks blood and provokes mild irritation and scratching. Heavy infestations may affect productivity.

Table 8.10 Parasitic genera most likely to be encountered on or in the skin of pigs

Host: PIG	
Ticks / nuisance and biting flies	Many
Myiasis flies	Screwworms etc. 2.2.6
Lice	*Haematopinus* 2.2.3
Fleas	*Tunga* 2.2.2
Subsurface mites	*Sarcoptes* 3.3.2
	Demodex 3.3.2

Note: these lists are not comprehensive; other parasites do occur but less frequently or are of more restricted distribution or importance; numbers in red cross-reference to section with more detailed information.

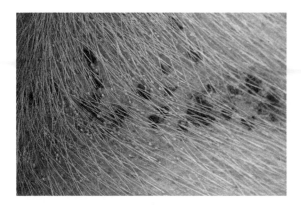

Figure 8.30 Adult lice (*Haematopinus suis*) and their eggs on a pig. Reproduced with permission of Merial GmbH.

Sarcoptic mange

Sarcoptes is extremely common in pigs. Infection is derived from the dam during the suckling period, although contact transmission can occur later in life. Many infestations go unnoticed but the frequency of scratching and rubbing in a group of seemingly healthy pigs can decline markedly following acaricidal treatment. As these behaviours expend considerable amounts of energy, effective mange control can enhance productivity.

Sarcoptic mange can manifest clinically with frequent scratching, hair loss, skin damage with secondary infection, and general loss of condition. Areas of papular lesions and erythema with scaly edges usually start on the ears, spread over the head and continue over the body. The skin later becomes thickened and crusty (see Figure 8.31). The condition is highly pruritic and rubbing the ear-edge may elicit a scratch

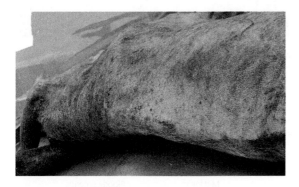

Figure 8.31 Sow showing the thickened and crusty skin associated with sarcoptic mange. Reproduced with permission of AHLVA, RVC Surveillance Centre © Crown copyright 2013.

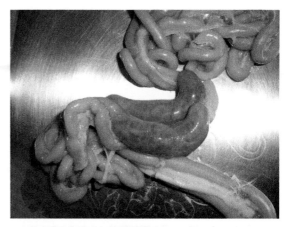

Figure 8.32 Caecal coccidiosis (*Eimeria tenella*). Reproduced with permission of L. Canseco.

reflex. Mites (see Figure 9.32) or their eggs may be found in skin scrapings or ear-wax. If they are difficult to find, response to treatment with an appropriate topically applied acaricide or systemic ML will confirm diagnosis. Control can be achieved by treating each sow as it is moved into the farrowing house to break the transmission cycle to piglets. The boar should be treated regularly to ensure it does not reinfect the sows.

8.4 Poultry

Intensive poultry farming is practised on an enormous scale, often with batches of 10 000 or more birds in a single house. The economic framework of such enterprises is finely balanced and small variations in feed consumption or daily mortality rates can be critical. It can be said without exaggeration that this type of poultry production would be impossible if planning, management and execution did not take full account of coccidiosis control requirements.

At the other end of the scale, the village chicken plays a vital role in subsistence farming, providing much needed protein for the family and a means of cash generation. As these birds are kept on earthen yards or allowed to roam freely and scavenge, they are prone to a wide variety of parasitic conditions, ranging from argasid tick infestation to spiruroid eye-worms and avian malaria. A recent survey in Tanzania, for example, revealed no fewer than 19 nematode species and 10 cestodes.

Table 8.11 Parasitic genera most likely to be encountered in the internal organs of poultry

	Cestodes	Nematodes	Protozoa
Host: **POULTRY**			
Pharynx to gizzard		*Capillaria* 7.1.6	*Trichomonas* 4.5.2
Small intestine	*Davainea* 5.3.5	*Capillaria* 7.1.6	*Eimeria* 4.6.2
	and other tapeworms	*Ascaridia* 7.1.3	*Cryptosporidium* 4.9.1
Caeca / large intestine / cloaca		*Capillaria* 7.1.6	*Eimeria* 4.6.2
		Heterakis 7.1.3	*Histomonas* 4.5.2
		Trichostrongylus 6.3.2	*Cryptosporidium* 4.9.1
			Trichomonas 4.5.2
Liver			*Histomonas* 4.5.2
Trachea/ lungs		*Syngamus* 6.3.3	

Note: these lists are not comprehensive; other parasites do occur but less frequently or are of more restricted distribution or importance; numbers in red cross-reference to section of book with more detailed information.

8.4.1 Internal organs

The internal parasites most commonly encountered worldwide are listed in Table 8.11.

Avian coccidiosis

Large-scale poultry production is dependent upon the scientific knowledge and technology needed to control coccidiosis. Even in the absence of overt disease, sub-clinical infection can have significant financial impact in terms of weight gain and feed conversion.

There are at least seven *Eimeria* species in chickens of varying pathogenicity. The most damaging are, predictably, those that cause haemorrhagic lesions (see Table 8.12). The first indication of a coccidiosis problem in large units is often an increase in daily mortality.

Diagnosis is based on autopsy of dead or culled birds and takes into consideration the region of intestine affected, the appearance of the lesions and whether or not there is evidence of haemorrhage. For example:

a - *E. tenella:* deaths from caecal coccidiosis occur commonly in back-yard chickens. Such cases are easily diagnosed as the caeca are swollen, thickened and dark (see Figure 8.32). When opened, they are found to contain a core of necrotic tissue and blood.

b – *E. necatrix:* the mid-gut is typically ballooned and blood is present in the lumen (see Figure 8.33).

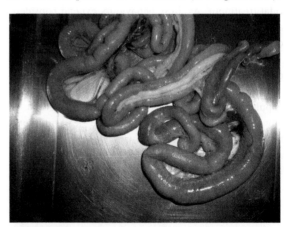

Figure 8.33 Haemorrhagic coccidiosis of the mid-gut due to *Eimeria necatrix*. Reproduced with permission of L. Canseco.

Table 8.12 Characteristics of the main *Eimeria* species of chickens

	Pathogenesis	Pathogenicity	Immunogenicity	Location in gut	Lesion type
E. tenella	Haemorrhagic	▼▼▼	▼	Caeca	Bloody core in caeca
E. necatrix	Haemorrhagic	▼▼▼	▼	Mid-gut	'Salt and pepper'
E. brunetti	Haemorrhagic	▼▼	▼▼	Mid/lower	Bloody enteritis
E. acervulina	Malabsorption	▼▼	▼▼	Proximal	'White ladder'
E. maxima	Malabsorption	▼▼	▼▼▼	Mid-gut	Pink exudates

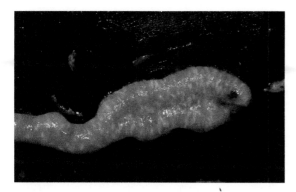

Figure 8.34 Proximal gut of chicken opened to show *Eimeria acervulina* 'ladder' lesions on mucosa. Reproduced with permission of L. Canseco.

Examination of the mucosa in the proximal intestine reveals 'salt and pepper' lesions due to the presence of multiple white spots (which mark the presence of second generation schizonts) interspersed with brownish-red petechiae.

c – *E. acervulina*: the proximal gut is thickened at intervals with lines of gamonts and oocysts giving the appearance of a white 'ladder' (see Figure 8.34).

d – *E. maxima*: petechial haemorrhages are present on the mid-gut wall (see Figure 8.35). Blood from these mixes with other excretions to form a pink exudate in the lumen of the intestine.

A well-defined system exists for lesion scoring with charts and tables readily available to assist with this task. The sizes of the schizonts and oocysts found in mucosal scrapings provide useful data for confirmation.

In an emergency, appropriate antiprotozoal drugs are added to the water supply (see Section 4.10.2), but the general aim must always be to prevent any such incidents from occurring. Buildings must be designed so that they can be thoroughly disinfected between batches of birds and management systems fine-tuned to ensure that the bedding is kept dry. In this way, numbers of sporulated oocysts can be kept at minimal levels.

Even so, it may be necessary to keep broilers on medicated feed for most of their short lives to attain maximum growth. As might be expected with a parasite of such enormous reproductive potential, resistance to many coccidiostats has become commonplace. Different strategies can be employed to prolong the life of still-useful compounds. For this purpose, available products are currently divided into 'ionophores' and 'chemicals'

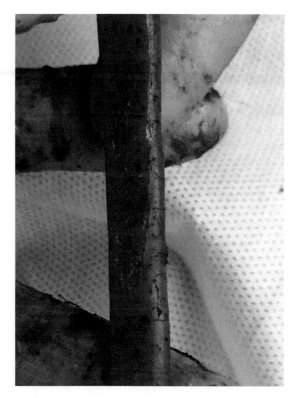

Figure 8.35 Patechial haemorrhages on the mid-gut wall due to *Eimeria maxima*. Reproduced with permission of L. Canseco.

(i.e. other synthetic anticoccidials). If reliance is placed mainly on 'ionophores' then, at appropriate intervals, a batch of birds can be medicated with a 'chemical' to curtail ('clean up') any trend towards ionophore-resistance. Alternatively, a 'chemical' may be used in the starter phase of each new batch of broilers to be replaced by an 'ionophore' for the remainder of the growth-cycle. This is an example of a 'shuttle programme'. Each scheme has to balance risk (of resistance developing), productivity and cost. Medication has to be withdrawn a statutory number of days prior to slaughter to avoid meat residues.

Growth-rate is less important for layer replacements (i.e. future egg-layers) and in this case a 'step-down' medication programme may be used to allow the birds to develop immunity. Such schemes have to be skilfully planned so they do not exert too much selection pressure on the parasite population.

An alternative or adjunct to medication is employment of an attenuated vaccine (see Section 1.6.5). Chicks are vaccinated on a single occasion by suspending the vaccine-dose in the drinking system or by spraying attenuated oocysts onto feed. There is no cross-immunity between *Eimeria* species, so exposure to one species does not protect against subsequent exposure to others. Vaccines, therefore, have to be multivalent and tailor-made to match regional variations in the spectrum of species or genotypes. A practical problem associated with vaccination is the difficulty on large farms of ensuring that feed in automated systems does not contain traces of any medication which might interfere with the development (and consequently immunogenicity) of attenuated organisms in the birds.

Helminths and histomonosis

With the exception of *Ascaridia*, which may become established in deep-litter systems, nematodes and cestodes are not normally of significance in intensively housed poultry. They can, however, be problematic in free-range birds. Scavenging birds are exposed to parasite eggs and larvae that have accumulated in soil or that are carried by intermediate or paratenic hosts (e.g. earthworms, molluscs or insects).

While mostly asymptomatic, helminths can affect appetite, growth rate or egg production if present in sufficient numbers. Heavy infestation may lead to loss of condition followed by emaciation and death. Diarrhoea may be a feature when the digestive system is affected.

The most informative method of diagnosis is recovery and identification of worms at autopsy. This procedure should include mucosal scrapings as some worms such as *Capillaria*, *Trichostrongylus tenuis* and the smaller tapeworms are otherwise easily overlooked. Fresh droppings can be examined for helminth eggs, but tapeworm segments are only passed intermittently. Eggs of the two ascarid genera, *Ascaridia* and *Heterakis*, are difficult to tell apart, although the latter are slightly smaller with straighter sides (see Figure 8.36). *Capillaria* eggs are recognised by their double-plugged appearance.

Syngamus

The gape-worm, *Syngamus*, has a wide host range including wild birds such as starlings. These contaminate the ground with eggs. Earthworms subsequently accumulate infective larvae and are eaten by free-range birds or by chicks and poults kept in pens with earthen floors. Young pheasants and turkeys of all ages are

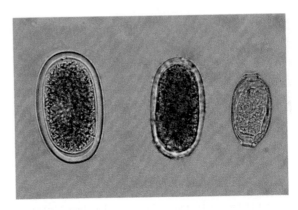

Figure 8.36 Eggs of *Ascaridia* (left), *Heterakis* (centre) and *Capillaria* (right). Reproduced with permission of C.A. Tucker and T.A. Yazwinski.

particularly vulnerable. Larvae migrating through the lungs can cause pneumonia, while adult worms induce the formation of mucus in quantities that can partly or completely occlude larger air passages. Consequently, affected birds breathe heavily with their neck extended and they can die of asphyxia. *Syngamus* also sucks blood and so chronic infection can lead to anaemia, weakness and emaciation.

At autopsy, the 'Y' shaped pairs of worms in the trachea are unmistakable (see Figure 8.37 and Figure 6.44).

Their eggs have an operculum at either end (see Figure 8.38) and so are easily differentiated from the typical strongyle appearance of the *T. tenuis* egg.

Histomonas

Histomonas, the cause of 'black-head' in turkeys, is not a helminth but is included here as it is transmitted by the

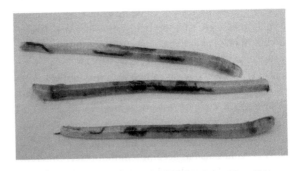

Figure 8.37 *Syngamus*: adult worms within the trachea (from three pheasants). Reproduced with permission of D.G. Parsons.

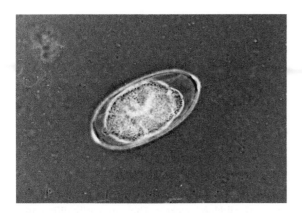

Figure 8.38 *Syngamus* egg. Reproduced with permission of the Institute of Parasitology, Justus Liebig University, Giessen.

ascarid, *Heterakis*. Currently, control of the worm is the only feasible method for preventing black-head disease as the antiprotozoal drugs previously used for this purpose are no longer available in many countries. (This is because of their potential toxicity to humans.) Turkeys affected by this disease go off their food, become listless, look dishevelled and may die. Some have cyanotic wattles and the droppings are characteristically yellow (see Figure 8.39). *Histomonas* also infects chickens and game birds, but these act mostly as symptomless carriers.

At autopsy, the caeca are enlarged and thickened (see Figure 8.40). The mucosa is ulcerated and covered with a yellow exudate which coagulates to form a caecal core. Multiple necrotic lesions are seen on the liver surface (see Figure 8.41). These are circular, yellowish-grey and can be more than 1 cm across.

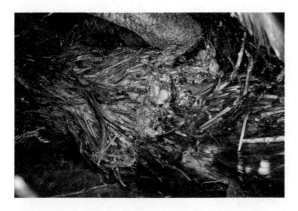

Figure 8.39 Histomonosis: turkey with yellow-coloured droppings typical of this disease around the vent. Reproduced with permission of D.G. Parsons.

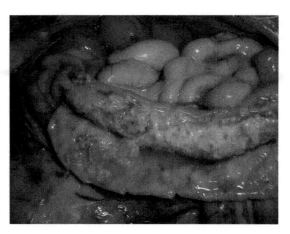

Figure 8.40 Histomonosis: caecum cut to show thickened wall and coagulated exudate. Reproduced with permission of D.G. Parsons.

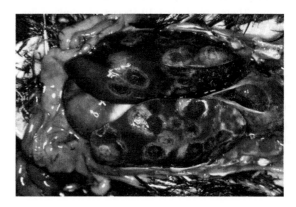

Figure 8.41 Histomonosis: lesions on liver. Reproduced with permission of D.G. Parsons.

Worm control

Handling individual birds is often impractical but anthelmintics and other parasiticides can be administered to a flock in medicated feed, although water has to be used as the treatment vehicle if appetite is depressed. Free-roaming game birds can be treated by offering medicated grit that, if taken, will remain for a time in the gizzard.

Management also plays an important role in the prevention of disease. For example, relocating rearing pens at intervals before *Syngamus* builds up to critical levels in the soil, or ensuring that turkey poults are not placed on ground previously used by chickens that might have been symptomless *Histomonas* carriers.

8.4.2 Integument

In general, small numbers of ectoparasites (see Table 8.13) pass unnoticed on chickens but heavy infestations provoke restlessness with parasite-induced and/or self-afflicted feather damage. Reduced productivity follows and, in severe cases, emaciation and death. Younger age-groups are particularly vulnerable. Some ectoparasites produce specific damage, e.g. female stick-tight fleas (*Echidnophaga*) burrow into the bare skin of the wattles and head, provoking small wounds that may become ulcerated and secondarily infected.

Lice, mites and mange

Lice

Louse infestation (pediculosis) in chickens is often associated with an underlying problem such as overcrowding, inadequate housing, poor hygiene or intercurrent disease. There are at least 10 species of chewing lice found on poultry worldwide. English names for the most important of them describe their appearance and/or favoured location (e.g. 'yellow body louse', 'wing louse', 'shaft louse'). The most pathogenic is the body louse, *Menacanthus*, which causes a reddening of the skin on the breast, thighs and around the vent. Like other chewing lice it feeds mainly on skin debris but it also attacks the base of new feathers while the shaft is still soft.

Close inspection of the skin and feathers may reveal lice 2–5 mm in length (depending on species), although sometimes it is easier to find their eggs stuck onto feathers. The eggs of the body louse are partly covered with frills and are laid in clusters at the base of feathers, often around the cloaca (see Figure 8.42). The clusters are easily visible with the naked eye. Lice are permanent parasites and so pediculosis control involves dusting affected birds with an appropriate insecticide and correcting management deficiencies.

Mites

Dermanyssus, the poultry red mite, and *Ornithonyssus* (a genus that includes the northern and tropical fowl mites) are all blood suckers. They are easily differentiated from lice as they are smaller (< 1 mm) and more spider-like. Heavy mite infestations cause anaemia. Birds become restless and egg production can drop. *Ornithonyssus*, which is the 'hairier' of the two genera,

Table 8.13 Parasitic genera most likely to be encountered on or in the skin of poultry

Host: **POULTRY**	
Ticks	*Argas* etc. 3.2.3
Nuisance and biting flies	many
Myiasis flies	Screwworms etc. 2.2.6
Chewing lice	*Lipeurus* 2.2.3
	Menacanthus etc. 2.2.3
Fleas	*Ceratophyllus* 2.2.2
	Echidnophaga 2.2.2
Surface mites	*Dermanyssus* 3.3.3
	Ornithonyssus 3.3.3
Subsurface mites	*Knemidocoptes* 3.3.2

Note: these lists are not comprehensive; other parasites do occur but less frequently or are of more restricted distribution or importance; numbers in red cross-reference to section with more detailed information.

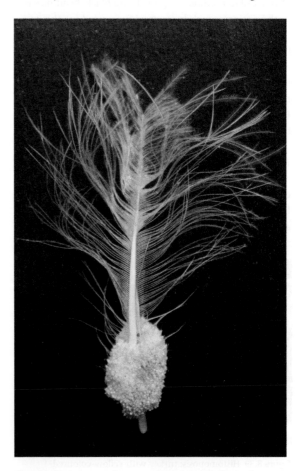

Figure 8.42 A cluster of *Menacanthus* eggs at the base of a feather.

spends much of its time on its host and can therefore be found on birds during the day. In contrast, *Dermanyssus* visits birds only at night and can spend considerable periods between feeds hiding in dark cracks and crevices. Consequently, bird treatments will be more effective against *Ornithonyssus* than *Dermanyssus*. In the latter case, control has to focus on cleaning and treating the surroundings. Creosote may be necessary in wooden buildings that can otherwise be difficult to disinfect. A neat idea for use on organic farms is to entice the mites to hide in strategically placed traps made of corrugated cardboard which can be collected and burnt.

Knemidocoptic mange

Different species of the microscopic (0.5 mm) subsurface mite *Knemidocoptes* are responsible for the following conditions:

a – Scaly leg in poultry: Mites burrow beneath leg scales provoking inflammation and exudation and causing the scales to loosen and rise, starting from the toes, giving a ragged appearance to legs and feet (see Figure 8.43). Chronically affected birds may have distorted feet and claws and show signs of lameness.

b – Depluming itch in poultry: Mites burrow into feather shafts producing intense pain and irritation causing birds to pull out body feathers.

c – Scaly face/ scaly beak in cage birds: Mites attack bare or lightly feathered parts of the beak, nostrils, face and body. Scaliness is first seen at the base of the beak and may spread across the face and sometimes the body. Despite this appearance there is apparently little pruritus.

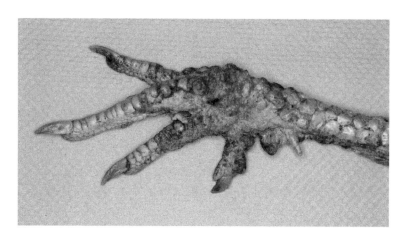

Figure 8.43 Scaly leg. Reproduced with permission of D.G. Parsons.

CHAPTER 9

Clinical parasitology: companion animals and veterinary public health

9.1 Equine parasitology

Horses and other equine species are simple stomached animals but also herbivores. Consequently, there are similarities with ruminants with regard to both the epidemiology and control of major gastrointestinal parasitic infections (see Section 8.2.1).

9.1.1 Digestive system

The equine digestive system is large and complex. It provides a home for many parasites, both in numbers and species diversity (see Table 9.1). Dominant amongst these are the strongyloids (*Strongylus* spp. and the cyathostomins) in the caecum and colon. An important feature of equine parasitology is that horses remain vulnerable to these infections throughout their lives as the immunity they develop provides only partial protection.

If faecal samples are monitored as foals grow older, a succession of parasitic infections becomes apparent. The sequence is determined by the epidemiological characteristics of each parasite. Foals acquire *Cryptosporidium* from their immediate environment within the first few days of life while *Strongyloides* is transmitted via the mare's colostrum and milk. *Parascaris* eggs can contaminate both stables and pasture, so initial infection may occur early in life but the prepatent period of *Parascaris* is at least 10 weeks. Exposure to infective strongyloid larvae does not usually occur until foals start to graze. Strongyle eggs from cyathostomin species appear in

Principles of Veterinary Parasitology, First Edition. By Dennis Jacobs, Mark Fox, Lynda Gibbons and Carlos Hermosilla.
© 2016 John Wiley & Sons, Ltd. Published 2016 by John Wiley & Sons, Ltd.
Companion website: www.wiley.com/go/jacobs/principles-veterinary-parasitology

Table 9.1 Parasitic genera most likely to be encountered in the gastrointestinal tract and liver of equidae

	Cestodes	Trematodes	Nematodes	Protozoa	Insects
Host: HORSE					
Mouth					*Gasterophilus* 2.2.6
Stomach			Spiruroids 7.1.5		*Gasterophilus* 2.2.6
			Trichostrongylus 6.3.2		
Small intestine	*Anoplocephala* 5.3.5		*Strongyloides* 7.1.2	*Cryptosporidium* 4.9.1	*Gasterophilus* 2.2.6
			Parascaris 7.1.3	*Eimeria* 4.6.2	
				Giardia 4.5.2	
Caecum / large intestine	*Anoplocephala*[1] 5.3.5		*Strongylus* 6.3.3		*Gasterophilus*[2] 2.2.6
			Cyathostomins 6.3.3		
			Oxyuris 7.1.4		
Liver	*Echinococcus*	Fasciola	*Strongylus*		
	(cyst) 5.3.4	5.6.2	(larvae) 6.3.3		

Note: these lists are not comprehensive; other parasites do occur but less frequently or are of more restricted distribution or importance; numbers in red cross-reference to section of book with more detailed information.
[1] ileocaecal junction; [2] rectum.

faeces some 6–12 weeks later, but *Strongylus* spp., because of their long migrations through the body, do not start to produce eggs until 9–12 months have elapsed.

Eggs of the different species, starting with *Strongyloides*, disappear from faeces as immune processes become effective. Patent *Parascaris* infections are seldom found in horses over a year old. In contrast, some individuals continue to shed strongyle eggs throughout their lives. Typically, a group of untreated adults will include a few with high strongyle egg-counts, some with low values and some registering zero. Egg-output tends to be higher in the spring than at other times. The risk of overt disease attributable to strongyloid worms diminishes after 2–5 years of age.

Similarly, the tapeworm, *Anoplocephala*, can be found in grazing horses of any age but clinical cases are less common after 3–4 years. Eggs of *Oxyuris*, the pin-worm, are not found in faeces as they are deposited onto the perineal skin. Large accumulations of eggs are itchy and horses respond by rubbing the tail-base.

The wormy horse

Every equestrian will be familiar with the 'wormy horse'. Such animals are generally unthrifty and their coat lacks the 'bloom' characteristic of healthy animals. They may have low grade anaemia and soft faeces. Parasitism is often a significant contributor to such cases but there are frequently other underlying factors that need to be investigated, such as poor pasture management.

The debilitation displayed by the wormy horse is due to the additive effect of multiple parasitic infections producing a range of pathologies. Prominent amongst these are the cyathostomins, with tens of thousands of adult worms and even greater numbers of mucosal larvae being a common occurrence. The adult cyathostomins are shallow plug feeders (see Section 6.2.2) producing superficial microinjuries to the gut wall. The greatest damage, however, occurs at an earlier stage in the life-cycle, when larvae emerge from their development sites within the mucosa.

The number of larvae in the mucosa depends, of course, on how many cyathostomin L_3 there were on the pastures being grazed. Seasonal fluctuations in pasture larval counts follow the same general pattern as that seen in the epidemiology of ruminant PGE (see Figure 6.18), with large numbers accumulating during the summer and autumn. Cyathostomin L_3 (see Figure 9.1) survive average winters relatively well but they die when temperatures rise in spring.

When horses are allowed to express natural behavioural patterns, they defecate onto some parts of a field (the 'roughs') while other areas (the 'lawns') are reserved for grazing. This provides some natural protection from parasitism. If overstocked, horses are forced to eat the highly contaminated grass as well.

As horses remain vulnerable to parasitism throughout their lives, they have by tradition been wormed at regular intervals to keep them healthy, but this has inevitably

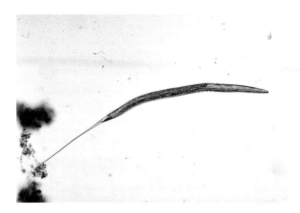

Figure 9.1 Infective cyathostomin larva: note the very long tail typical of many horse strongyle third stage larvae.

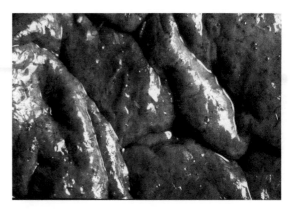

Figure 9.2 Intestinal mucosa of a horse that died of larval cyathostominosis note oedema, inflammation and numerous larvae (appearing at this magnification as black dots). From Jacobs, 1986 with permission of Elsevier.

given rise to resistance problems. Only three types of anthelmintic are currently available for broad-spectrum worm control in horses – benzimidazoles (BZDs), macrocyclic lactones (MLs) and pyrantel. It is therefore of paramount importance that control schemes should comply with best practice for maintaining the usefulness of those anthelmintics still effective on a property (by applying the principles outlined under '*Ovine PGE*' in Section 8.2.1). Some options for horse owners are discussed in the next section.

Larval cyathostominosis

During the summer, the intestinal damage suffered by the 'wormy horse' is associated mainly with cyathostomins that complete their parasitic life-cycle without interruption (Type I disease). Many larvae, however, become arrested in the early third stage of their development. These are termed 'EL_3'. A serious condition, known as larval or Type II cyathostominosis, occurs if large numbers of EL_3 resume their development to the early fourth stage (EL_4) and break out of the mucosa simultaneously. This tends to happen in the late winter or early spring (but occasionally at other times) in horses up to 5 years old. It is a sporadic disease but appears to be increasing in incidence. Dramatic weight-loss is often, but not always, accompanied by sudden-onset severe diarrhoea and sometimes peripheral oedema. Prognosis has to be guarded as affected animals often succumb despite intensive anthelmintic and supportive therapy.

Diagnosis is difficult as faecal egg-counts give no information on larval development. Large numbers of small (4–8 mm) red L_4 may be passed in faeces or be seen

adhering to the clinician's glove after rectal examination. Haematology will show hyperglobulinaemia (mainly IgE), hypoalbuminaemia and leukocytosis. At autopsy, enormous numbers of EL_4 can be seen as brown flecks in the inflamed and oedematous luminal mucosa of the caecum and colon (see Figure 9.2).

Larval cyathostominosis is an unpredictable disease which can destroy valuable or well-loved horses with little warning. Arrested larvae protected within their nodules are insusceptible to most anthelmintics and so the most effective way to prevent this disease is to ensure that EL_3 do not accumulate in the mucosa. Thus, the primary objective of worm control programmes must be to maintain pasture contamination within safe limits.

One useful way of doing this is by mechanical removal of faecal material from paddocks at intervals of no more than a week. Although labour intensive, this approach has the twin advantages of reducing the number of worming treatments needed during the year and increasing the amount of palatable grass, allowing better utilisation of the pasture.

Anthelmintic usage can be further reduced by performing faecal egg-counts at intervals. This determines when the overall faecal egg-output reaches a level justifying intervention and identifies which individuals have high egg-counts and should be treated. Those with low egg-counts contribute little to pasture contamination and their worm-burdens can therefore be left *in refugia* (see Section 1.6.3).

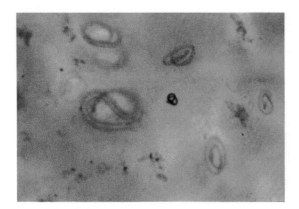

Figure 9.3 Magnified view of the intestinal mucosa of a pony that died of larval cyathostominosis showing larvae in various stages of development. Reproduced with permission of T.R. Klei.

The cyathostomin population in a horse comprises five distinct developmental stages with different anthelmintic susceptibilities. These are:

a – Within the mucosa: arrested third-stage larvae (EL_3); developing (late) third-stage larvae (LL_3); early fourth-stage larvae (EL_4) (see Figure 9.3).

b – Within the intestinal lumen: late fourth-stage larvae (L_4) and adults.

Some anthelmintics such as pyrantel are active mainly against luminal forms. Others, such as fenbendazole at normal dose-rates, will kill luminal forms and the more advanced mucosal larvae. The macrocyclic lactones impact earlier larvae as well, but to different degrees depending on the compound and conditions of use. Fenbendazole when given daily for at least five consecutive days also has good effect against earlier larvae. The clinical relevance of this information has two facets:

a – Egg reappearance period: when given to healthy horses, anthelmintics will suppress faecal egg-output for different lengths of time depending upon how many mucosal life-cycle stages are killed (see Figure 9.4). The 'ERP' for different products varies from around 5–14 weeks and is an important factor in determining treatment intervals. The first sign of an impending resistance problem is often a shortening of the ERP.

b – Choice of anthelmintic: for treating clinical cases of larval cyathostominosis or for protecting 'high risk' horses (e.g. those that have grazed heavily contaminated pasture) it is, of course, imperative to choose an anthelmintic that kills as many mucosal larval stages as possible.

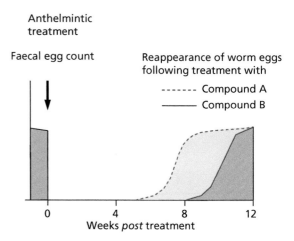

Figure 9.4 Egg reappearance time (EPR): graph comparing the faecal strongyle egg-output of two groups of horses treated on Day 0 with a different anthelmintic.

Other parasitic infections

Stomach

There are three main species of the stomach bot fly, *Gasterophilus*. Their larvae have periods of development in the mouth and stomach before exiting the horse in its faeces. Some also attach to the pharynx, pylorus or rectum (see Table 2.4). The burrowing activities of the small newly-arrived larvae in the gums and tongue, although seldom recognised, must nevertheless be detrimental to welfare. Otherwise, stomach bots are rarely responsible for obvious disease despite their size (growing to 2 cm) and rows of hooks (see Figure 2.49). MLs are active against *Gasterophilus* should treatment be required.

Trichostrongylus axei is the only nematode species common to horses and other herbivores. Strains of *T. axei* appear to be host-adapted with only limited cross-infectivity between hosts. In any event, *T. axei* is generally of low pathogenicity in horses, although hyperplastic gastritis can occur.

Similarly, the gastric spiruroid nematodes are only infrequently associated with overt disease. *Habronema* stimulates the production of thick mucus in the stomach while *Draschia* induces the formation of large submucosal granulomas which can occasionally affect the functioning of the pylorus.

Small intestine

Strongyloides infections are generally asymptomatic and high faecal egg-counts can be recorded from healthy foals. Alternative causes of diarrhoea should

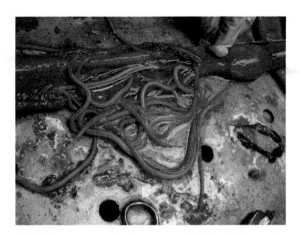

Figure 9.5 *Parascaris*: the small intestine has been opened to display the worms that were within. Reproduced with permission of M.K. Nielsen.

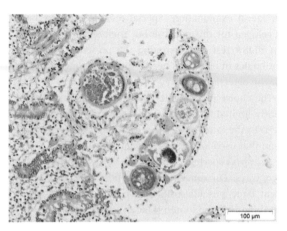

Figure 9.6 *Eimeria leuckarti* macroschizont and gametocytes at the tip of an intestinal villus.

be investigated before *Strongyloides* is judged to be the culprit. *Parascaris* usually does no more than contribute to the 'wormy horse' syndrome although blockage, and even perforation, of the small intestine is possible in heavy infections on account of its impressive size, up to 50 cm long (see Figure 9.5).

The eggs of *Strongyloides* (see Figure 7.2) and *Parascaris* are easily detected and identified in faecal samples, the latter being similar to *Ascaris* eggs (see Figure 8.28). *T. axei* produces typical strongyle ova. These can be differentiated from those of the cyathostomins and *Strongylus* spp. by faecal culture as *T. axei* L$_3$ lack the long filamentous tail characteristic of the others (see Figure 9.1). Spiruroid eggs have a characteristic appearance (see Figure 7.21) but are rarely seen on faecal examination.

Horses have just one significant coccidian species, *E. leuckarti*. This produces large subepithelial gametocytes at the tips of intestinal villi, which become disrupted, stunted and oedematous (see Figure 9.6). The nucleus of the swollen host cell is pushed to one side, giving a 'signet ring' appearance. The clinical significance of *E. leuckarti* infection is uncertain, but it is sometimes associated with intermittent diarrhoea in foals. The oocysts are unlike those of other *Eimeria* species in that they are much larger (80 μm long) and dark brown in colour (see Figure 9.7). They are ovoid with a distinct 'gap' (the micropyle) at the narrow end. *E. leuckarti* is often overlooked in routine diagnosis as the oocysts are heavy structures that do not rise in commonly used flotation fluids.

Caecum and colon

The commonest tapeworm species, *Anoplocephala perfoliata*, clusters around the ileocaecal valve. Although the resulting inflammation and ulceration are not severe, larger numbers (> 20) can sometimes interfere with the coordination of gut motility, thereby predisposing to dysfunctions such as spasmodic colic, ileal impaction and some forms of intussusception.

Diagnosis of tapeworm infection can be problematic as segments and eggs are shed only intermittently. To add to the difficulty, the eggs, although easily recognised by their shape and internal structure (see Figure 5.26), do not float well in the flotation fluids used routinely

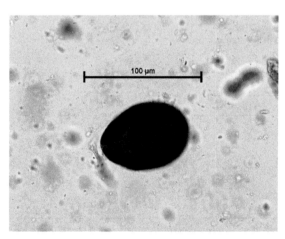

Figure 9.7 *Eimeria leuckarti* oocyst. Reproduced with permission of M.K. Nielsen.

for faecal examination. Special techniques have been developed for this purpose but their sensitivity is low. An ELISA test demonstrating the presence of specific antibodies in blood has been shown to be more reliable for the detection of heavy infection.

The choice of cestocide for tapeworm control is currently limited to praziquantel or pyrantel (see Section 5.5). In the latter case, the required dose-rate is higher than that used for general worm control.

Strongylus species contribute to the 'wormy horse' in two ways. On completing their body migration, they form large pus filled nodules in the gut wall before breaking into the lumen. Like cyathostomins, they are plug feeders but, having much larger buccal cavities, they bite more deeply into the mucosa. They create bleeding ulcers that are large enough to be seen with the naked eye at autopsy. Heavy infestations can cause anaemia.

Liver

In the British Isles and Ireland, the dog-horse strain of *Echinococcus granulosus* is host specific and is not thought to be a zoonotic hazard. Hydatid cysts can grow to the size of a tennis ball in the horse liver. They appear to have no discernible effect on health or welfare and the same applies to the liver nodules associated with migrating larvae of *Strongylus edentatus* and *S. equinus*.

9.1.2 Respiratory and circulatory systems

The lungworm *Dictyocaulus arnfieldi* is the main parasitic problem affecting the respiratory system (see Table 9.2). A nasal discharge may sometimes be observed in young

Table 9.2 Parasitic genera most likely to be encountered in the lung and circulatory system of equidae

	Trematodes	Nematodes	Protozoa
Host: HORSE			
Lung		Dictyocaulus 6.3.5	
		Parascaris 7.1.3	
Circulation	Schistosoma 5.6.3	Strongylus 6.3.3	Trypanosoma 4.5.1
			Babesia 4.8.1

Note: these lists are not comprehensive; other parasites do occur but less frequently or are of more restricted distribution or importance; numbers in red cross-reference to section with more detailed information.

horses on pasture grossly contaminated with embryonated *Parascaris* eggs. This coincides with large numbers of ascarid larvae passing through the lungs. Like *Parascaris*, *Strongylus vulgaris* is a gastrointestinal parasite but it, too, has a place in this section because of the injuries that its migrating larvae cause to the wall of the cranial mesenteric artery. Schistosomosis and trypanosomosis are other parasites associated with the circulatory system but they are not discussed here as major aspects of these diseases were highlighted in Sections 5.6.3 and 8.2.3. Another troublesome condition is equine piroplasmosis, different forms of which are caused by *Babesia caballi* and *B. equi* (although technically, it may be more correct to call the latter *Theileria equi*). Equine piroplasmosis is a major constraint on the international movement of horses for trade and sporting activities.

Lungworm

Horses exposed to *D. arnfieldi* infection often develop a chronic cough. The diagnosis can be difficult to confirm as the causal worms usually succumb to immunity while still immature. If adult worms do establish, mainly in animals younger than 1 year, then embryonated eggs are passed in faeces. These soon hatch, so the Baermann apparatus is used to detect the L_1 which are similar in appearance to those of *D. viviparus* (see Figure 8.11) except that the tail has a small spike. If larvae are not found, endoscopy of the trachea may reveal globules of greenish mucus, while sediment from tracheal washings will contain numerous eosinophils.

In contrast to horses, infected donkeys rarely show clinical signs but often shed eggs (see Table 9.3). They can therefore act as asymptomatic carriers and it is prudent to check that donkeys are free of lungworm before allowing horses onto pastures that they have grazed. The *D. arnfieldi* life-cycle can, however, continue in horses in the absence of donkeys.

Table 9.3 Comparison of *D. arnfieldi* infections in donkeys and horses

	Donkey	Horse
Prevalence	High	Low
Adult worms	Many	Few
Eggs in faeces	Many	Often zero
Patency	> 5 yrs	< 8 months
Clinical signs	Rarely	Sometimes

Verminous endarteritis

Strongylus vulgaris is known to be a significant risk factor in the aetiology of colic in horses as the incidence of this condition often declines when an effective worm control programme is introduced. This correlation is linked to parasite-induced damage to the cranial mesenteric artery which disturbs blood-flow dynamics and predisposes to thrombo-embolism (Figure 6.36). The gross enlargement of the cranial mesenteric artery associated with verminous endarteritis can be detected by rectal palpation. The prevalence of *Strongylus* species has declined markedly in many areas where ML anthelmintics are commonly used for general worm control.

Equine piroplasmosis

Equine piroplasmosis may be acute or chronic. Clinical signs are mostly nonspecific – malaise, inappetence, weight-loss, exercise intolerance – but *Babesia* should be suspected if these are combined with anaemia, jaundice and fever. Death can occur in previously naive animals.

Giemsa-stained blood smears are useful only in acute *B. equi* infections. The complement fixation test (see Section 1.5.2) is widely used in endemic areas but it does not pick up early infections and it may give false negative results for a small proportion of symptomless carrier animals. Consequently, IFAT or ELISA methods are often preferred. The importation of horses into many nonendemic countries is strictly regulated. This is because epidemics could easily occur if infected animals were allowed into regions where the presence of potential tick vectors coexists with a local absence of herd immunity.

Drugs such as imidocarb (see Section 8.2.3) may restore health but often do not completely eliminate the parasite, which can still be taken up by feeding ticks or transferred to other horses via blood transfusions, inadequately sterilised needles, instruments etc. There is currently no vaccine available for equine use.

9.1.3 Integument

Horses at grass in the summer are plagued with a multitude of flies and, to a lesser extent, other types of ectoparasite (see Table 9.4). Still worse hazards exist in warmer climates, e.g. screwworm myiasis and the plethora of arthropods that transmit debilitating or fatal protozoal, bacterial and viral diseases (including African horse sickness).

Table 9.4 Parasitic genera most likely to be encountered on, in or under the skin of horses

Host: **HORSE**			
Ticks	Many including: *Dermacentor* 3.2.2 *Otobius* 3.2.3	Surface mites	*Chorioptes* 3.3.3 Trombiculids 3.3.3
Biting and nuisance flies	Many including: *Culicoides* 2.2.5 Muscids incl. *Stomoxys* 2.2.5 Tabanids 2.2.5 *Hippobosca* 2.2.5	Ear mites	*Psoroptes* 3.3.3
Myiasis flies	*Gasterophilus* (eggs) 2.2.6 *Hypoderma* (aberrant larva) 2.2.6 Screwworms etc. 2.2.6	Subsurface mites	*Demodex* 3.3.2 *Sarcoptes* 3.3.2
Lice	*Bovicola** 2.2.3 *Haematopinus* 2.2.3	Nematodes	*Habronema* 7.1.5 *Parafilaria* 7.1.5 *Onchocerca* 7.1.5 *Oxyuris* (eggs) 7.1.4

Note: these lists are not comprehensive; other parasites do occur but less frequently or are of more restricted distribution or importance; numbers in red cross-reference to section with more detailed information.

* *Bovicola* is also known as *Damalinia*.

Fly worry

Flies can worry horses in a number of ways. The non-biting muscid flies that cluster round the eyes, lips, genitalia and open wounds to sponge-feed on secretions and exudates are an obvious annoyance. They disturb grazing and induce head shaking, tail switching and other protective behaviours. Biting flies inflict different degrees of discomfort. The stabbing action of the stable fly, *Stomoxys*, provokes irritable reactions such as stamping. But most painful are the rasping bites of the tabanids (horse flies). These can elicit sudden alarm that may result in a rider becoming unseated. The simuliids (blackflies) are much smaller but attack in persistent swarms and can cause considerable distress, especially those species that crawl into the nose or ear (see Figure 9.8). All the flies so far mentioned are transient visitors but *Hippobosca*, once it has found a host, adopts a parasitic lifestyle and remains on the thin skin of the upper hindquarters until it is ready to give birth to the fully grown larva it has been nurturing. Other flies feeding on horses include midges, phlebotomine sand-flies and mosquitoes. The bot fly, *Gasterophilus*, does not bite but upsets horses by hovering nearby and darting in to deposit eggs onto hairs.

Many ectoparasites have specific predilection sites (see Figure 9.9). Some species of *Culicoides*, for example, feed along the line of the mane and tail, while other species attack the ventral midline or other parts of the body. As well as the physical damage they cause, biting flies can induce allergic reactions in some horses. Self-trauma may follow and lesions can become secondarily infected and attract myiasis flies such as calliphorine blowflies or screwworms. Flies also transmit skin pathogens such as the nematode parasites *Habronema* and *Parafilaria*.

Equine seasonal allergic dermatitis

This is an intensely pruritic condition that recurs seasonally when certain species of *Culicoides* are biting. It is known by a variety of local names, including 'sweet-itch' in the UK. There is as yet no reliable remedy and painstaking management is required to ameliorate suffering. The disease is confined to individuals that develop hypersensitivity to allergens in midge saliva. There is a hereditary component and some breeds are more susceptible than others.

Lesions occur initially on the skin of the forelock, mane and tail-head (see Figure 9.10), but can progress along the spine and may, in very severe cases, affect other parts of the body surface. The itching provokes vigorous rubbing and hair loss. The skin becomes thickened, corrugated and scaly. There may be secondary infection if the skin becomes broken. The lesions resolve in the winter (or the dry season in the tropics if midges are not biting).

Management of the condition falls into three parts (although desperate owners often attempt alternative strategies that are not evidence-based):

a – Decrease exposure: by stabling affected horses during periods of greatest midge activity, i.e. from late afternoon through early morning. Fine mesh screens may be necessary over ventilation gaps. While grazing, vulnerable parts of the body can be covered with light blankets etc. (see Figure 9.11).

b – Repel midges: insect repellents, such as some pyrethroids, can have beneficial effects if used according to label recommendations, but results are sometimes disappointing.

c – Supportive therapy: aimed at moderating immune responses and promoting healing.

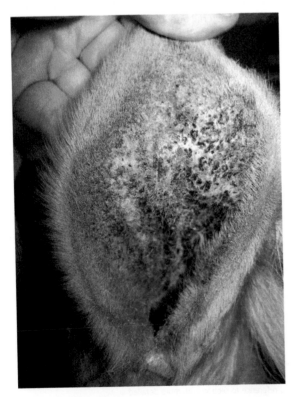

Figure 9.8 Damage in the ear of a horse induced by *Simulium* bites. Reproduced with permission of D.C. Knottenbelt.

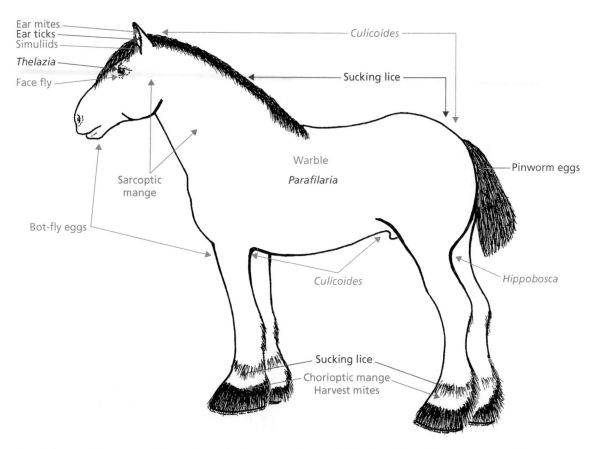

Ear mites
Ear ticks
Simuliids
Thelazia
Face fly

Culicoides

Sucking lice

Sarcoptic
mange

Warble
Parafilaria

Pinworm eggs

Bot-fly eggs

Culicoides

Hippobosca

Sucking lice
Chorioptic mange
Harvest mites

Figure 9.9 Some skin parasites of horses that tend to favour certain parts of the body. Redrawn after Jacobs, 1986 with permission of Elsevier.

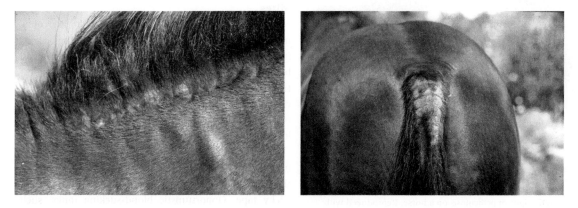

Figure 9.10 Sweet itch lesions on mane (left) and base of tail (right). Reproduced with permission of R. Bond.

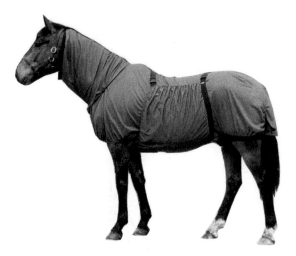

Figure 9.11 Sweet itch: vulnerable horse wearing protective blanket to prevent *Culicoides* bites. Reproduced with permission of E. Greaves.

Lice, mange and ticks

Lice

Louse infestations generally become apparent in winter causing horses to lose their 'bloom'. Hair loss may follow from licking, biting and rubbing (see Figure 9.12). Horses have a sucking louse, which favours areas of the body with long coarse hair, but heavy infestations may spread over the body (see Figure 9.13). There is also a chewing louse which prefers finer hair cover. Lice and their nits (eggs) are not always obvious but can often be found by parting the hair. The chewing louse, however, will try to move out of sight. Nits are

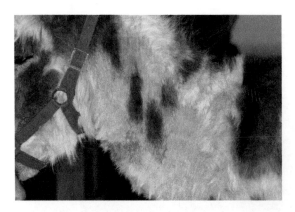

Figure 9.12 Signs of pediculosis on a horse. Reproduced with permission of D.C. Knottenbelt.

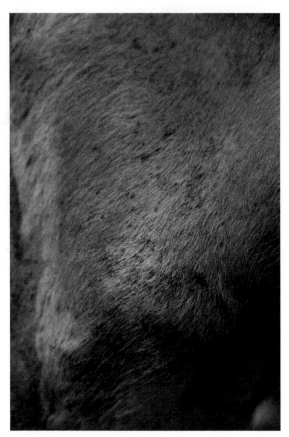

Figure 9.13 Close-up of a horse with a heavy infestation of sucking lice. Reproduced with permission of D.C. Knottenbelt.

cemented onto the hairs (see Figure 2.24) and can be distinguished from bot eggs which are larger and held in place with a clasp.

Mites

Body mange (caused by a *Psoroptes* species) and sarcoptic mange are severe equine conditions but both are becoming rare in the modern world. *Demodex* is uncommon and benign, so leg mange (chorioptic mange) is now the most troublesome mite infestation (see Figure 9.14). Papules, crusty lesions and hair-loss appear on the lower limbs of heavier breeds, particularly if this site is cloaked with long hair ('heavily feathered').

For diagnosis, a wooden spatula is adequate for taking scrapings and is preferred to a scalpel blade (in case the horse kicks). Mites can sometimes be captured on sticky tape. Opportunistic blood-sucking mites, such as the poultry red mite or trombiculid larvae, can also

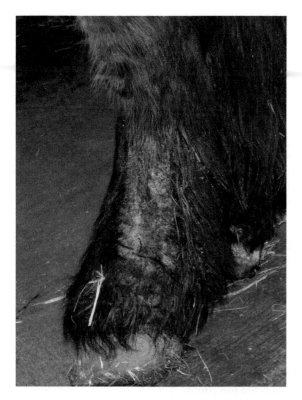

Figure 9.14 Chorioptic mange on the hind leg of a horse. Reproduced with permission of B. Losson

be detected in this way. Finally in this category, horses occasionally become infested with the rabbit ear-mite (a *Psoroptes* species) which induces head-shaking.

Ticks

Of the many ticks that bite horses, the tropical horse tick, *Dermacentor nitens*, is of particular note as the vector of equine piroplasmosis in the Americas. It attacks the ears, as does the spinose ear tick, *Otobius*, which is confined to hot, dry climatic regions. The latter can cause considerable damage to the aural canal and eardrum of horses and other animals. Early infestations are easily overlooked as *Otobius* larvae are small and move deep into the ear, which can later become blocked by engorging ticks and waxy exudate. Secondary infection and myiasis flies can complicate the condition. *Otobius* eggs are deposited in crevices in stable buildings where hatched larvae can survive for more than two years. Foals are susceptible to paralytic toxins in the saliva of some ticks, including *Ixodes holocyclus* in Australia.

Nematode conditions

The most common filarial infection of horses is *Onchocerca*. The adults live in connective tissues including tendons and ligaments where they provoke painless swellings. Their microfilariae congregate in subdermal tissues along the ventral abdominal mid-line, which is the predilection site for the intermediate host, *Culicoides* (a different species from those causing sweet-itch). This is usually without detriment, although there may be some local dermatitis. Abdominal oedema develops occasionally when ML anthelmintics are used for general worm control (presumably due to a sudden release of antigen from dead microfilariae).

Although not endemic in the USA or western European countries, parafilariosis does occur sporadically in horses that have been imported during the winter (when the subcutaneous lesions are least obvious). In the summer, the parasitic nodules start to ooze blood to attract muscid flies. These act as intermediate hosts for the causal filarial worm.

Broken hairs and alopecia at the base of the tail may indicate sweet itch hypersensitivity, pediculosis or it could be due to the presence of pinworm (*Oxyuris*). Large clusters of eggs on the perineal skin appear as greyish streaks. Infection is common but usually inapparent. *Oxyuris* egg masses can be washed off the skin with a cloth (which should then be destroyed).

Practical tip box 9.1

Diagnosis of 'Seat-itch'

Pinworm eggs are about the same size as strongyle eggs but differ in appearance as they are flattened on one side and have an operculum (see Figure 7.17). As they are stuck to the perineal skin, they are unlikely to be found in faecal samples. If a pinworm infection is suspected, a piece of transparent adhesive tape (e.g. Sellotape or Scotch tape) is applied to the skin around the anus, pulled off and stuck onto a slide for microscopic examination. Take care – the condition causes pruritus, so the horse may be irritable.

Avoid common mistakes!

Don't confuse 'seat itch' (anal pruritus caused by pinworm infection) with 'sweet itch' (hypersensitivity reaction to midge bites).

Cutaneous and ocular habronemosis

Although only sporadic in occurrence, cases of cutaneous habronemosis in horses are difficult to manage. Infective

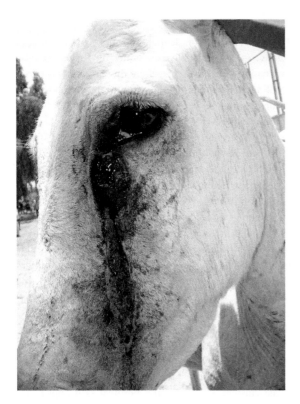

Figure 9.15 A case of cutaneous habronemosis. Reproduced with permission of D.C. Knottenbelt.

larvae of *Habronema* or *Draschia* after deposition by feeding muscids can survive in an open wound for prolonged periods. Their presence prevents the wound from healing (see Figure 9.15). As this condition is initiated by fly activity, it is seasonal in occurrence and known as 'summer sores'. Larvae deposited around the eye can cause a swelling of the third eyelid or median canthus. Diagnosis is based on history and appearance, but biopsy may be necessary to exclude other possible causes.

9.1.4 Other body systems

Just three parasites come under the spotlight in this category (see Table 9.5). The prevalence of the eyeworm, *Thelazia*, is quite high in many areas but, as with the corresponding conditions in cattle and dogs, clinical signs are usually minimal. Dourine, caused by *Trypanosoma equiperdum*, was once widespread but has been eradicated from some countries, including the USA and most of Europe, while equine protozoal myeloencephalitis, caused by *Sarcocystis neurona*, is an emerging disease in the Americas.

Table 9.5 Parasitic genera most likely to be encountered in other body systems of horses

	Urogenital	CNS	Eye
Host: HORSE			
Nematodes			*Thelazia* 7.1.5
Protozoa	*Trypanosoma* 4.5.1	*Sarcocystis* 4.7.1	

Note: these lists are not comprehensive; other parasites do occur but less frequently or are of more restricted distribution or importance; numbers in red cross-reference to section with more detailed information.

Dourine

Dourine is a venereal disease important as a serious equine welfare issue. It is also capable of disrupting breeding programmes. It is highly contagious. Treated horses or those in remission can act as symptomless carriers, as can male donkeys. Seropositive animals, therefore, should not be used for breeding. Countries that are free from the disease have strict regulations governing importation and suspected infections.

Clinical signs are nonspecific and highly variable depending on the virulence of the strain, the condition of the horse and stress factors. The only pathognomonic sign is the presence of raised 2–10 cm diameter plaques on the skin (see Figure 9.16), but these

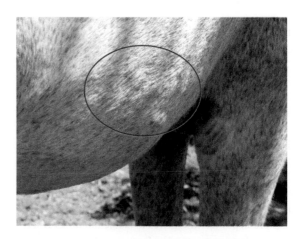

Figure 9.16 Dourine: skin plaques (circled). Reproduced with permission of Istituto Zooprofilattico Sperimentale dell'Abruzzo e del Molise 'G. Caporale', Teramo, Italy.

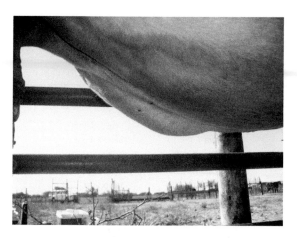

Figure 9.17 Dourine: ventral oedema. Reproduced with permission of Istituto Zooprofilattico Sperimentale dell'Abruzzo e del Molise 'G. Caporale', Teramo, Italy.

are transitory and do not always occur. Oedema of the genitalia spreads to the ventral abdomen and mammary gland or scrotum (see Figure 9.17). This may be followed by conjunctivitis, facial paralysis, progressive weakness, emaciation, incoordination and death (see Figure 9.18).

Serology is used for diagnosis as demonstration of the parasite is extremely difficult. The most widely used method is the complement fixation test although false positives may occasionally occur. In endemic areas, dourine is controlled by using artificial insemination or by ensuring that only seronegative animals are used

for breeding. If a case is suspected all venereal contacts must be traced and isolated until their infection-status can be determined.

Equine protozoal myeloencephalitis

EPM is confined to the Americas where it is the most commonly diagnosed neurological condition of horses. Cases are sporadic but appear to be increasing in frequency. It is a necrotising encephalomyelitis affecting both grey and white matter in the CNS. It leads to a slowly progressive condition. The first sign is often stumbling or an abnormal gait, sometimes accompanied by head-tilt, depression or difficulty in swallowing.

Diagnosis is largely dependent on neurological examination supported by complement fixation and immuno-blotting tests (see Section 1.5.2). Horses can be seropositive without showing any sign of disease. Long-term sulphonamide treatments (see Section 4.10.2) have been employed with moderate success and newer anticoccidials are being evaluated. Advice on prevention is currently incomplete as the risk factors associated with the disease are as yet poorly understood. The final host is the opossum and so contamination of horse feed with their faeces should be prevented wherever this is feasible.

9.2 Small animal parasitology

Parasitic problems in farm livestock, and to a lesser extent equine species, are regarded as herd problems, but small animal practice focuses on the individual animal. Although rabbits, ferrets, reptiles and more unusual creatures are increasing in popularity, dogs and cats still predominate and provide the basis for most of the illustrative examples in this section.

Increasing human mobility, global trade and more relaxed quarantine restrictions have substantially increased the risk of diseases occurring outside their normal endemic range. For example, canine babesiosis and canine heartworm disease are now diagnosed regularly in the UK, even though transmission is not as yet known to occur locally.

9.2.1 Digestive system

Diarrhoea is the most frequent parasite-related digestive condition in small animals, although some of the parasites listed in Table 9.6 can cause other signs such as vomiting, haemorrhage, blockage and intussusception.

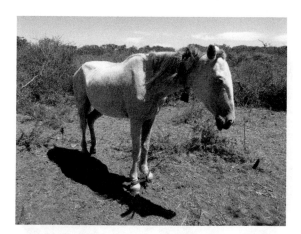

Figure 9.18 Dourine: a chronic case with paralysis of the lower lip. Reproduced with permission of Istituto Zooprofilattico Sperimentale dell'Abruzzo e del Molise 'G. Caporale', Teramo, Italy.

Table 9.6 Parasitic genera most likely to be encountered in the gastrointestinal tract and liver of dogs and cats

	Cestodes	Trematodes	Nematodes	Protozoa
Host: DOG				
Oesophagus			*Spirocerca* 7.1.5	
Stomach			*Spirocerca* 7.1.5	
			Spiruroids 7.1.5	
Small intestine	*Echinococcus* 5.3.4	*Alaria* 5.6.3	*Toxocara* 7.1.3	*Giardia* 4.5.2
	Taenia 5.3.3	*Nanophyetus* 5.6.3	*Toxascaris* 7.1.3	*Isospora* 4.6.1
	Dipylidium 5.3.5	etc.	*Ancylostoma* 6.3.4	*Cryptosporidium* 4.9.1
	Spirometra 5.4.2		*Uncinaria* 6.3.4	*Sarcocystis* 4.7.1
			Strongyloides 7.1.2	*Neospora* 4.7.4
Caecum			*Trichuris* 7.1.6	
Liver			*Capillaria* 7.1.6	*Leishmania* 4.5.1
Host: CAT				
Small intestine	*Taenia* 5.3.3	*Alaria* 5.6.3	*Toxocara* 7.1.3	*Giardia* 4.5.2
	Dipylidium 5.3.5	*Nanophyetus* 5.6.3	*Toxascaris* 7.1.3	*Isospora* 4.6.1
	Spirometra 5.4.2	etc.	*Ancylostoma* 6.3.4	*Cryptosporidium* 4.9.1
				Toxoplasma 4.7.3
				Sarcocystis 4.7.1
Liver			*Capillaria* 7.1.6	

Note: these lists are not comprehensive; other parasites do occur but less frequently or are of more restricted distribution or importance; numbers in red cross-reference to section with more detailed information.

Intestinal infections, such as *Toxoplasma, Neospora* and *Sarcocystis* are unlikely to cause alimentary problems but, by shedding oocysts into the environment, they play an important role in the epidemiology of disease in other hosts or organ systems.

Spirocercosis

Dogs will, if opportunity arises, eat beetles and small vertebrates. In tropical and subtropic climates, some of these act as intermediate and paratenic hosts for *Spirocerca lupi* (see Figure 7.23). Infection is therefore common but fortunately mostly asymptomatic. Large oesophageal lesions (see Figure 9.19) may hinder the passage of food or induce persistent vomiting. Red 3–8 cm long worms are sometimes regurgitated. Faecal egg-counts are of limited value as *S. lupi* eggs are not passed in the early developmental stages of the disease and, in any event, are similar to those of the stomach spiruroids. Endoscopy or radiography, possibly aided by a barium meal, may confirm diagnosis. Neoplastic transformation of the lesion or sudden death due to rupture of an aortic aneurism are occasional sequelae.

Toxocarosis

Heavy infestations of *Toxocara canis* can easily accrue in young puppies if appropriate precautions are not taken. Most of the worms will have been derived from the dam by transplacental transfer (see Figure 7.9). Affected puppies fail to thrive, have a dull coat and a distended

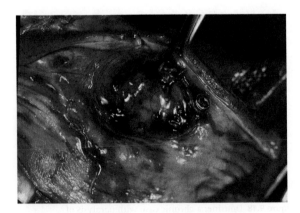

Figure 9.19 Dog with spirocercosis: oesophagus opened to show adult worms and nodular lesion. Reproduced with permission of R.C.Krecek and K. Snowden.

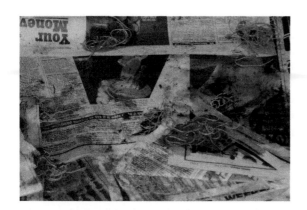

Figure 9.20 *Toxocara canis* expelled by a puppy in faeces. Reproduced with permission of J. Bowman and A. Gray.

abdomen ('pot-belly'). They may have diarrhoea and ascarid worms are often seen in faeces or vomit (see Figure 9.20). More serious signs of intestinal dysfunction may occur in severe cases. Respiratory signs and nasal discharge are indicative of continuing larval migration. Faecal examination will register high egg-counts after the pups are about two weeks of age. The adult worm population is expelled spontaneously after about six weeks but in the meantime growth and development can be affected, with stunting or even death in the worst cases.

Although disease can be prevented by using a single anthelmintic treatment prior to the expected onset of clinical signs, this empirical approach does little to reduce the overall faecal egg-output of an infected litter. There are several reasons for this:

a – large numbers of eggs can be shed before infection becomes obvious;

b – reinfection occurs during suckling and later by ingestion of embryonated eggs from the environment;

c – few canine anthelmintics kill ascarid life-cycle stages migrating through the body at the time of treatment.

If egg-production is not eliminated completely, environmental contamination will continue and bitches will accumulate more somatic larvae. The clinical problem is thereby perpetuated for future litters. To break this cycle, a routine worming programme must be initiated when puppies are two weeks old with treatments repeated every two weeks. A longer dosing interval is possible if the chosen anthelmintic has good activity against migrating larvae. Nursing bitches should also be

treated. This is because a relaxation of their immunity at this time sometimes allows the establishment of *T. canis* in the intestine. A scrupulous level of kennel hygiene is needed. This is particularly important as few commonly used disinfectants are capable of killing the thick-walled *Toxocara* eggs.

Transmission of *T. cati* from the queen to her offspring occurs only via the transmammary route and so associated events occur rather later in the life of kittens than they do in puppies.

Toxocara is not usually a clinical issue in older dogs as adult worm burdens are generally small or absent. Nevertheless, eggs shed by dogs with patent infections into gardens and public places can constitute a potential zoonotic hazard (see Section 9.3.2). Adult dogs should therefore be wormed if they have positive egg-counts. At the time of writing, no routine treatments are licensed for killing somatic larvae in bitches and special anthelmintic therapies (e.g. multidose fenbendazole) are required to prevent transplacental and transmammary transmission.

Other helminth infections

Hookworms and whipworms

Diarrhoea during puppyhood in warmer regions can be due to *Ancylostoma caninum* acquired via the transmammary route. Both larvae and adults are avid blood-suckers so profound anaemia is a prominent presenting sign and usually the cause of death when it occurs. Other hookworms, such as *A. braziliense* and *Uncinaria* in dogs and *A. tubaeforme* in cats, are less pathogenic. They are not transferred in milk and so tend to occur most frequently in adolescent animals. An effective attenuated vaccine was developed against *A. caninum* but it was not a commercial success and is no longer available.

Trichuris vulpis can cause bloody diarrhoea, especially in warmer climates where the long-lived eggs are more likely to embryonate and accumulate. Dogs of any age with access to contaminated soil may be affected. Infection can easily be overlooked as the eggs do not always float well in routine faecal examinations. Not all canine anthelmintics are effective against whipworm infections.

Tapeworms

Although tapeworm infections can cause digestive upset and provoke pruritus in the perineal region, they are usually relatively innocuous. Of greater importance is

Table 9.7 Relative activity of some anthelmintics used for tapeworm control in dogs

	Dipylidium	Taenia	Echinococcus Adult	Immature
Praziquantel	+++	+++	+++	+++
Fenbendazole	–	+++	–	–
Dichlorophen	++	++	–	–
Niclosamide	+	++	–	–
Nitroscanate	+++	+++	++	–

the role that infected dogs play in the epidemiology of conditions associated with the establishment of metacestodes in intermediate hosts (e.g. hydatidosis). When selecting a cestocidal treatment for dogs or cats, it has to be remembered that few anthelmintics expel all tapeworm genera (see Table 9.7).

Protozoan infections

A number of protozoan infections can cause diarrhoea, especially in younger animals, but *Giardia* is probably the commonest of these. It is also the most difficult to diagnose. Trophozoites and cysts are shed intermittently and so repeat faecal samples over 3–5 days increase chances of detection. Microscopy requires patience as the organisms are often few in number. They are also

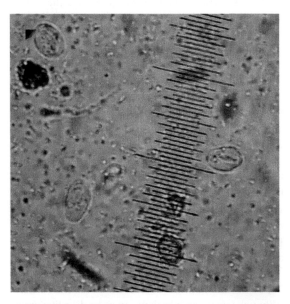

Figure 9.21 *Giardia* cysts in faecal preparation. (Scale: 1 large division = approx. 20 μm.) Reproduced with permission of T. Geurden and E. Claerebout.

small (see Figure 9.21) and easily confused with pollen grains and yeasts. The cysts are relatively heavy objects and so concentration techniques using high density flotation fluids have to be employed (although sugar solutions are not appropriate as they cause *Giardia* to collapse). Commercially available coproantigen tests are easier to use and generally reliable. Some BZD compounds are effective against this protozoan and provide an alternative to the older drugs used for this purpose. Although many routes of infection exist, contaminated water is a common source.

Cryptosporidium oocysts are even smaller than *Giardia*, but are often present in large numbers in clinically affected animals. They show up clearly on Ziehl-Neelsen stained faecal smears (see Figure 8.5) and immunodiagnostic tests are also available. There is still no completely effective treatment and so reliance has to be placed on strict hygiene and supportive therapy.

Dogs and cats can each harbour several host specific *Isospora* species. High oocyst counts often occur in apparently healthy animals and so the pathogenicity of these infections is uncertain. *Isospora* oocysts at 20–40 μm, are much larger than those of the tissue cyst-forming coccidia that also occur in canine and feline faeces.

9.2.2 Respiratory and circulatory systems

While lungworms can be troublesome in some localities, canine heartworm disease and canine babesiosis are major veterinary problems affecting many warmer regions. Dogs may sometimes become infected with fox lungworms such as *Crenosoma* (see Table 9.8).

Lungworms

The presence of *Oslerus* nodules close to the bifurcation of the trachea in dogs may provoke a chronic dry cough which can be stimulated by gently pinching the throat. Eggs and larvae can sometimes be found in sputum (see Figure 9.22) or larvae in faeces, but they are often few in number and difficult to recover. In such cases, diagnosis is best confirmed by endoscopy. Transmission occurs directly from dam to pup and clinical cases are therefore often linked to particular breeding kennels. *Aelurostrongylus* is rarely a problem in cats unless there is an underlying immunodeficiency.

Angiostrongylosis

Although commonly known as the canine lungworm, *Angiostrongylus vasorum* actually resides in the pulmonary

Table 9.8 Parasitic genera most likely to be encountered in the respiratory and circulatory systems of dogs and cats

	Trachea/bronchi	Lung	Pulmonary arteries and heart	Blood
Host: DOG				
Nematodes	*Oslerus (Filaroides)* 6.3.5	*Capillaria* 7.1.6	*Angiostrongylus* 6.3.5	*Dirofilaria* (mf*) 7.1.5
		Crenosoma	*Dirofilaria* 7.1.5	
Protozoa				*Babesia* 4.8.1
Host: CAT				
Nematodes		*Aelurostrongylus* 6.3.5	*Dirofilaria* 7.1.5	

Note: these lists are not comprehensive; other parasites do occur but less frequently or are of more restricted distribution or importance; numbers in red cross-reference to section with more detailed information.

* mf = microfilariae.

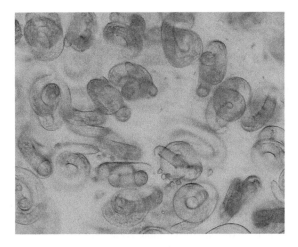

Figure 9.22 Unhatched *Oslerus* eggs recovered by tracheal lavage. Reproduced with permission of J.W. McGarry.

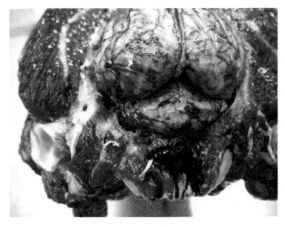

Figure 9.23 Angiostrongylosis: head of dog dissected to show large haemorrhage in spinal canal (at base of brain). Reproduced with permission of B. Smyth.

artery and right side of the heart. The alternative name of 'French heartworm' is perhaps more accurate but leads to confusion with canine heartworm disease caused by *Dirofilaria immitis*. Use of the technical term, angiostrongylosis is therefore preferable.

Clinical presentation is very variable as there are at least two disease processes developing simultaneously:

a – Release of anticoagulant factors: These worm secretions make affected dogs prone to bruising and internal haemorrhage. Clinical consequences will, of course, depend on where the internal bleeding occurs but include subcutaneous haematoma and epistaxis (nose-bleed). Neurological signs result if there is haemorrhage into the brain or spinal cord (see Figure 9.23).

b – Lung damage: A microinjury is caused every time an *A. vasorum* egg is caught in a lung capillary and the hatched larva migrates to the air passages. Damage accumulates leading eventually to exercise intolerance and coughing, followed by lethargy, weakness, dyspnoea and, in extreme cases, right-sided heart failure.

The highly motile first-stage larvae are usually easy to find in the faeces of infected dogs (see Figure 9.24) but cases can be missed. Earlier efforts to develop an immunological test were thwarted by cross-reactions with other pathogens, but recent developments suggest that a more reliable test may soon become available. Haematology will often show a thrombocytopaenia (reduced platelet count), prolonged clotting times and sometimes anaemia.

Historically, angiostrongylosis was confined to defined endemic areas, but the condition is spreading as dogs travel greater distances with their owners. Control is difficult as foxes act as a reservoir host and the molluscan

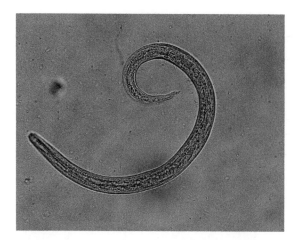

Figure 9.24 *Angiostrongylus vasorum*: first stage larva (L₁) recovered from faeces. Reproduced with permission of J.W. McGarry.

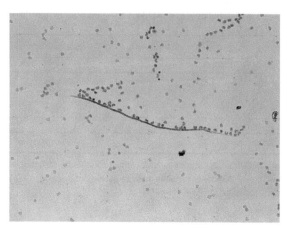

Figure 9.25 Knott's test: stained microfilaria of *Dirofilaria immitis*. (White blood cells also present but no RBCs as these have been lysed.)

intermediate hosts are plentiful in all but the driest localities. Moxidectin is effective against larval and adult *A. vasorum* and can be used to protect dogs at high risk.

Canine heartworm disease

Like *A. vasorum*, *D. immitis* lives in the pulmonary artery and right side of the heart. It is a much bigger worm and its pathogenesis is even more complex (see Section 7.1.5). Canine heartworm disease (HWD) can appear in a number of different forms including:

a – acute prepatent HWD: immature worms in pulmonary arteries induce coughing, seen mainly on exercise;

b – chronic HWD: accumulating lung damage and the consequent onset of heart failure produces progressive exercise intolerance or fainting, sometimes with ascites and other signs of multiple organ dysfunction;

c – acute caval syndrome: venous stagnation in the right side of the heart can lead to hepatic failure and sudden collapse accompanied by increased erythrocyte fragility, haemolytic anaemia and haemoglobinuria.

Thus the clinical signs of HWD are variable and non-pathognomonic, thereby presenting a diagnostic challenge to the veterinarian. Consequently, clinical judgment has to be supported by reliable laboratory back-up together with an appreciation of the strengths and limitations of each diagnostic test (see Section 1.5.3).

In some parts of the world, diagnosis is still dependent on parasite detection. This can be achieved by finding

motile microfilariae (mf) during microscopic examination of a wet blood film. Greater sensitivity can be obtained by forcing blood through a micropore filter to capture the mf, which can then be fixed and stained. Alternatively, the RBCs can be lysed with 2% formalin and the mf (see Figure 9.25) concentrated by centrifugation – this is known as Knott's test. Whichever method is used the mf of *D. immitis* have to be distinguished from those of less pathogenic filarial parasites such as *Dipetalonema* (see Table 9.9).

Experience in endemic areas shows that mf cannot be demonstrated in the blood of up to 40% of infected dogs. This happens if:

a – infection comprises only immature worms: therefore, no mf-producing females;

b – only one adult worm present: so fertilisation cannot take place;

Table 9.9 Diagnostic characteristics of *D. immitis* microfilariae

	D. immitis	*Dipetalonema*
Behaviour in wet blood film	Motile but stays in same place	Swims through blood
Shape in dried, fixed blood film	Body slightly curved along whole length	Posterior body strongly curved ('hooked')
Length in dried, fixed blood film*	At least 315 µm	Up to 290 µm

* Exact length may be influenced by fixation method.

c – adult worms all the same sex: again, fertilisation cannot occur;

d – mf succumbing to immune attack: this happens in about 15% of infected dogs;

e – inadequate chemotherapy: this can sterilise female worms without killing them.

Consequently, other approaches such as immuno-diagnostic techniques are preferred where they are available and affordable. There are a number of commercial kits employing different methodologies (see Figure 9.26). Antigen-detection is generally the most reliable as antibody-detection systems sometimes give false positives. Even so, heartworm antigen tests will not give an accurate result on every occasion as they are based on a glycoprotein originating from the female reproductive tract. Hence they will not detect all-male infections, nor will they pick up immature infections until about one month prior to patency. This antigen also lingers in the blood for some 10–12 weeks after worms have been expelled by chemotherapy.

Treatment can be hazardous as dying worms up to 30 cm long will be swept into the lungs and trapped as emboli (see Figure 9.27). This can cause coughing, haemoptysis (expectorating blood) and an exacerbation of cardiac and pulmonary signs. This can be serious or fatal in a dog already weakened by its clinical condition. A comprehensive physical examination, radiography (see

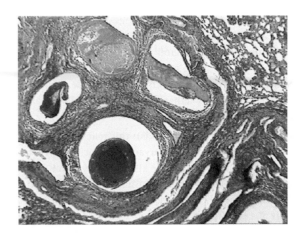

Figure 9.27 Canine heartworm disease: a large thrombus formed by dying worms within a pulmonary artery. Reproduced with permission of L.H. Kramer.

Figure 9.28), echocardiology, an electrocardiogram and a full clinical pathology profile are therefore required to establish the degree of heart failure and organ dysfunction. This will determine the treatment strategy (e.g. whether hospitalisation is necessary) and prognosis. Symptomatic supportive therapy is essential in advanced cases.

The use of chemotherapeutic drugs in HWD has three distinct objectives requiring different approaches, although these can be combined in some cases:

a – Adulticidal: drugs are used to kill adult worms slowly. In this way, the body is able to deal with the pulmonary emboli one by one, increasing the chances of a favourable outcome.

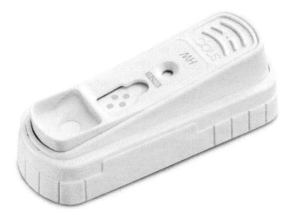

Figure 9.26 An example of a heartworm immunodiagnostic test kit: a prepared blood sample is placed in the well (left). The blue spots in the centre 'results window' represent positive and negative controls together with low and high heartworm antigen level indicators. These change colour if the corresponding reaction occurs. Reproduced with permission of IDEXX Laboratories Europe BV.

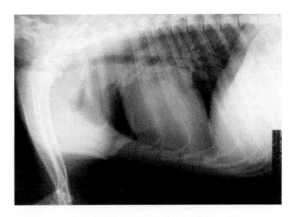

Figure 9.28 Canine heartworm disease: radiograph showing enlarged main pulmonary artery and perivascular inflammation in lungs. Reproduced with permission of L.H. Kramer.

b – Microfilaricidal: not all drugs are active against both adults and mf. It may be an advantage in some circumstances to delay microfilaricidal treatment until the risk of embolism from adulticidal therapy has receded. Some dogs develop a hypersensitivity to dead microfilariae indicated by lethargy, retching, tachycardia and circulatory collapse.

c – Prevention (prophylaxis): this relies on the fact that migrating *D. immitis* larvae are very sensitive to ML anthelmintics and can be killed by very small doses given at appropriate intervals (usually monthly). Microfilaraemic dogs should be cleared of infection before the start of a prophylactic programme.

It can be appreciated from the preceding paragraphs that the treatment and prevention of HWD is a complex topic and sophisticated protocols have been developed to assist veterinarians. These, however, are the domain of specialist texts on veterinary cardiology.

Extra information box 9.1

Heartworm treatments

The developmental stages of *D. immitis* vary in their susceptibility to chemotherapy and so different anthelmintics or different dose-rates are required for each treatment objective.

Adulticides: Adult *D. immitis* are difficult to kill and an arsenical drug (melarsamine) is still used for this purpose. It is potentially toxic and so label instructions should be followed exactly. Ivermectin has no immediate effect on adult *D. immitis*, but monthly treatments at an appropriate dosage rate will cause their eventual demise, although this may take 24 months. A concern with the widespread use of any such long-term treatment is possible induction of anthelmintic resistance in local parasite populations, although few cases have been reported at the time of writing. Recent research has indicated a possibility that anthelmintic therapy could be synergised by antibiotics that kill bacterial symbionts (*Wohlbachia*) in the tissues of *D. immitis*.

Microfilaricides: Milbemycin oxime and some other MLs are effective and safer to use than diethylcarbamazine, which was formerly the drug of choice.

Prevention: Monthly dosing during the mosquito season with ivermectin or some other MLs gives virtually 100% protection from HWD at doses too low for there to be any risk of canine toxicity (Section 7.3.2). Moxidectin can achieve a similar result when administered at six-monthly intervals. Successful prophylaxis does, however, depend on a high level of owner compliance.

Heartworm in cats and ferrets

Cats and pet ferrets can both become infected with *D. immitis* although they are not natural hosts. Few worms establish and these produce only small numbers of mf over a short period. Consequently, and in contrast to canine practice, diagnostic tests employing antibody-detection are more useful than antigen-recognition methods. Echocardiography can be useful for diagnosing infection in cats. Coughing can result from lung pathology similar to that in the dog and just one displaced adult can give rise to an acute crisis or fatal embolism. Adulticidal treatments can therefore be risky.

Canine babesiosis

The impact of babesiosis on dogs depends on their immunity, which is often incomplete, and the *Babesia* species and strain. There is much antigenic variation and strains vary in virulence. The main presenting signs are those associated with intra- and extravascular haemolysis including fever, pallor, jaundice, splenomegaly, weakness and collapse. More virulent infections may involve neurological disturbances and organ damage.

The parasites are intraerythrocytic and usually relatively easy to find in blood smears from acute infections. Samples are best taken from a capillary bed such as the tip of the ear. Parasitized RBCs are most plentiful just below the buffy coat in a haematocrit tube after centrifugation. Differentiation into 'large' and 'small' morphological types (see Figure 4.42) is straightforward and necessary for the selection of appropriate chemotherapy, but confirmation of species identification needs DNA technology. If no parasites are found, serological techniques, such as IFAT and ELISA, may sometimes aid diagnosis but, in endemic areas, most dogs will show evidence of prior exposure.

Treatment options are limited and vary with locality depending on the *Babesia* species and local regulations. The best method of prophylaxis is to protect dogs from the tick vector and, if this is impractical, to remove attached ticks as quickly as possible (since there is a delay of 2–3 days between attachment and transmission). A vaccine providing partial protection against *B. canis* is available in some countries.

9.2.3 Integument

Pets, like other animals, are subject to the irritation and annoyance associated with a variety of visiting arthropods including flies, ticks, harvest mites etc. Some of these transmit vector-borne diseases (e.g. Lyme disease carried by some ticks). Fleas, lice, burrowing and ear mites have a more intimate relationship with their host and are often associated with dermatological problems. Cutaneous myiasis can also occur, although the flies responsible for this condition prefer animals with denser coats, such as rabbits.

Not all integumentary parasites are arthropods (see Table 9.10). A protozoan infection, leishmaniosis, is clinically challenging and has serious animal welfare and zoonotic implications. There are also several filarial worms which are minor pathogens but their presence can complicate the diagnosis of canine heartworm disease.

Flea infestations

Fleas can invoke a spectrum of effects ranging from minor irritation through to flea allergic dermatitis (FAD) characterised by severe pruritus, hair-loss from excessive licking, extensive papular lesions (usually with overlying crusting) and, in cats, miliary dermatitis.

Table 9.10 Parasitic genera most likely to be encountered on, in or under the skin of dogs and cats

Host:	**DOG**	**CAT**
Ticks / biting flies	many	many
Lice	*Trichodectes* 2.2.3 *Linognathus* 2.2.3	*Felicola* 2.2.3
Fleas	*Ctenocephalides* etc. 2.2.2	*Ctenocephalides* etc. 2.2.2
Surface mites	*Cheyletiella* 3.3.3 *Neotrombicula* etc. 3.3.3	*Cheyletiella* 3.3.3 *Neotrombicula* etc. 3.3.3
Ear mites	*Otodectes* 3.3.3	*Otodectes* 3.3.3
Subsurface mites	*Sarcoptes* 3.3.2 *Demodex* 3.3.2	*Notoedres* 3.3.2 *Demodex* 3.3.2
Myiasis flies	Screwworms etc. 2.2.6	Screwworms etc. 2.2.6
Protozoa	*Leishmania* 4.5.1; 9.3.2	*Leishmania* 4.5.1
Helminths	*Dipetalonema* etc. 7.1.5	

Note: these lists are not comprehensive; other parasites do occur but less frequently or are of more restricted distribution or importance; numbers in red cross-reference to section with more detailed information.

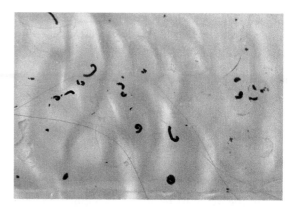

Figure 9.29 Flea faeces brushed from the coat of an infested animal. Reproduced with permission of L. Cornegliani.

Flea infestations are not always obvious unless large numbers of parasites are present. Running a fine-toothed comb (as used for hair-lice in children) vigorously through the animal's coat is a good way of trapping fleas, but they move fast and are good at hiding. So, light infestations are easily missed. If no fleas are caught, the animal may be brushed and any dislodged debris examined for eggs and flea dirt (see Figure 9.29). If there is any doubt, brushings can placed onto wet filter paper or similar substrate. A red stain appears if flea dirt is present (see Figure 9.30).

Fleas can be difficult to control and success depends on having clear treatment objectives appropriate to the circumstances of each case. A clinical scenario in which fleas are just a nuisance is much easier to deal with than the management of an FAD patient. In the former case, flea numbers need only be suppressed to a tolerable level but to protect a hypersensitive pet the aim has to be to stop flea-bites from occurring altogether.

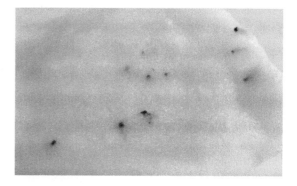

Figure 9.30 Red stains left by flea dirt on a wet substrate. Reproduced with permission of L. Cornegliani.

From a veterinary perspective it is natural to focus on the patient when confronted with disease, but this ignores the fact that the fleas on the animal are only a tiny proportion of the total population. The vast majority are developing forms and newly-emerged host-seeking adults in the household environment. Thus, single or occasional animal treatments will give no more than temporary respite as reinfestation will quickly occur. Control strategies have to eliminate the domestic reservoir of off-host life-cycle stages.

Effective flea control is a three stage process:

a – Rid the pet of its resident flea population: this provides immediate relief from discomfort and aids the resolution of skin lesions due to self-trauma or allergy.

b – Protect the pet from reinfestation, originating:

i) within the home – eggs deposited before the start of the control programme will give rise to new host-seeking fleas for a period of weeks or months;

ii) from external sources – e.g. fleas picked up when visiting other contaminated places; or originating from untreated visiting pets or wild animals that drop eggs in the house or garden.

c – Eliminate the domestic reservoir of infestation: This can be approached in two ways:

i) by directly treating flea-development 'hotspots' in the home, outbuildings and garden with insecticides, suitable inorganic compounds or insect growth regulators (see Sections 3.5.2 and 3.5.3), or, if available, entomophagous nematodes (see Section 1.6.6);

ii) by treating all animals in the household at appropriate intervals with persistent insecticides or IGRs, thereby stopping the deposition of eggs or preventing the subsequent development of larvae. By doing this, the environmental reservoir becomes progressively depleted and the domestic flea population is driven towards extinction (a process that usually takes about 2–3 months).

Historically, flea populations have developed resistance to several insecticidal classes and, to avoid this happening with currently effective treatments, control programmes should not depend on the use of a single chemical group for prolonged periods (see Section 1.6.3).

The importance of removing as many flea eggs as possible from the domestic environment by regular and vigorous vacuum cleaning, laundering pet's blankets etc., should be self-evident.

Mites and lice

Sarcoptic mange

Sarcoptic mange is a common condition in dogs worldwide. It is highly contagious, so single cases are unlikely in kennels. A particularly virulent strain may sometimes be acquired from foxes. The burrowing activity of the mites and the antigenic substances in their saliva and faeces cause intense pruritus. Gentle stroking of an ear will generally cause a back leg to make involuntary scratching movements (the 'pinna-pedal reflex'). Lesions include papules, erythema, scaling and alopecia. The edges of the ears are most commonly affected, followed by the muzzle, face, hock and elbows (see Figure 9.31). In neglected cases, the condition may become generalised with thickening of the skin, crusting and emaciation. The owners of infected dogs may themselves sometimes exhibit papular or more chronic lesions.

Confirmation of diagnosis is usually obtained by the microscopic examination of material collected from the edge of lesions (see Figure 9.32). The mites can be very few in number, so multiple samples may be required. As sarcoptic mites are mostly buried within the stratum corneum, it is necessary to scrape the skin lightly with a scalpel blade until capillary blood starts to ooze out. Collected material can be viewed directly in liquid paraffin on a glass slide or, more satisfactorily, after the skin debris has been dissolved in a few drops of 10%

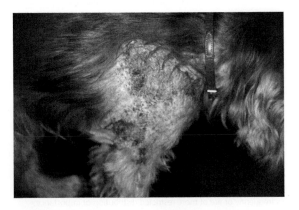

Figure 9.31 Dog suffering from sarcoptic mange. Reproduced with permission of R. Bond.

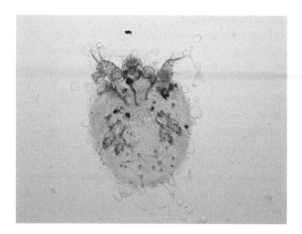

Figure 9.32 *Sarcoptes* mange mite recovered from skin scrape.

potassium hydroxide solution (caution – also corrosive to living animal and human skin). Eggs and faecal pellets may sometimes be seen in the absence of adult or immature mites. Current serological tests may provide useful supportive evidence but do not detect early cases.

Effective topical and systemic therapies are available for sarcoptic mange. Even with a good clinical response, repeat treatments are necessary to ensure that all mites are killed. For the same reason, in-contact animals should also be treated. Measures to ameliorate the pruritus may also be required initially to prevent further self-injury.

Demodectic mange

Demodectic mange is seen mostly in dogs, clinical cases being associated with inherited or acquired immunodeficiency. The condition is not considered to be contagious, transmission taking place only during the suckling period. Lesions are first seen on the muzzle, face and forelimbs, appearing initially as a slight loss of hair which may resolve spontaneously or spread over the entire body (see Figure 9.33). Generalised infestations occur in two manifestations:

a – Squamous demodicosis: This is characterised by a dry reaction with skin thickening, desquamation and alopecia; pruritus is absent or moderate.

b – Pustular (or follicular) demodicosis: This form of the disease is complicated by secondary staphylococcal infection. The skin becomes wrinkled and thickened and contains numerous pustules which ooze serum, blood or pus. Affected animals may be severely disfigured.

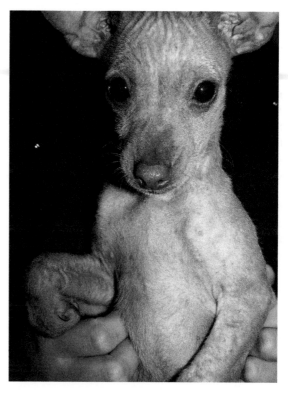

Figure 9.33 Puppy with demodectic mange. Reproduced with permission of L.H. Kramer.

Deep skin scrapings or hair plucks are required for diagnosis which is confirmed by finding numerous cigar-shaped mites (see Figure 9.34) or their diamond-shaped eggs. Small numbers may indicate no more than an incidental commensal infection. The management of advanced cases can take many weeks and requires

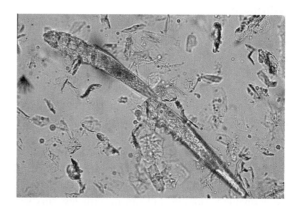

Figure 9.34 Demodex mites in skin scrape. Reproduced with permission of R. Bond.

clinical expertise as demodicosis responds poorly to most standard acaricidal treatments. Underlying immunological factors and secondary infections have also to be addressed.

Ear mites

Most cats harbour *Otodectes* but few show clinical signs. In contrast, dogs are less likely to be infested but more likely to develop inflammatory reactions in the outer ear (a condition known as 'otitis externa'). The severity of the reaction varies considerably between individuals, but there is often a brown waxy exudate which later becomes crusty. This can be complicated by secondary bacterial and fungal infections producing a purulent otitis. Irritation and discomfort leads to frequent head shaking and ear scratching which can result in an aural haematoma.

Otodectic mites live on the surface of the skin and can be seen with an auroscope in the external ear canal as motile white specks. If hidden under waxy exudate, a sample can be removed gently with a cotton bud and examined microscopically. Treatment may require a combination of acaricidal, antibiotic, antifungal and supportive therapy.

Cheyletiella

Dogs, cats and rabbits each have their own species of *Cheyletiella* that lives in the fur. These can cause minor irritation and skin scaling, but their main significance is that they can be transmitted to humans. If a suspect animal is brushed while standing on a dark surface the mites, if present, appear as 'walking dandruff' amongst the fallen debris.

Pediculosis

Dogs have both a broad-headed chewing louse and a narrow-headed sucking species. Cats have just a chewing louse. Heavy infestations tend to be sporadic and associated with a failure to groom efficiently, which may indicate neglect or other underlying health problems. The coat appears rough and eggs ('nits') may be seen stuck to hairs. Severe cases may exhibit eczema with evidence of scratching and rubbing.

The presence of lice can be demonstrated by parting the hair or fur. Pediculosis is easily treated with topical insecticides, including many flea control products. Lice are permanent parasites, but can nevertheless survive off the host for a short time and so treatment has to be accompanied by cleaning blankets, brushes etc.

Canine leishmaniosis

Leishmaniosis is generally restricted to the Mediterranean region and parts of Asia, South America and Africa. It has a very long incubation period and can appear unexpectedly in transported dogs many months after they have left an endemic area. The disease affects multiple bodily functions, but skin manifestations are often prominent, including alopecia around the eyes (popularly known as 'spectacles' – see Figure 9.35) and over other parts of the body, together with shallow ulcers on the nose, lips, ear-tips, tail or feet.

In the visceral form of the disease, signs are nonspecific, highly variable and indicative of chronic damage to many body systems, including: exercise intolerance, lameness, ocular lesions, polydipsia/polyuria, weight-loss etc. Most infected dogs, however, remain as asymptomatic carriers.

There is a wide choice of serological tests for detecting infection but these vary in sensitivity and specificity. Diagnosis is usually confirmed by demonstrating *Leishmania* amastigotes in Giemsa-stained skin scrapings or, preferably, biopsy samples taken from lymph nodes or bone marrow. The organisms are found inside macrophages (see Figure 9.36) or in extracellular tissue fluid. They are oval, up to 6 µm long, with a dark-stained rod (the kinetoplast) close to the nucleus (see Figure 4.11). PCR tests provide the most reliable results and are likely to be used more frequently as this technology advances.

There are as yet no wholly satisfactory treatments for this condition and medication programmes span periods

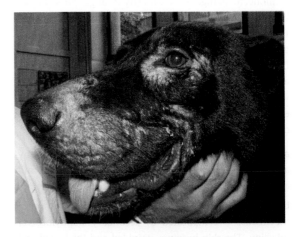

Figure 9.35 Leishmaniosis: advanced case showing alopecia around the eyes and ulceration. Reproduced with permission of A.F. Koutinas.

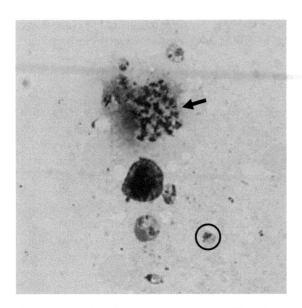

Figure 9.36 Lymph node biopsy smear showing *Leishmania* amastigotes in macrophages (arrow) and free in tissue fluid (circle).

of weeks or months. Even then, chemotherapeutic agents such as pentavalent antimony compounds may not eliminate the parasite completely, so relapses are common. The potential risk of onward zoonotic transmission has to be considered (see Section 9.3.2) and, in some circumstances, euthanasia of an infected animal may be deemed a more responsible option than an attempted cure.

Some products containing a synthetic pyrethroid (e.g. dog collars impregnated with deltamethrin or spot-ons containing permethrin) can be used in endemic regions to reduce (but not eliminate) the risk of new infections happening. These compounds are insect repellents (see Section 3.5.2) that deter potential vectors from feeding, thereby reducing the number of bites. Further protection can be attempted by keeping dogs indoors at dusk and dawn when phlebotomine sandflies tend to be most active. Controlling the stray dog population can reduce transmission rates significantly, although there may also be wild-life reservoir hosts.

Vaccines are starting to become available in some countries but their development has been hindered by the considerable evolutionary diversity between and within *Leishmania* species, the complexity of associated pathogenic mechanisms and variation in individual host responses.

9.2.4 Other body systems

Thelazia (see Table 9.11) is a fly-transmitted nematode in the conjunctival sac that can cause lacrimation, conjunctivitis and corneal opacity. One canine species, *T. californiensis* in western USA, is also found in mule deer and some other animals. Another, *T. callipaeda*, appears to be becoming more prevalent in parts of Asia and has recently been reported in southern Europe. Both occasionally infect humans.

The finding of double-plugged nematode eggs in urine samples indicates the presence of *Capillaria plica* in the bladder.

The granulomata surrounding somatic *Toxocara* larvae and *Toxoplasma* cysts, both found in many different tissues, are rarely a clinical problem in dogs and cats unless they impinge upon a particularly sensitive tissue. Active *Neospora* infections in dogs, however, can be very damaging.

Table 9.11 Parasitic genera most likely to be encountered in other body systems of dogs and cats

	CNS	Eyes	Urogenital	Musculature
Host: **DOG and CAT**				
Nematodes	*Toxocara* 7.1.3	*Thelazia* 7.1.5	*Capillaria* 7.1.6	*Toxocara* 7.1.3
Protozoa	*Toxoplasma* 4.7.3 *Neospora*[1] 4.7.4			*Toxoplasma* 4.7.3

Note: these lists are not comprehensive; other parasites do occur but less frequently or are of more restricted distribution or importance; numbers in red cross-reference to section with more detailed information.

[1] Dog only.

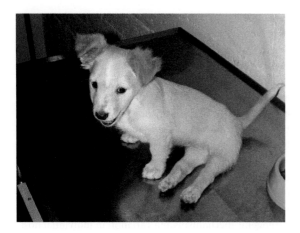

Figure 9.37 Canine neosporosis: paralysis of hind limbs. Reproduced with permission of L. De Risio.

Canine neosporosis

Dogs become infected with *Neospora* most frequently by eating raw meat, offal or foetal membranes from infected cattle. Prevalence is therefore highest in farm and hunting dogs. Infected bitches can transmit the parasite to successive litters. Typically, around half the pups will be affected and about half of these will succumb to disease between the third week and the sixth month of life. The most common presentation is an ascending paralysis, especially of the hind limbs (see Figure 9.37), accompanied by muscle atrophy and contracture, although other neurological effects can occur. Clinical signs are more variable when dogs contract neosporosis later in life.

Faecal examination is not used for diagnosis as *Neospora* oocysts are shed for only a brief period. Serology or PCR techniques, if available, are preferred. Chemotherapy is often only partially successful, unless given in the very early stages of the disease process.

The incidence of disease in puppies can be substantially reduced by not using seropositive bitches for breeding.

9.3 Veterinary public health

Dozens, if not hundreds, of parasites can be transmitted from animals to humans. The medical conditions associated with these are often multifaceted and their control on a national or global basis requires input from many disciplines including medical and veterinary professionals, scientists and epidemiologists, the pharmaceutical and food industries, water engineers, agriculturalists, sociologists, educationalists and politicians.

The ecological relationships that draw mankind into this wider web of nature were outlined in Section 1.2.3. Some zoonoses are associated with the food we eat; others are derived from environmental sources such as soil or water. Some may be present in our homes while others are vector-borne. Examples of these various routes of transmission are given in the remaining sections of this text.

9.3.1 Food-borne zoonoses

Zoonotic parasites can be associated with a number of food-stuffs including plants, marine life and meat (see Table 9.12).

Salad crops can be contaminated with a variety of helminth eggs and protozoon cysts. These pathogens can originate from the soil in which the plants grow or from water used to wash them. Trematode cysts (metacercariae) can be a particular hazard on plants growing in wetter areas where snail intermediate hosts flourish. Human fasciolosis is prevalent in some high Andean valleys where edible plants become accessible as water courses

Table 9.12 Some food-borne zoonoses

Source:	Cestodes	Trematodes	Nematodes	Protozoa
	Host: HUMAN			
Plants		*Fasciola* 5.6.2		
Fish	*Diphyllobothrium* 5.4.2	Various intestinal and liver flukes 5.6.3	*Anisakis*	
Meat	*Spirometra* 5.4.2 *Taenia* 5.3.3		*Trichinella* 7.1.6	*Toxoplasma* 4.7.3 *Sarcocystis* 4.7.1

Note: these lists are not comprehensive; other zoonoses do occur; numbers in red cross-reference to section of book with more detailed information.

and lakes recede in the dry season. In Britain, sporadic cases are usually associated with eating wild water-cress harvested from muddy snail habitats. In Asia, the cercariae of a number of zoonotic trematodes invade the tissues of fish or crabs where they become metacercariae awaiting ingestion by dogs, cats or humans.

The fish tapeworm, *Diphyllobothrium*, has a wide range of final hosts in northern regions (see Figure 5.31) and causes vitamin B_{12} deficiency in some human carriers. Species of another pseudophyllidean tapeworm, *Spirometra*, occur in dogs or cats in warmer parts of the world. Humans become involved in the life-cycle either by drinking water contaminated with infected copepod intermediate hosts or by eating undercooked meat containing the plerocercoid larval stage. This can grow to a length of several cm in human tissues causing a disease known as 'sparganosis'.

The anisakids are a nematode family within the Ascaridoidea. Adult worms are found in the stomach of seals or dolphins where they aggregate in groups protruding from large ulcerated nodules. Eggs pass into the sea and larvae ascend the marine food chain, starting in crustacea and moving to bigger and bigger fish, as one host is eaten by the next. The larvae are normally coiled in the body cavity (see Figure 9.38), but may move into the musculature after infected fish are caught and die. They are of public health importance as they can provoke the formation of an intensely painful eosinophilic intestinal swelling in people who eat raw or inadequately marinated fish (particularly herring). This zoonotic hazard can be significantly reduced by gutting the fish at sea

before the larvae move into the musculature. Alternatively, fish can be deep frozen before they are marinated.

Veterinary involvement is greatest with meat-borne zoonoses. This can be at two levels: on the farm, by maintaining healthy livestock; and in food hygiene, by detecting contaminated carcasses so they can be made safe or removed from the human food chain. Meat inspection is of prime importance for controlling some human diseases, including trichinellosis and *Taenia solium* infections. There are, however, anomalies based on tradition, feasibility or aesthetics. In some countries, for example, lamb or mutton harbouring metacestodes (cysticerci) of *Taenia ovis* is condemned as unfit for human consumption even though this parasite is incapable of infecting people. At the other extreme, few regulatory protocols adequately address the possible occurrence in meat of 'invisible' zoonotic parasites such as *Toxoplasma*.

Trichinellosis

Human trichinellosis is a very unpleasant condition. Patients suffer from muscle pains and heart disease (myositis and myocarditis), sometimes accompanied by facial oedema, encephalitis and other signs. The disease can last many months and some patients may die.

In fatal cases, there may be more than 100 *Trichinella spiralis* larvae per gram of muscle, equivalent to more than 50 million larvae in the body. In contrast, a pig of equivalent body-weight can harbour three times this number without clinical effect. Farmers can therefore unknowingly send infected pigs for slaughter.

Undercooked meat from infected pigs is the most common, but not the only, source of human infection. Recent cases in France and Italy, for example, were traced to *T. spiralis*-infected meat from horses. People are also vulnerable if they fail to cook meat from wild animals (e.g. bears, wild-boar) adequately over the camp fire or barbeque. Inuit communities are at particular risk as the arctic *Trichinella* species, unlike *T. spiralis*, survives storage in a freezer.

In countries with well regulated, intensive pig husbandry systems, the transmission risk to both pigs and humans is very low. Nevertheless, after a pig has been butchered and divided into pork cuts, chops, mince, bacon, ham, salami, sausages etc., muscle tissue from this one carcase may be consumed by a thousand or more people. Consequently, a single infected pig has the potential to start a mini-epidemic. Until the mid-20th century, such 'common-source outbreaks' were relatively common in Europe, North America and elsewhere.

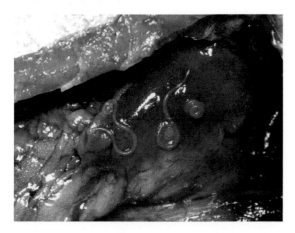

Figure 9.38 *Anisakis* larvae in body cavity of a Mediterranean mackerel. Reproduced with permission of L.H. Kramer.

Rigorous meat inspection and other measures have gone a long way towards eliminating this public health hazard in many regions. Infected pigs are hardly ever found to originate from intensive production systems in the USA, Canada or Western Europe and schemes for auditing and accrediting *Trichinella*-free herds are being evaluated. Over the whole European Union, including recently admitted eastern countries, just 430 of over 200 million pigs tested in 2009 (0.0002%) were found to be positive for *Trichinella*. Even so, 748 confirmed human cases were recorded, mostly associated with uninspected pigs or wild boar that had been slaughtered for home consumption.

The main principles for the prevention of trichinellosis are:

a – Control the diet of the pig population:

  i)   scavenging must be prevented to stop ingestion of infected food waste, rodent carcases etc.;

  ii) swill or kitchen scraps, if fed, must be boiled long enough to kill all *T. spiralis* larvae.

b – Meat inspection: The detection and destruction of infected carcasses removes hazardous meat from the human food-chain and prevents contaminated food-residues getting into swill or scraps eaten by pigs.

c – Food preparation: All pork products should be properly cooked or otherwise processed to ensure that any *T. spiralis* larvae that may have escaped detection at meat inspection are killed.

Methods for the detection of *T. spiralis* in pigs at the slaughter-house include:

a – Trichinoscopy: A muscle snip taken from the diaphragm (where larval densities tend to be highest) is squashed between glass plates and examined microscopically for the presence of larvae (see Figure 7.34).

b – Pepsin digest: A pooled sample of diaphragm muscle from a batch of pigs is subjected to enzymatic digestion and the sediment examined microscopically. If larvae are found, each pig is investigated individually.

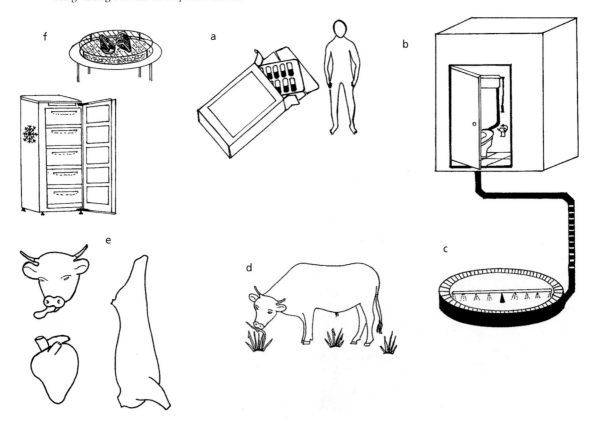

Figure 9.39 Control of *Taenia saginata*, the beef tapeworm – possible intervention points in life-cycle: a – human infection; b – sanitation; c – sewage; d – bovine infection; e – meat inspection; f – food preparation (details in text).

c – Serology: Automated tests based on ELISA technology have been developed for large scale screening, but to date they are better suited for epidemiological surveillance than for detection of individual carcases at meat inspection.

Taenia saginata and T. solium

The adult beef tapeworm, *T. saginata*, and the pork tapeworm, *T. solium*, are both relatively innocuous parasites in the human small intestine. Similarly, their metacestode stages are well tolerated by their natural intermediate hosts, cattle and pigs, respectively. With *T. solium*, however, there is the complication that the metacestode of this species is capable of invading the human body (see Section 5.3.3). When this happens, the aberrant parasite becomes disorientated and can establish in the CNS as well as in musculature, provoking neurological disease. This hazard persists in parts of Latin America, Africa and Asia where scavenging pigs have access to human waste.

Taenia saginata

Consideration of the *T. saginata* life-cycle indicates a number of points where beneficial interventions are possible (see Figure 9.39), although none is fully effective in breaking the life-cycle:

a – Treat human carriers: Safe and effective anthelmintics are available for human treatment but not all infected people seek, or have access to, medical advice.

b – Sanitation: The provision of toilets removes the need for humans to defecate directly onto agricultural land but such facilities are not yet universally available.

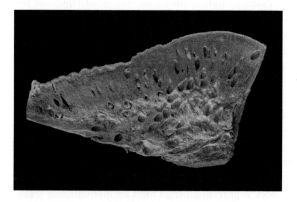

Figure 9.40 Museum specimen: ox tongue cut to show numerous *T. saginata* cysticerci in muscle. Reproduced with permission of The Royal Veterinary College.

c – Sewage disposal: Human effluent should not be applied to grassland unless it has been composted or treated to kill or remove *Taenia* eggs. Not all sewage works have this capability even in advanced countries.

d – Prevent or treat bovine infection:

i)   An effective recombinant vaccine has been developed but commercial availability is currently inhibited by inadequate demand. Bovine cysticercosis is not of sufficiently high public health priority in developing countries and is generally of sporadic and unpredictable occurrence in wealthier regions.

ii) Chemotherapy in the bovine intermediate host is currently impractical because: (i) serology is required to identify which animals need treatment; (ii) available drugs are prohibitively expensive and may leave tissue residues; and (iii) dead cysticerci also diminish the value of the carcase to the meat trade.

e – Meat inspection: The greatest density of cysticerci is found in the heart, masseter and tongue (see Figure 9.40). Inspection is performed by making a series of incisions into these which, fortuitously, are the least valuable muscle masses in the carcase. The risk of an infected carcase escaping detection is related to the number of cysticerci present. One study showed a > 90% chance of detection when there were around 70 cysticerci in a carcase, but the probability of detection fell to just 15%, if there were only four.

f – Food preparation: In the knowledge that meat inspection can never be 100% effective, all beef products should be prepared in a manner that will kill cysticerci: for example, cooking so that the centre of the meat reaches a temperature of at least 57°C, or freezing to below -10°C for at least 14 days. (Note: precise regulations and recommendations for meat inspection and food preparation vary from country to country.)

Taenia solium

Application of the control principles described above for *Trichinella* and *T. saginata* would theoretically be effective for *T. solium* also, but this infection is prevalent particularly in deprived communities where such measures are difficult to implement. Education is therefore the main weapon for enabling people to take steps that will reduce the risk to themselves and their families. A recombinant vaccine which prevents the establishment

Table 9.13 Some environmental zoonoses and sources of infection

Source:	Trematodes/ cestodes	Nematodes	Protozoa	Arthropods
	Host: HUMAN			
The ground	*Echinococcus* (hydatid and alveolar cysts) 5.3.4	*Ascaris* 7.1.3 *Strongyloides* 7.1.2 Larva migrans: *Toxocara* 7.1.3 *Baylisascaris* 7.1.3 Hookworms 6.3.4	*Toxoplasma* 4.7.3 *Giardia* 4.5.2 *Cryptosporidium* 4.9.1 *Sarcocystis* 4.7.1	Many fleas, ticks etc. 2.2.2, 3.2.2, 3.2.3
Water-borne	*Schistosoma* 5.6.3		*Giardia* 4.5.2 *Cryptosporidium* 4.9.1	
Air-borne	Faecal-derived eggs, oocysts etc. in dust			Many biting and myiasis flies 2.2.5, 2.2.6
The home environment	Faecal-derived eggs, oocysts etc. on shed hairs and skin debris			Fleas 2.2.2 *Rhipicephalus* 3.2.2 *Dermanyssus* 3.3.3
Handling pets, litter trays etc.	*Echinococcus* (hydatid and alveolar cysts) 5.3.4	*Toxocara* (larva migrans) 7.1.3	*Toxoplasma* 4.7.3 *Giardia* 4.5.2 *Cryptosporidium* 4.9.1	*Sarcoptes* 3.3.2 *Cheyletiella* 3.3.3
Vector-borne		*Dirofilaria* (larva) 7.1.5	*Leishmania* 4.5.1 *Trypanosoma* 4.5.1 *Babesia* 4.8.1	*Dermatobia* 2.2.6

Note: these lists are not comprehensive; other zoonoses do occur; numbers in red cross-reference to section of book with more detailed information.

of cysticerci in pigs is being evaluated and may be employed if the cost can be borne by international and governmental agencies.

Heavy porcine infection can sometimes be detected *in vivo* by inspecting the surface of the tongue for underlying cysticerci. While this practice has obvious diagnostic benefits, it also encourages illegal slaughter (to avoid condemnation at meat inspection) and the illicit distribution of unsafe meat.

9.3.2 Environmental zoonoses

Zoonotic hazards can be present in water, soil and even in the home. They can be carried by pets or transmitted by biting flies, ticks and other vectors (see Table 9.13).

Eggs, larvae, cysts and other infective stages originating from parasites of domesticated and wild animals exist all around us in astronomic numbers. When taken into the human body, most find themselves in an alien environment and fail to establish. Many are expelled immediately, while others may start to develop but later succumb

prematurely or are halted in their progress. Just a few are well-enough adapted to reach maturity in both animal and human hosts. Sometimes this is a very rare event; for example, human infections with adult *Dipylidium* or the metacestode of *Taenia multiceps*. Other zoonoses are of more frequent occurrence and some of these have serious consequences for human health, especially if the affected person is immunocompromised.

Epidemiological relationships can be ambiguous if humans and animals harbour the same or closely related parasites. It can be difficult to determine whether or not infections are host-specific or, if not, to what extent cross-transmission occurs and in which direction. Such knowledge is needed to determine zoonotic risk and to formulate appropriate control strategies. Molecular biology is providing useful tools for disentangling these interrelationships. Evidence is accumulating, for example, to support the contention that *Ascaris* populations in pigs and humans are genetically separate, but that cross-infections do nevertheless occur in some circumstances.

Another example is *Giardia duodenalis* which has been shown to comprise several host-associated genotypes. This is of relevance as only some of these have zoonotic potential (Table 4.3). Genotyping can also be used to help determine sources of contamination, e.g. *Cryptosporidium* in water-supplies.

Soil-transmitted zoonoses

Human toxoplasmosis

A significant proportion of humans, domesticated animals and wildlife are seropositive for *T. gondii*, indicating prior exposure to the parasite and the probable continuing presence of tissue cysts. Prevalence in human populations is dependent on climatic and cultural factors, especially eating habits, but is typically between 30% and 70%.

Fortunately, most human infections are asymptomatic. The more virulent strains produce acute 'flu-like symptoms or longer term malaise, sometimes with marked lymphadenopathy. Even avirulent strains, however, can induce fatal encephalitis in immunocompromised patients.

Humans can become infected in three ways (see Figure 4.35):

a – By ingesting sporulated oocysts: e.g. from licking dirty fingers or eating contaminated salad crops. The oocysts will have originated from a cat or other felid. They can survive in the environment for many months. The pivotal role of the cat in the epidemiology of toxoplasmosis is evidenced by the observation that strict vegetarians are sometimes seropositive for *T. gondii*.

b – By eating undercooked meat: The risk to humans varies with the type of meat and the production system. Many more tissue cysts accumulate in the flesh of pigs and small ruminants than in beef. Rabbit meat, venison and chicken fall between these extremes. On the other hand, pigs and poultry reared in biosecure indoor units are unlikely to be exposed to oocyst infection. Cured or smoked meats are safe unless only lightly processed. Unpasteurised goats milk has also been identified as a significant risk factor.

c – Congenital infection: This happens when infection occurs for the first time during pregnancy. (Infection earlier in life confers immunity which will prevent tachyzoites from multiplying and crossing the placenta.) The outcome depends on the virulence of the parasite and the stage of pregnancy, but may involve miscarriage, still-birth or a congenitally infected child.

Congenitally infected children often lead normal or near-normal lives, but a small number are born with disorders such as hydrocephalus, learning difficulties, epilepsy, ophthalmitis or hearing problems.

Public health issues concerning human toxoplasmosis are complex and beyond the scope of this text. General advice for reducing risk includes:

a – Avoid ingestion of oocysts:

i) Wash potentially contaminated raw food thoroughly (e.g. salad crops);

ii) Wash hands after gardening or handling cats, especially before eating;

iii) Clean out cat litter trays thoroughly every day (i.e. before oocysts sporulate) and dispose of the refuse securely.

iv) Wearing gloves when engaged in these activities will provide an extra level of protection.

b – Avoid ingestion of tachyzoites or tissue cysts:

i) Do not eat undercooked meat;

ii) Wash hands after handling raw meat; wash all pans, knives etc. immediately after contact with raw meat;

iii) Do not drink unpasteurised goats milk.

c – At lambing time: Veterinarians, farm-staff and laboratory diagnosticians should assess risk and take appropriate precautions when handling ewes at lambing time or when dealing with material from sheep abortions or stillbirths. Women should avoid such activities altogether if they could be pregnant.

Hydatid disease (cystic echinococcosis)

Hydatid cysts in the human lung or liver are generally asymptomatic and only discovered incidentally during medical examination. Problems may arise, however, in these and other sites from pressure being exerted on neighbouring structures. In remote geographical regions lacking medical facilities, hydatid cysts can become large enough to distend the abdomen. Rupture of a cyst (e.g. as a result of trauma in a traffic accident) can cause an anaphylactic reaction, while dissemination of brood capsules in the blood circulation (e.g. as an unintended result of a surgical procedure) can give rise to secondary cysts.

The only way humans are likely to become infected with *E. granulosus* is by swallowing an egg from an infected dog (see Figure 9.41). The contents of hydatid cysts are infective only for dogs and other canids (except in the rare event of a person in the abattoir or kitchen accidentally rubbing a brood capsule or protoscolex into an open wound).

E. granulosus has been eradicated from New Zealand but this took more than 20 years of intensive effort.

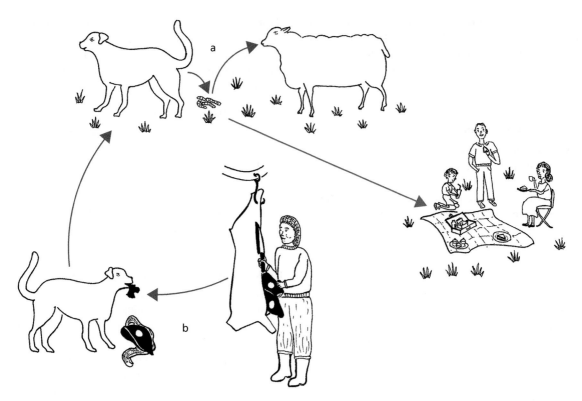

Figure 9.41 Hydatid disease: a – humans and sheep are infected by eggs from dog faeces; b – dogs are infected by eating undercooked offal from sheep.

Schemes are well advanced in several other countries. The following approach is usually adopted:

a – Define local epidemiology: the relative roles of different final and intermediate hosts vary considerably between localities. Effort and expense can be wasted if these interrelationships are not understood. This exercise also produces base-line data essential for measuring subsequent progress.

b – Registration of dogs: This is needed to ensure complete compliance. The campaign will be undermined if even a small proportion of dogs escape inclusion.

c – Regular treatment of all dogs: the objective is to prevent *E. granulosus* eggs being shed into the environment (see Figure 9.41a). A treatment interval of 6 weeks is used (based on the prepatent period of the parasite). Praziquantel (or other equally effective compound) is used as it is necessary to kill tapeworms at all stages of maturity in the dog (see Table 9.7).

d – An intensive educational programme: Schemes will fail without the cooperation and compliance of both farmers and dog owners.

e – Regular testing of dogs: This is necessary for monitoring progress (necessary to maintain political momentum) and to identify noncompliance or other difficulties. This task has become much easier since the introduction of coproantigen tests. (Previously, an arecoline purge was used and the faeces examined for expelled tapeworms.)

f – Dietary restrictions for farm dogs: Farm casualties should be buried or otherwise destroyed so they cannot be scavenged. Any offal fed to dogs must be previously boiled or frozen.

g – Meat inspection: To ensure offal containing hydatid cysts is destroyed so that it cannot be fed to dogs.

h – Legislation: To ensure that all the measures listed above can be enforced.

Alveolar echinococcosis

Alveolar echinococcosis caused by *Echinococcus multilocularis* is a serious, inoperable and potentially fatal human infection. Fortunately, effective chemotherapy is now available but treatment has to be continued over a prolonged period. Risk levels are rising in several European countries as foxes (the final host of *E. multilocularis*) become more plentiful in and around urban areas. Control is impossible unless reliable methods can be developed to entice foxes to take medicated baits. It is important that nonendemic countries maintain their *E. multilocularis*-free status. For this reason, all dogs and cats coming into the UK have to be treated with praziquantel.

Human toxocarosis

Toxocara canis eggs passed by dogs or foxes take two or more weeks to embryonate in humid summer conditions, although many remain unembryonated for prolonged periods in cooler or drier circumstances. They accumulate in city parks, suburban gardens and similar places and can survive for 4–5 years. As the eggs are sticky, there is always a possibility of one being transferred to the mouth on dirty fingers, especially by children. Serological surveys suggest a relatively high prevalence of infection in the general population (2.5% in Britain, for example). Fortunately, an infective *T. canis* larva is less than a half-millimetre long and its presence in the human body is normally of no consequence. Clinical concerns arise, however, should a large number of embryonated eggs be swallowed over a short time-span, or if a single larva migrates through or settles by mischance in a sensitive tissue (such as the retina of the eye). Such cases are relatively infrequent in temperate climates (20–50 diagnosed per year in the UK, for example) but the incidence-rate can be much higher in communities where social deprivation coincides with a hot, humid climate.

Large numbers of *T. canis* larvae passing through human tissues provoke a condition known as 'visceral larva migrans' or 'VLM' characterised by eosinophilia, enlargement of the liver and fever along with skin rash, asthmatic and neurological signs. Sometimes high *T. canis* antibody levels are associated with nonspecific signs such as cough, abdominal pains, headaches and behavioural disturbance. As the causal relationship is often ill-defined and unproven, this is called 'covert toxocarosis'. Partial impairment of vision in one eye can follow if a single larva settles in or passes through the retina or nearby tissues ('ocular larva migrans' or OLM). The degree of impairment depends on the host response and size of the resulting lesion but unilateral blindness may occur in severe cases. There is only a remote statistical chance of both eyes being affected.

Ways of minimising the number of *T. canis* eggs shed into the environment by well-cared-for dogs were outlined in Section 9.2.1. Stray dogs and urban foxes present a much greater challenge.

Help box 9.1

Clinical syndromes associated with *Toxocara canis* recognised in human medicine

Visceral larva migrans (VLM):	many larvae ⇒ swollen liver and allergic signs.
Ocular larva migrans (OLM):	one larva in retina ⇒ unilateral impairment of vision.
Covert toxocarosis:	nonspecific signs, high antibody titres.

Cutaneous larva migrans

Infective larvae (L_3) of most hookworm species are capable of penetrating skin. If they find themselves in the wrong host they quickly succumb. Antigens released during this process provoke inflammatory reactions in some individuals, usually in the form of a meandering red track tracing the movements of the dying parasite (see Figure 9.42). This condition is termed *cutaneous larva migrans* and is seen most commonly in warmer climates, often in people who walk barefoot.

Extra information box 9.2

Baylisascaris procyonis

B. procyonis is the common raccoon ascarid. It is an important zoonosis. It is most prevalent in the northern United States but is also found in other localities where raccoons occur, including parts of Germany and Japan where captive specimens escaped to establish breeding colonies. Its life-cycle resembles that of *Toxascaris* (see Section 7.1.3). *B. procyonis* larvae in paratenic hosts are aggressively invasive and grow to a length of almost 2 mm. The larvae are therefore more damaging than those of other somatic ascarids (which do not grow). As well as causing visceral and ocular larva migrans, *B. procyonis* larvae in the brain can produce acute or chronic neurological signs (neural larva migrans, NLM). Deaths and severe disability due to NLM have been diagnosed in infants and pet dogs in the USA, and OLM has been recognised in both North America and Germany. Raccoons often establish latrines close to human habitation with a correspondingly high local transmission risk. The egg is typically ascarid in appearance but has a finely granular surface.

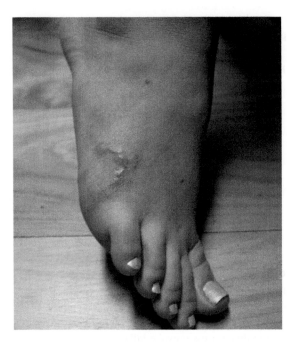

Figure 9.42 Cutaneous larva migrans. Reproduced with permission of R.C. Krecek.

Water-borne zoonoses

A condition similar to *cutaneous larva migrans*, called 'swimmer's itch', occurs when people bathe in water polluted with the cercariae of some avian *Schistosoma* species. This can happen in cooler climates, as well as in the tropics where schistosome infections are more frequently found.

Human schistosomosis

On the league table of misery-inducing human parasites, schistosomes are second only to malaria. The diseases they cause are mostly chronic. They impair growth and cognitive development in children, and give rise to malaise and lethargy in adults. Species inhabiting hepato-peritoneal venous networks, such as *S. mansoni* and *S. japonicum*, can induce serious pathological changes in the liver and intestine (see Figure 9.43) provoking diarrhoea, a swollen liver and ascites. *S. haematobium* affects the urogenital system with the resulting pathology developing into cancer of the bladder in some long-term sufferers.

There are eight human *Schistosoma* species belonging to three groups:

a – The *S. haematobium* group: These occur in Africa and the Middle East and are almost entirely confined to primates and rodents.

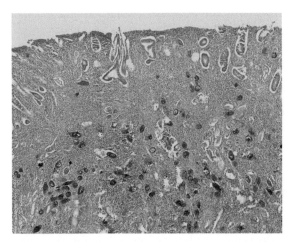

Figure 9.43 Schistosomosis: many eggs in severely affected intestinal wall.

b – The *S. mansoni* group: Originally endemic only in Africa and the Middle East, but *S. mansoni* has established in some Latin American and Caribbean countries. Again, they are associated mostly with primates and rodents.

c – The *S. japonicum* group: Found in China, The Philippines and Indonesia. Domesticated animals play an important role in the epidemiology of human disease by acting as reservoirs of infection (water buffalo for *S. japonicum* itself and dogs for a related species).

Intermediate hosts for schistosomes are aquatic snails. The cercariae that are released penetrate the skin of people or animals wading in contaminated water. Changes in water management and agricultural practice can alter the dynamics of ecological relationships. Engineering works, such as dams and irrigation canals, can increase opportunities for transmission unless they are designed to discourage snail colonisation (e.g. by ensuring a vigorous flow-rate or by periodically drying out the littoral zones where the snails are found).

Efforts are being made to control the human disease in many countries. Japan achieved eradication in 1976 and considerable progress has been made in some others, including parts of China. Consideration has to be taken of the schistosome species involved, the ecology of the local snail intermediate host(s) and the possible involvement of reservoir hosts, as well as specific community risk factors. Targeted mass treatments of the human population with praziquantel are widely practised, coupled with educational programmes and improvements in sanitation. The use of molluscicides has been largely superseded, where feasible, by manual modification of the banks of waterways to minimise the extent of snail habitats.

Pets and the home

Even the domestic environment can be a potential source of zoonotic infection. Flea-bites can be a considerable annoyance (see Figure 9.44) and can transmit microbial pathogens such as that causing cat-scratch fever. Flea eggs drop off the pet and the photophobic larvae develop in 'hotspots' around the house, outbuildings and even in the car. Control has to be based on an understanding of flea biology as discussed in Section 9.2.3. The brown dog tick, *Rhipicephalus sanguineus*, is another ectoparasite capable of biting humans that thrives in houses and kennels.

Two parasitic mites, *Cheyletiella* and *Sarcoptes*, are readily transmitted to humans in close contact with infested pets. *Cheyletiella* can pass through clothing with ease. The resulting skin rash is often transient but can be persistent with intense pruritus and vesicular or pustular eruptions. Pets are sometimes presented for veterinary inspection because of their owner's skin problem. The dog strain of *Sarcoptes* will not establish on humans but it can provoke a transient rash or a more hyperkeratotic lesion if there is prolonged exposure. When people in their homes are bitten by the poultry red mite, *Dermanyssus*, or a hippoboscid fly, the source is usually an abandoned bird nest in the roof.

Parasite eggs and cysts have a propensity to stick to animal hair. Tapeworm segments crawl out of the anus and may deposit eggs directly onto the skin or fur before dropping to the floor. *Toxocara* eggs have also been recovered from coat brushings. These presumably originate from adherent faecal material.

As noted earlier in this chapter, the cat litter tray is hazardous as a potential source of *Toxoplasma* oocysts.

Vector-borne zoonoses

Biting arthropods, such as mosquitoes (see Figure 9.45), are vectors for many human as well as animal pathogens. An unusual biological association in this category involves the human bot fly, *Dermatobia*, which occurs in parts of Central and South America. This attaches its eggs onto mosquitoes and other flies (apparently without affecting their aerodynamics) and relies on them to find a suitable host (mostly cattle, dogs and humans). The bot larvae hatch while their transport host is feeding. Each enters the skin and produces a swelling with a breathing hole. Here they stay for up to five months before emerging to pupate.

Another mosquito-transmitted zoonotic parasite is the canine heartworm, *Dirofilaria*. In humans, a larva may get as far as the lungs before becoming entrapped. Fortunately, this is a relatively rare event. Such cases are usually detected as a radio-opaque plaque on a routine chest X-ray examination, necessitating further tests to reveal the causal aetiology.

Bovine and rodent *Babesia* species can be hazardous to people lacking a spleen (e.g. as a result of a traffic accident) if they are bitten by a tick vector.

African trypanosomosis

Sixty million people living in tsetse fly infested regions of sub-Saharan Africa are exposed to infection with *Trypanosoma brucei*. A red sore ('chancre') develops at

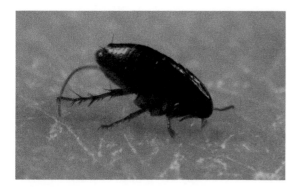

Figure 9.44 Cat flea biting human. Reproduced with permission of D.-H. Choe.

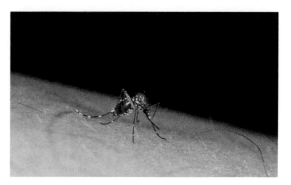

Figure 9.45 Mosquito (*Aedes*) replete after feeding on human. Reproduced with permission of J.G. Logan.

the site of the tsetse bite followed by a period with fever, swollen lymph nodes and pain in muscles and joints. Later still, there is neurological involvement including disruption of circadian rhythms (hence the term 'sleeping sickness'). Death may ensue if treatment is not given. This sequence of events extends over months in the case of the form of *T. brucei* found in eastern and southern regions. This subspecies has game animals and cattle as reservoir hosts.

Another subspecies produces an even more protracted form of the disease and predominates in central and western parts of the continent. It is primarily a human parasite, although pigs and some other mammals can become infected. (A third subspecies affects cattle but not humans.)

Aggressive control policies substantially reduced disease transmission by the mid-20th century but complacency and political instability allowed a recrudescence. Control now depends on effective surveillance (to ensure early detection and treatment of human cases), alongside the widespread use of insecticide-treated baits and traps (to reduce the density of the tsetse population). The incidence of new human cases has fallen dramatically in many countries in recent years.

Chagas disease

Trypanosoma cruzi is a serious zoonotic infection in parts of Latin America. It has wild-life reservoirs and is transmitted by biting reduviid (assassin) bugs. In humans, it may cause an initial local swelling at the site of entry accompanied by mild fever and malaise, sometimes with swelling of an eyelid. Thereafter, infection may be asymptomatic but a small proportion of patients develop potentially fatal heart problems and/or debilitating dilatation of the oesophagus or colon. Transmission can also occur via blood transfusion and across the placenta to the unborn child.

There is no vaccine and it is impossible to control infection in wild-life reservoirs, so control is reliant upon improvements in home construction to eliminate places where the nocturnal vector can hide, together with interior insecticidal treatments.

Human leishmaniosis

Human leishmaniosis mainly affects the underprivileged and is a barrier to socio-economic progress in some remote regions. The most serious, but least common, form of the disease is visceral leishmaniosis ('kala-azar') with fever, weight-loss, swelling of liver and spleen and eventually death if untreated. There are also cutaneous forms of the disease.

Leishmania spp. are transmitted by phlebotomine sandflies. Reservoir hosts include dogs and a range of wild animals. Humans can acquire infection from dogs:

a – Directly, by physical contact: if, for example, a person with a skin abrasion handles a dog with an open skin lesion;

b – Indirectly, via the intermediate host: i.e. by receiving a bite from a sandfly that has previously fed on an infected canid.

There is as yet no human vaccine and the drugs needed for chemotherapy are difficult to administer. Consequently, the main preventative measures are control of the sandfly population with persistent insecticides and reduction of the infected canine population in areas where they are a significant reservoir host (see Section 9.2.3).

References

Abbott, K.A., Taylor, M.A. and Stubbings, L.A. (2012) *Sustainable Worm Control Strategies for Sheep: A Technical Manual for Veterinary Surgeons and Advisors* (SCOPS 4th edn). Santa Rosa, CA: Context Publications.

Ackert (1931) cited in Mozgovoi, A.A. (1953) Ascaridata of animals and man and the diseases caused by them. Part I. In K.I.Skrjabin (ed.), *Essentials of Nematodology, Vol. II.* Moscow: Izdatel'stvo Akademii Nauk SSR (in Russian).

Antipin (1940) cited in Mozgovoi, A.A. (1953) Ascaridata of animals and man and the diseases caused by them. Part I. In K.I.Skrjabin (ed.), *Essentials of Nematodology, Vol. II.* Moscow: Izdatel'stvo Akademii Nauk SSR (in Russian).

Bedford, G.A.H. (1928) South African mosquitoes. *13th and 14th Reports of the Director of Veterinary Services and Animal Industry, Union of South Africa,* pp. 883–990.

Bedford, G.A.H. (1932) A synoptic check-list and host-list of the ectoparasites found on South African Mammalia, Aves and Reptilia (2nd edn). *18th Report of the Director of Veterinary Services and Animal Industry, Union of South Africa,* **18**(2): 223–523.

Bray, R.A., Gibson, D.I. and Jones, A. (eds) (2008) *Keys to the Trematoda, Volume 3.* London: CAB International and The Natural History Museum.

Cali, A. (1991) General microsporidian features and recent findings on AIDS isolates. *Journal of Protozoology* 38: 625–30.

Castellani, A. and Chalmers, A.J. (1913) *Manual of Tropical Medicine,* 2nd edn. London: Baillière, Tindall and Cox (cited in Wall and Shearer, 1997).

Carpenter, S.J. and Lacasse, W.J. (1974) *Mosquitos of North America (North of Mexico).* Berkeley, CA: University of California.

Cheng, T.C. (1986) *General Parasitology,* 2nd edn. New York: Academic Press Inc.

Chinery, M. (1977) *A Field Guide to the Insects of Britain and Northern Europe,* 2nd edn. Glasgow: Collins.

Dean, R. (2013) How to read a paper and appraise the evidence. *In Practice* **35**(5): 282–5.

Deplazes, P., Eckert, J., von Samson-Himmelstjerna, G. and Zahner, H. (eds) (2013) *Lehrbuch der Parasitologie für die Tiermedizin,* 3rd edn. Stuttgart: Enke Verlag.

Dubey, J.P. (1976) A review of *Sarcocystis* of domestic animals and other coccidia of cats and dogs. *American Veterinary Medical Association* **169**: 1061–78.

Dunn, A.M. (1978) *Veterinary Helminthology,* 2nd edn. London: Heinemann.

Eckert, J. (2013) World Association for the Advancement of Veterinary Parasitology (WAAVP): the 50th anniversary in 2013 – history, achievements and future perspectives. *Veterinary Parasitology* **195**: 206–17.

Eckert, J., Friedhoff, K.T., Zahner, H. and Deplazes, P. (eds) (2008) *Lehrbuch der Parasitologie für die Tiermedizin,* 2nd edn. Stuttgart: Enke Verlag.

Edwards, K.T., Goddard, J. and Varela-Stokes, A.S. (2009) Examination of the internal morphology of the ixodid tick, *Amblyomma maculatum* Koch (Acari: Ixodidae); 'How to' pictorial dissection guide. *Midsouth Entomologist* **2**: 28–39.

FAO (1994) *Diseases of Domestic Animals Caused by Flukes: Epidemiology, Diagnosis and Control of Fasciola, Paramphistome, Dicrocoelium, Eurytrema and Schistosome Infections of Ruminants in Developing Countries.* Rome: Food and Agriculture Organization of the United Nations.

Garcia, L.S. and Bruckner, D.A. (1988) *Diagnostic Medical Parasitology.* New York: Elsevier Scientific Publishing Co., Inc.

Gardiner, C.H., Fayer, R. and Dubey, J.P. (1988) *An Atlas of Protozoan Parasites in Animal Tissues.* United States Department of Agriculture, Agriculture Research Service, Agriculture Handbook Number 651, p. 36.

Gerichter, C.B. (1949) Studies on the nematodes parasitic in the lungs of Felidae in Palestine. *Parasitology* 39(3-4): 251–262.

Gibbons, L.M. (1986) SEM guide to the morphology of nematode parasites of vertebrates. Wallingford: CAB International, UK.

Grove, D.I. (1989) *Strongyloidiasis: A Major Roundworm Infection of Man.* London, New York and Philadelphia, Taylor & Francis.

Hegner, R.W., Root, F.M. and Augustine, D.L. (1929) *Animal Parasitology.* New York: Appleton-Century (cited in Cheng, 1986).

Hewitt, C.G. (1914) *The House Fly.* Cambridge: Cambridge University Press (cited in Lapage, 1962).

Hirst, S. (1922) Mites injurious to domestic animals (with an appendix on the acarine disease of hive bees). *British Museum (Natural History) Econ. Ser.* **13**: 1–107 (cited in Roberts and Janovy Jr, 1996).

Imms, A.D. (1957) *A General Textbook of Entomology,* 9th edn. London: Methuen & Co. Ltd.

Jacobs, D.E. (1986) *A Colour Atlas of Equine Parasites.* London: Baillière Tindall; London and New York, Gower Medical Publishing.

James, M.T. and Harwood, R.F. (1969) *Herms's Medical Entomology,* 6th edn. New York: Macmillan (cited in Cheng, 1986).

Jones, A. (2005) Family Fasciolidae Railliet, 1895. In A.Jones, R.A.Bray, and D.I.Gibson, et al. (eds), *Keys to the Trematoda,*

Volume 2, Chapter 6, London: CAB International and The Natural History Museum.

Krämer, F. and Mencke, N. (2001) *Flea Biology and Control. The Biology of the Cat Flea: Control and Prevention with Imidacloprid in Small Animals*. New York: Springer.

Lacey, E. (1990) Mode of action of benzimidazoles. *Parasitology Today* **6**: 112–15.

Lapage, G. (1962) *Mönnig's Veterinary Helminthology and Entomology*, 5th edn. London: Baillière, Tindall and Cox Ltd.

Lichtenfels, J.R. (1975) Helminths of domestic equids. Illustrated keys to genera and species with emphasis on North American forms. *Proceedings of the Helminthological Society of Washington*, 42, special issue.

MAFF (1986) *Manual of Veterinary Parasitological Techniques*, 3rd edn. Reference Book 418. London: Her Majesty's Stationery Office.

Miyazaki, I. (1991) *An Illustrated Book of Helminthic Zoonoses*. Tokyo: International Medical Foundation of Japan.

Mönnig, H.O. (1962) *Mönnig's Veterinary Helminthology and Entomology*, 5th edn (G.Lapage, ed.). London: Baillière, Tindall and Cox Ltd.

Morgan, B.B. and Hawkins, P.A. (1953), cited in I. Miyazaki (1991) *An Illustrated Book of Helminthic Zoonoses*. Tokyo: International Medical Foundation of Japan, p. 307.

Mozgovoi, A.A. (1953) Ascaridata of animals and man and the diseases caused by them. Part I. In K.I.Skrjabin (ed.), *Essentials of Nematodology, Vol. II*. Moscow: Izdatel'stvo Akademii Nauk SSR (in Russian).

Nicolson, M. (2010) 'Death and Doctor Hornbook' by Robert Burns: a view from medical history. *Journal of Medical Ethics: Medical Humanities* 36: 23–6.

Oldham, J.N. Unpublished drawings in the Parasitology Collection of The Royal Veterinary College (University of London).

Perdue, K.A., Copeland, M.K., Karjala, Z., *et al.* (2008) Suboptimal ability of dirty-bedding sentinels to detect *Spironucleus muris* in a colony of mice with genetic manipulations of the adaptive immune system. *Journal of the American Association of Laboratory Animal Science* 47(5): 10–17.

Poluszynski, Von G. (1930) Morphologisch-biologische Untersuchungen über die freilebenden Larven einiger Pierdestrongyliden Vorläunge Mittelung. Sonderdruck aus der Tierärztlichen Rundschau 36, Jahrgang, 1930, Nr. 51, Seite 871–3.

Roberts, L.S. and Janovy Jr., J. (1996) *Gerald D. Schmidt and L.S. Roberts' Foundations of Parasitology*, 5th edn. New York: Wm. C. Brown Publishers, Time Mirror Higher Education Group Inc.

Robertson, J. cited in Roberts, L.S. and Janovy Jr., J. (1996) *Gerald D. Schmidt and L.S. Roberts' Foundations of Parasitology*, 5th edn. New York: Wm. C. Brown Publishers, Time Mirror Higher Education Group Inc.

Skrjabin, K.I. and Evranova, V.G. (1952) Family Dicrocoeliidae Odhner, 1911. In: Skrjabin, K.I. [editor] *Trematodes of Animals and Man. Osnovy Trematodologii* **7**: 33–604. [In Russian]

Sloboda, M. (2008) cited in J. Votýpka, *Babesia*. Version 18 May 2011 (under construction). http://tolweb.org/Babesia/68087/2011.05.18 in The Tree of Life Web Project, http://tolweb.org/

Smart, J. (1943) *A Handbook for the Identification of Insects of Medical Importance*. London: British Museum (Natural History).

Smit, F.G.A.M. (1957) *Handbooks for the Identification of British Insects. Siphonaptera*. Royal Entomological Society of London, **1** (16).

Smyth, J.D. (1994) *Introduction to Animal Parasitology*, 3rd edn. Cambridge: Cambridge University Press.

Soulsby, E.J.L. (1965) *Textbook of Veterinary Clinical Parasitology. Vol. I: Helminths*. Oxford: Blackwell Scientific Publications.

Soulsby, E.J.L. (1982) *Helminths, Arthropods and Protozoa of Domesticated Animals*, 7th edn. London: Baillière Tindall.

Stewart, T.B. (1954) The life history of *Cooperia punctata*, a nematode parasitic in cattle. *Journal of Parasitology* **40**: 321–7.

Taylor, E.L. (1964) *Fascioliasis and the Liver Fluke*. FAO Agricultural Studies No. 64.

Taylor, M.A., Coop, R.L. and Wall, R.L. (2007) *Veterinary Parasitology*, 3rd edn. Oxford: Blackwell.

Thomas, R.J. (1959) Field studies on the seasonal incidence of *Nematodirus battus* and *N. filicollis* in sheep. *Parasitology* **49**: 387–410.

Urquhart, G.M. and Armour, J. (1973) *Helminth Diseases of Cattle, Sheep and Horses in Europe*. Glasgow: Glasgow University Press.

Urquhart, G.M., Armour, J., Duncan, J.L., *et al.* (1987) *Veterinary Parasitology*, 1st edn. Harlow: Longman Scientific and Technical.

Urquhart, G.M., Armour, J., Duncan, J.L., *et al.* (1996) *Veterinary Parasitology*, 2nd edn. Oxford: Blackwell Science.

Varma, M.G.R. (1933) Ticks and mites (Acari). In R.P.Lane and R.W.Crosskey (eds), *Medical Insects and Arachnids*, London: Chapman & Hall, pp. 597–658 (cited in Wall and Shearer, 1997).

Wall, R.S. and Shearer, D. (1997) *Veterinary Entomology*, 1st edn. London: Chapman & Hall.

Weinrich, D.H. and Emmerson, M.A. (1933) Studies on the morphology of *Tritrichomonas foetus* (Riedmuller) from American cows. *Journal of Morphology* **55**: 129.

Zumpt, F. (1965) *Myiasis in Man and Animals in the Old World*. London: Butterworths.

Index

abomasal worms 215
acanthocephalan worms 205–6
acaricide 75
Ascaris 189
acute toxicity 79
adulticides 268
Aedes 42–3
Aelurostrongylus 174
aesthetic considerations and
        parasites 11
aetiology/aetiological agent 2
African trypanosomosis 283–4
agriculture and parasites 11
albendazole 223
allergic dermatitis, seasonal 256
alopecia 68
alternative parasite control
        technologies 21
  biological control 23
  breeding for resistance/resilience 22
  delaying parasite resistance 22–3
  enhancing host resistance 22
  nutrition 22
alveolar cyst 121
alveolar hydatid disease 129–30
amastigote 87
Amblyomma 63–4
American dog tick 63
amino-acetonitrile derivatives
        (AADs) 211
amitraz 78
amoebae 82, 85–6
Ancylostoma 171–2
Ancylostomatoidea *see* hookworms
angiostrongylosis 264–6
Angiostrongylus 173–5
animal welfare and parasites 11
Anisakis 275
Anopheles 42–3
Anoplocephala 130–1
antennae of insects 29
anthelmintic drugs 207
  benzimidazoles (BZDs) 209
    activity 209–10

general spectrum 210
  mode of action 209–10
  pharmacokinetics 210–11
combination and multiple active
    parasiticides 211
levamisole group 207–8
  general spectrum 208
macrocyclic lactones (MLs) 208
  activity 208
  general spectrum 208
  pharmacokinetics 209
newer chemical groups
  amino-acetonitrile derivatives
    (AADs) 211
  depsipeptides 211
  spiroindoles 211
antibodies 7
anticoccidial drugs 115
  ionophores 115–16
  sulphonamides 116
antifeeding effects 76
antigens 7
antiprotozoan drugs 115
apical complex 83
apicomplexa 82–3
  blood-borne 107–8
    Babesia 108–12
    Theileria 112–13
apoptosis
  definition 7
  parasite influence upon 10
Argas 65
Argasidae (soft ticks) 58, 65
  life-cycle 60
arthropods 25, 57
  ectoparasiticides 75
    basic concepts 75–6
    important examples 77–9
    insect growth regulators (IGRs) 79
    problems associated with
      use 79–80
  insects 26
    body structure 26–32
    bugs (Hemiptera) 39–40

fleas (Siphonaptera) 32–6
flies (Diptera) 40–55
lice (Phthiraptera) 36–8
naming conventions 26
major parasitic groups 25
mange mites 65–6
  infestation range 74
  subsurface 66–9
  surface 69–74
other arthropods 74–5
skin parasites 26
ticks 57
  body structure 57–62
  hard ticks 62–5
  soft ticks 65
ascarid nematodes 184
  Ascaris 189, 278
  Ascaridia 192
  characteristics 184
  epidemiology 188
  hepatotracheal migration 186
  Heterakis 94, 189, 192, 242,
    244
  important examples 189
  infective stage 185
  life-cycle 185, 186
  Parascaris 190
  pathogenicity 188
  poultry 192
  somatic infection 187
  Toxascaris 191–2
  Toxocara 190–1
    T. canis 187–8, 190–1, 262–3, 273,
    280
    T. vitulorum 190, 217
Ascaridia 189, 192
Ascaris 189
  in pigs 239
  in humans 278
Ascarops 195, 197
assassin bugs 39
attenuated vaccines 20–21
avian coccidiosis 98–9, 242–4
axostyle 92

Principles of Veterinary Parasitology, First Edition. By Dennis Jacobs, Mark Fox, Lynda Gibbons and Carlos Hermosilla.
© 2016 John Wiley & Sons, Ltd. Published 2016 by John Wiley & Sons, Ltd.
Companion website: www.wiley.com/go/jacobs/principles-veterinary-parasitology